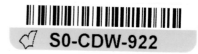

COLON CANCER
GENETICS

COLON CANCER GENETICS

Edited by

PATRICK M. LYNCH, J.D., M.D.

Department of Medicine
University of Arkansas for Medical Sciences

and

HENRY T. LYNCH, M.D.

Professor and Chairman
Department of Preventive Medicine
Creighton University School of Medicine

VNR **VAN NOSTRAND REINHOLD COMPANY**

Published by Van Nostrand Reinhold Company Inc.
135 West 50th Street
New York, New York 10020

Van Nostrand Reinhold Company Limited
Molly Millars Lane
Wokingham, Berkshire RG11 2PY, England

Van Nostrand Reinhold
480 Latrobe Street
Melbourne, Victoria 3000, Australia

Macmillan of Canada
Division of Gage Publishing Limited
164 Commander Boulevard
Agincourt, Ontario MIS 3C7, Canada

15   14   13   12   11   10   9   8   7   6   5   4   3   2   1

Library of Congress Cataloging in Publication Data
Main entry under title:
Colon cancer genetics.
   Includes index.
   1. Colon (Anatomy)—Cancer—Genetic aspects.   I. Lynch,
Patrick M.   II. Lynch, Henry T.   [DNLM: 1. Colonic
neoplasms—Familial and genetic.   WI 520 C7 172
RC280.C6C635   1984   616.99'4347   84-2398
ISBN 0-442-24918-7

Contents

Foreword

This is the first book devoted to the genetic aspects of colorectal cancer, so it is appropriate that it is edited by someone who has been responsible for so much valuable research work in this field. Henry Lynch is to be congratulated not only on his selection of authors but also on his choice of colleagues for the Omaha team.

Unlike lung and stomach cancer, colon cancer shows little sign of diminishing in frequency in the urban populations of North America and northern Europe. In fact, it may even be afflicting an increasing number of middle-aged people. The search for the environmental causes of colon cancer continues unabated, but although investigations in the dietetic field may someday give clues to external carcinogens, so far there is little indication of a single important factor similar to the relationship between smoking and lung cancer. Biochemical and microbiological studies of possible endogenous cocarcinogens have been more fruitful, particularly in the sphere of bile-salt metabolism. However, the outlook for prevention is bleak, and the medical profession will probably have to pursue a curative role for the foreseeable future. Success in cure depends on early diagnosis and, therefore, on education and screening of those at risk.

Who are the people at greatest risk of developing colon cancer? They may be those who have a particularly high intake of certain foods, but even within this group, experience with other human cancers and with experimental carcinogenesis indicates varying genetically based individual susceptibility. Hence, it is important to understand the genetics of the condition before formulating cost-effective screening programs. Family data suggest possible genetic explanations ranging from strong monogenetic influences in 10 to

20% of cases with the remainder largely environmental in etiology, to a wholly quantitative genetic basis in which people with a large number of the genes that contribute to susceptibility have more early-onset and multiple-site cancer than those with fewer of the susceptibility genes.

For a long time I was in favor of the second theory, so I was considerably skeptical when, 12 years ago, Henry Lynch started attributing familial aggregations of colon cancer to the effects of single genes. As time went on, he and his team assembled more and more data supporting his original concept. The finding of a preponderance of right-sided colon lesions not only in Nebraska cancer families but also in developing countries has completed my conversion to his view.

I wish this excellent book and its authors well in their lucid expositions on so many aspects of the subject. They have raised their sights to a broader horizon than the traditional view of medical genetics and have made a significant contribution to our understanding of this important disease. This book will prove a stimulating orientation course for those involved in the clinical care of colon cancer patients as well as those with responsibility for the planning of cancer prevention and detection programs.

RICHARD B. McCONNELL
Consultant Physician

Preface

To the practicing physician as well as to the clinical investigator, there are certain questions about hereditary colonic cancer (HCC) whose answers would aid immeasurably in surveillance/management programs. The answers to these questions would also enable a more clear comprehension of etiology. Among the specific questions to be addressed are the following: What sort of family history is required before one should suspect an HCC syndrome, and how common are such histories? What clinical or laboratory features are common to patients from such families, and how might these be used by clinicians for syndrome recognition? What differences exist between colon cancer-prone families that justify subclassification, and what clinical significance attaches to these differences? What available screening and management protocols are currently recommended? What promise does ongoing research hold for improving recognition and treatment of high-risk patients? These questions are addressed in this book, but considerably more research on each of them is needed.

The true frequency of hereditary colorectal cancer in the general population is not known. Based on the few reliable figures that exist, we estimate that a simply inherited predisposition to colon cancer may account for as many as 7 to 10% of *all* cases of colorectal cancer. Moreover, the hereditary, nonpolyposis, colorectal-cancer syndromes may occur more frequently than the hereditary, familial, polyposis-coli (FPC) varieties.

Historically, interest in the heritability of colon cancer was focused primarily on adenomatosis coli. In 1882, Cripps provided the first description of familial, multiple-adenomatous polyposis coli (FPC); its cancer association was established in 1890 by Handford. More than a quarter of a century later (1925), the St. Mark's group under the direction of Lockhart-Mummery established the first registry of FPC families—a registry that has been expanded by his successors until the present time. These pioneering efforts yielded significant etiologic insights. They also showed that this disease could be controlled through knowledge of its natural history and genetics, even to prophylactic colectomy in persons manifesting the phenotype (colonic polyposis). The necessity of vigilant programs for case detection and surveillance was demonstrated early on. Hereditary adenomatosis coli remains the undisputed model for colon cancer genetics.

As knowledge accrued, it became apparent that FPC was not the simple disease it was originally thought to be. A major breakthrough was made by Gardner in the early 1950s when he recognized the significance of extracolonic signs in FPC. Initially considered a distinct entity, Gardner's syndrome and perhaps even the polyposis-glioma complex (Turcot's syndrome), have come to be considered by many a continuous phenotypic expression of the FPC gene. The present controversy shows no sign of early resolution.

Work beginning in the mid-1960s suggested the existence of nonpolyposis colorectal-cancer syndromes. Some of this work was actually the prospective follow-up of Dr. Aldred Warthin's observations of a single family dating from 1895. The autosomal dominantly inherited predisposition to adenocarcinomas of the colon appeared complicated by the presence of other adenocarcinomas (predominantly of the female genitourinary system), a marked excess of multiple primary cancer, and an early age of cancer. Recently a tendency toward proximal localization of colon cancer has become a prominent distinguishing feature of the syndrome. In the past few years, patients with colon cancer in affected families have been noted to have improved survival, stage for stage, compared with the American College of Surgeons Audit Series on colorectal cancer. Unusual cutaneous lesions (sebaceous carcinoma, sebaceous adenoma, multiple keratoacanthoma) that mimic Torre's syndrome have been seen in a fraction of affected patients. Families expressing the above features have been said to have the "cancer family syndrome" (CFS). Unfortunately, this term has also been applied to families expressing a host of completely unrelated multi-tumor constellations.

Like FPC, CFS varies greatly in its expression. Possible syndrome variants include site-specific HCC with or without associated isolated adenomas, and colorectal cancer in association with carcinoma of the breast. Other colon cancer families with differing tumor combinations undoubtedly exist and may or may not prove to be genotypically distinct. The extent of extracolonic cancer expression in CFS and the etiologic factors influencing differential cancer expression remain matters for intensive investigation.

Certain biological markers in both the polyposis and nonpolyposis syndromes appear to hold promise for early identification of carriers and for syndrome subclassification. Tritiated thymidine labeling of upper colonic crypt compartments has been seen in patients with FPC syndromes and may prove to be a feature of nonpolyposis syndromes as well. Increased *in vitro* tetraploidy has been shown to appear in excess in Gardner's syndrome and in CFS. Chapters are devoted to each of these laboratory models as well as to the more speculative topics of immune perturbations and deoxyribonucleic acid (DNA) repair in HCC.

When the precise etiologic and pathogenetic mechanisms for HCC are elucidated, individualized programs for prevention may be possible. Pending such discoveries, both polyposis and nonpolyposis HCC-prone families must be regarded as significant clinical entities meriting meticulous early diagnostic measures tailored to the entities in question. The early age at onset and multiple organ susceptibility necessitate a long-term and well-informed relationship between the patient and physician. Several chapters are devoted to the screening and management of heritable colon cancer as well as to problem areas that remain in identifying affected families and specifying the high-risk members within them.

ACKNOWLEDGMENTS

The family studies that form the basis of the editors' contributions to this book required the devoted support of many persons. Some of the clinical data go back approximately 20 years to our original contact with "Family N," and these observations facilitated delineation of CFS.

We have continued to receive the unqualified support of our parent institution, the Creighton University School of Medicine, which has provided us with excellent facilities. Among the people warranting special recognition are our chief librarian, Marge Wannarka, M.L.S., and her devoted staff, as well as our dedicated secretaries Diane Stanley and Maggie Meston.

This book could not have been completed without assistance from highly skilled contributors, representing several specialized areas. We have had the opportunity to work closely with several of these contributors (William Albano, M.D., B. Shannon Danes, M.D., Ph.D., Eleanor Deschner, Ph.D., Martin Lipkin, M.D., Guy Schuelke, Ph.D., and Jane Lynch, B.S.N.) over the past several years in connection with an ongoing research project dealing with biomarkers in hereditary, nonpolyposis colorectal cancer.

Adequate funding is essential to any such endeavor, and expenses, including the many laboratory disciplines involved, may be enormous. We therefore consider ourselves fortunate in receiving generous support from the National Institutes of Health (currently supported by NCI Grant No. CA 27831). We also received donations from organizations such as the Fraternal Order of Eagles—Nebraska Division and the Veterans of Foreign Wars and from members of cancer-prone families.

PATRICK M. LYNCH
HENRY T. LYNCH

Contributors

William A. Albano, M.D., deceased

Thor Alm, M.D.
Department of Gastroenterology, St. Erik's Hospital, Stockholm, Sweden

Steffen Bulow, M.D.
Department of Surgical Gastroenterology, Bispebjerg Hospital, Copenhagen, Denmark

Edward A. Chaperon, Ph.D.
Department of Microbiology, Creighton University School of Medicine, Omaha, Nebraska 68178

B. Shannon Danes, M.D., Ph.D.
Laboratory for Cell Biology, Department of Medicine, Cornell University Medical College, New York, New York 10021

Eleanor E. Deschner, Ph.D.
Laboratory of Digestive Tract Carcinogenesis, Memorial Sloan-Kettering Cancer Center, New York, New York 10021

John A. Johnson, Ph.D.
Department of Biochemistry, University of Nebraska College of Medicine and Creighton University Omaha, Nebraska 68178

Jane Keathley, M.S.
Department of Pathology, Medical Center Hospital of Vermont, Burlington, Vermont 05401

Martin Lipkin, M.D.
Memorial Sloan-Kettering Cancer Center, New York, New York 10021

Henry T. Lynch, M.D.
Department of Preventive Medicine, Creighton University School of Medicine, Omaha, Nebraska 68178

Jane F. Lynch, B.S.N.
Department of Preventive Medicine, Creighton University School of Medicine, Omaha, Nebraska 68178

Patrick M. Lynch, J.D., M.D.
Department of Medicine, University of Arkansas for Medical Sciences, Little Rock, Arkansas 72205

Rulon W. Rawson, M.D.
University of Utah, School of Medicine, Salt Lake City, Utah 84112

Guy S. Schuelke, Ph.D.
Department of Preventive Medicine, Creighton University School of Medicine, Omaha, Nebraska 68178

Lars Bo Svendsen, M.D.
Department of Surgical Gastroenterology, Bispebjerg Hospital, Copenhagen, Denmark

A. M. O. Veale, M.D.
School of Medicine, University of Auckland, Auckland, New Zealand

COLON CANCER
GENETICS

1
Epidemiology of Colon Cancer

Henry T. Lynch, M.D.,
Patrick M. Lynch, J.D., M.D.,
and Jane Keathley, M.S.

The epidemiology of colorectal cancer shares certain similarities with the epidemiology of breast cancer. In each case, there are marked geographic, dietary, and socioeconomic differences and a striking increase in incidence with age.[1, 2]

Migrant studies have shown parallels between breast and colon cancer. Immigrants from Japan and black Africa, where the rates of both lesions are very low, have shown progressive increases in risk during the decades following arrival in the United States.[3] Such shifts are thought to negate primary genetics as being etiologic.[4]

Temporal variation in colorectal cancer has also provided clues to its etiology. However, high standards of case registration for periods of a decade or more have been available in just a few places in the world, and no useful frequency figures exist before this century. Incidence data for Connecticut, New York, and Denmark have covered the longest time frame. In these regions, little change during the past 30 years has been observed,[5] although an increase over the first half of the century has been well substantiated.[6] Japan has shown a substantial increase in colon cancer mortality, particularly among the elderly.[7] This increase appears to be associated with greater consumption of meat and milk products in Japan. Such shifts in age-specific incidence toward older patients are consistent with hypotheses that would demand many years of chronic exposure to moderately weak carcinogens.[8]

In the past, incidence and mortality data for colon and rectal cancers were customarily lumped together as "colorectal" or "large bowel" cancer. However, recent epidemiologic evidence suggests the need for a distinction between carcinomas of the colon and rectum.[9, 10] Figures 1-1 and 1-2 illustrate the dramatic international variation in mortality for both colonic and rectal carcinoma. Comparison of these figures, however, reveals only a moderate correlation of rankings within a given geography for colon versus rectal cancer. Colonic cancer frequency in the United States may be as much as

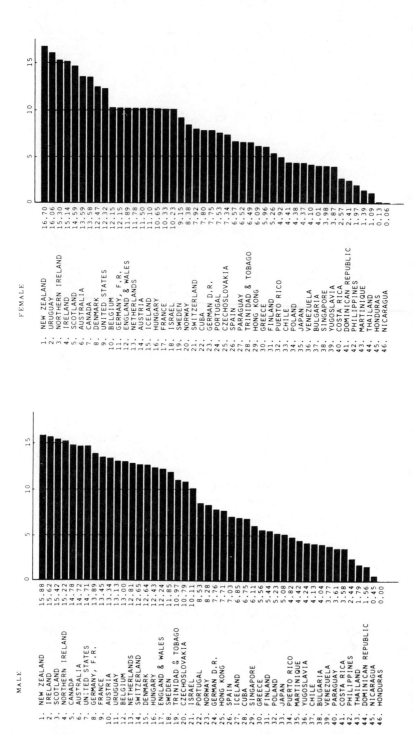

Figure 1-1. Age-adjusted death rates for malignant neoplasm of intestine except rectum (1975). *(From M. Segi, H. Hattori, and R. Segi: Age-Adjusted Death Rates for Cancer for Selected Sites (A-Classification) in 46 Countries in 1975. Segi Institute of Cancer Epidemiology, Japan, 1980, p. 11.)*

MALE

1.	NEW ZEALAND	15.88
2.	IRELAND	15.62
3.	SCOTLAND	15.42
4.	NORTHERN IRELAND	15.22
5.	CANADA	14.78
6.	AUSTRALIA	14.72
7.	UNITED STATES	14.71
8.	GERMANY, F.R.	13.89
9.	FRANCE	13.45
10.	AUSTRIA	13.34
11.	URUGUAY	13.13
12.	BELGIUM	13.00
13.	NETHERLANDS	12.81
14.	SWITZERLAND	12.65
15.	DENMARK	12.64
16.	HUNGARY	12.43
17.	ENGLAND & WALES	12.24
18.	SWEDEN	11.85
19.	TRINIDAD & TOBAGO	10.97
20.	CZECHOSLOVAKIA	10.79
21.	ISRAEL	10.11
22.	PORTUGAL	8.53
23.	NORWAY	8.28
24.	GERMAN D.R.	7.76
25.	HONG KONG	7.71
26.	SPAIN	7.03
27.	ICELAND	6.85
28.	CUBA	6.75
29.	SINGAPORE	6.11
30.	GREECE	5.56
31.	FINLAND	5.44
32.	POLAND	5.23
33.	JAPAN	5.08
34.	PUERTO RICO	4.82
35.	MARTINIQUE	4.42
36.	YUGOSLAVIA	4.24
37.	CHILE	4.13
38.	BULGARIA	4.04
39.	VENEZUELA	3.77
40.	PARAGUAY	3.61
41.	COSTA RICA	3.58
42.	PHILLIPINES	2.44
43.	THAILAND	1.79
44.	DOMINICAN REPUBLIC	1.56
45.	NICARAGUA	0.45
46.	HONDURAS	0.00

FEMALE

1.	NEW ZEALAND	16.70
2.	URUGUAY	16.06
3.	NORTHERN IRELAND	15.30
4.	IRELAND	15.14
5.	SCOTLAND	14.59
6.	AUSTRALIA	13.59
7.	CANADA	13.58
8.	DENMARK	12.47
9.	UNITED STATES	12.32
10.	BELGIUM	12.15
11.	GERMANY, F.R.	12.15
12.	ENGLAND & WALES	11.89
13.	NETHERLANDS	11.78
14.	AUSTRIA	11.50
15.	ICELAND	11.10
16.	HUNGARY	10.65
17.	FRANCE	10.33
18.	ISRAEL	10.23
19.	SWEDEN	9.15
20.	NORWAY	8.38
21.	SWITZERLAND	7.92
22.	CUBA	7.80
23.	GERMAN D.R.	7.75
24.	PORTUGAL	7.53
25.	CZECHOSLOVAKIA	7.34
26.	SPAIN	6.57
27.	PARAGUAY	6.52
28.	TRINIDAD & TOBAGO	6.49
29.	HONG KONG	6.09
30.	GREECE	5.96
31.	FINLAND	5.26
32.	PUERTO RICO	4.92
33.	CHILE	4.41
34.	POLAND	4.38
35.	JAPAN	4.37
36.	VENEZUELA	4.10
37.	BULGARIA	4.01
38.	SINGAPORE	3.98
39.	YUGOSLAVIA	3.87
40.	COSTA RICA	2.57
41.	DOMINICAN REPUBLIC	2.41
42.	PHILIPPINES	1.97
43.	MARTINIQUE	1.39
44.	THAILAND	1.09
45.	HONDURAS	0.13
46.	NICARAGUA	0.06

2

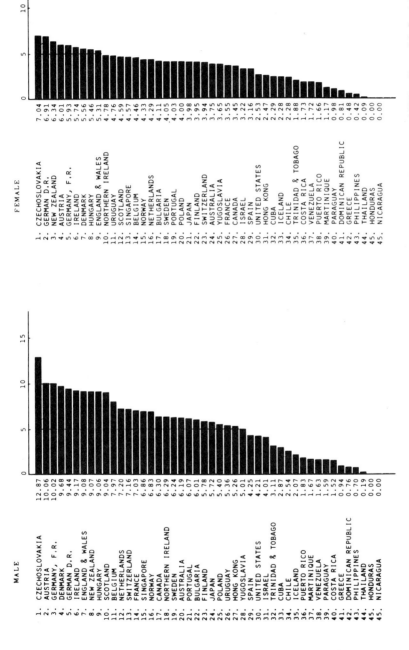

Figure 1-2. Age-adjusted death rates for malignant neoplasm of rectum and rectosigmoid junction (1975). *(From M. Segi, H. Hattori, and R. Segi: Age-Adjusted Death Rates for Cancer for Selected Sites (A-Classification) in 46 Countries in 1975. Segi Institute of Cancer Epidemiology, Japan, 1980, p. 12.)*

3

four times greater as in a lower-risk country such as Japan; however, rectal cancer incidence in these countries is roughly equal. These data, therefore, suggest differing etiologies for colonic and rectal carcinomas. In western countries, cancer occurs more frequently in the sigmoid and descending colon, while in low-risk countries, carcinoma of the proximal colon shows a higher relative incidence. The male to female ratio approaches unity for colon cancer but is 1 to 4 for rectal cancer. Curiously, despite accepted theories of carcinogen concentration and metabolic potentiation in the distal colon, recent studies have documented an increase in right-sided lesions over the past few years.[11]

SPECIFIC ENVIRONMENTAL AGENTS

Purgatives

In reviewing the subject of purgatives, Doll cited one study done 25 years ago of 614 patients with gastrointestinal cancer whose past histories were compared with those of matched patients with nongastrointestinal diseases.[4] No differences were found in purgative use in general. However, the proportion of patients with both gastric and intestinal cancer who had used liquid paraffin regularly for more than 5 years was about double that of the control group, and the relative excess was greater still for those few patients who had used it for more than 20 years. At the time of the study, liquid paraffin contained fluorescent substances that may have been carcinogenic. (Today, liquid paraffin is purified and no longer contains these substances.) But clearly, the role of such agents is limited to, at most, a small subset of the cancer-affected population.

Occupational Factors

There has been evidence, particularly in the United States, of increased mortality from cancer of the large bowel in asbestos workers.[12] However, other studies have not supported this association,[13] and a causal relationship cannot be inferred at this time.

Selenium

Studies in experimental animals have shown that selenium can reduce the incidence of spontaneous colorectal tumors as well as those that are chemically induced.[14] In humans, an inverse relationship appears to exist between serum levels of selenium and colorectal cancer, with colorectal cancer increased in the presence of low serum-selenium levels.[15, 16] Regarding selenium levels in crops, areas with low levels of selenium had higher rates of colorectal cancer mortality. It therefore appears that selenium may protect against colorectal cancer in both animals and humans.

Alcohol

Alcohol consumption, specifically beer, has been linked to colorectal carcinoma.[17] Enstrom's survey showed a correlation between beer consumption in 47 states and mortality from colorectal cancer. The association was greater for rectal than colonic cancer. A study by Dean et al. of blue-collar workers in a Dublin brewery has also supported the association.[18] Over a 20-year period, there were 32 deaths from carcinoma of the rectum versus an expected 13.2. How beer drinking contributes to carcinoma of the large bowel is not clear at this time, but one suggestion is that beer drinkers retain greater amounts of liquid stool in the rectosigmoid area, thereby providing greater contact over time for carcinogens to react with the mucosal surface. However, the distinction between colonic and rectal cancer in such epidemiological investigations may be difficult to establish because of the large number of lesions occurring at the rectosigmoid junction and the arbitrary, conflicting boundaries that have been drawn.

Diet

Extensive reviews of the role of nutrition in colon cancer have been published.[19-41] However, in spite of intensive searches for specific dietary factors that may initiate or promote colon cancer, there is no clear consensus as to the role of any given agent. Diet appears to play a major role in contributing to geographic differences in colon-cancer rates. For example, in high-risk areas, a major portion of the dietary fat is derived from meat, particularly beef. Typically, diets high in fat are correspondingly low in fiber. This undoubtedly has contributed to the attention given to dietary fat and fiber in many epidemiologic studies.[21-24]

Many experts have suggested that the most fruitful etiologic hypotheses are those concerned with diet, in spite of the extreme difficulties in investigating foods with available epidemiologic methods. While the components of diet change during a person's lifetime, a given patient may not recall what specific foods he ate early in life. In developed countries such as the United States, consumed foods vary from day to day, and it becomes very difficult to systematically recall one's dietary history. Thorough evaluation of dietary practices requires complete chemical analysis of food consumed—a very expensive and time-consuming process, particularly when conducted on the extremely large population samples that are required. Consequently, many researchers have resorted to less thorough and less accurate methods of obtaining dietary information, such as interviews or questionnaires. It is, therefore, not surprising that epidemiologic studies of specific dietary items have given conflicting results.

Burkitt has emphasized that the distribution, both geographic and socioeconomic, of high-fat diets is almost the same as for low-fiber diets.[21, 40] In virtually all communities, 10 to 15% of the energy requirements are derived from protein and the remaining 85 to 90% come from fats and carbohydrates. Burkitt states that these two main sources of energy are reciprocally related, in that carbohydrate-rich diets are almost invariably fiber rich and high-fat diets are fiber poor. Studies by Antonis and Bersohn relate Burkitt's position to the potential role of dietary fats and bile acids in colon tumorigenesis.[32] These investigators presented evidence that reducing the fat in a low-fiber diet or increasing the fiber in a high-fat diet would each decrease the fecal bile-acid concentration.

N-nitroso compounds in stools may have carcinogenic properties, and these have been reduced in stools by reducing fat intake or by adding large quantities of wheat bran to the daily diet.[25-28] Mutagenic activity due to N-nitroso compounds was observed more frequently in feces from patients with colorectal cancer than in laboratory personnel.

In addition to environmental factors such as high dietary intake of animal fats and proteins and low dietary intake of unrefined fiber, some other dietary factors correlate with the incidence of colon cancer. These include nonnutritive substances in food such as bacterial or fungal metabolites,[42] food additives such as nitrosamines and nitrosamides, and by-products arising from frying or barbecuing fish and meat.[43]

Indirect effects of diet may also be important in intestinal carcinogenesis. For example, diet can alter the metabolism of the intestinal microflora and the resulting altered bacterial-metabolic patterns can lead to either an increased or decreased conversion of procarcinogens to proximal carcinogens.[44, 45] Dietary components may also influence the level of intestinal-epithelial microsomal-enzyme systems involved in the activation of carcinogens.

If the risk of colorectal cancer is diminished by a vegetarian diet, it may be due to the excess of vegetables, not the absence of meat. Bjelke[19] suggests that vegetables in particular may have a protective effect against colorectal cancer. Case-control studies in Scandinavia and the United States showed the risk of colon cancer to be reduced by about 25% in men who ate large amounts of vegetables.[23-24] Graham et al. also concluded that vegetables conferred protection against colon cancer.[20]

Experiments on the possible protective effect of dietary fiber on 1,2 dimethylhydrazine [DMH] injected animals have shown a significant benefit.[25, 26, 48] In rats receiving DMH, the amount of stool bulk and the fiber consumed was inversely related to large-bowel-tumor frequency.[26, 48] The addition of cellulose to an otherwise fiber-free diet in DMH-treated rats also reduced colonic tumors. However, Cruse et al.[27] concluded that fiber was not protective against DMH-induced tumors. Others believe that these results may have been caused by the way the test animals received injected carcinogens, and that this is not a suitable model for demonstrating the effect of diet on humans.[28]

Dietary fiber might protect against colorectal cancer by increasing fecal volume with resulting dilution of carcinogens or cocarcinogens in the gut; reducing intestinal transit time thereby lessening the period of physical contact between fecal carcinogens and intestinal mucosa; and adsorbing potentially carcinogenic particles in the bowel.

The pH of the stool may also be related etiologically to colorectal cancer incidence. Dietary fiber consumed with milk can carry lactose into the colon and diminish the pH of the stool.[29] It has further been shown that the colorectal-cancer risk decreases as stool pH declines. Low pH diminishes the gut bacteroides population—a notable consideration since these bacteria have been implicated in colorectal carcinogenesis.[29]

MacDonald and associates have shown *in vitro* that increasing pH significantly enhances bacterial activity on bile acids.[29, 30] Such activity may play a role in the promotion of colonic tumors. Population data point to consistent differences in average stool pH in geographies with high rates of colon cancer (e.g., America) and low rates (e.g., Africa). Burkitt concludes that fiber has an important function in lowering fecal pH and that this may in turn protect against colon cancer.[21, 40]

Bile Acids

Hill et al. have suggested that diet significantly influences large bowel flora and digestive enzymes.[44] Their hypothesis is that biochemically active bowel flora may degrade the intestinal substrate, in turn producing carcinogens or cocarcinogens. Bile acids are considered central to this entire scheme in that their fecal levels are related to fat intake and their acid-steroid–chemical structure is somewhat similar to the polycyclic, aromatic carcinogens.[40] In a report by Hill, 82% of colorectal cancer patients had fecal-bile-acid (FBA) levels that were above an arbitrarily selected value; only 17% of the control group were above the same value.[37] The same percentage of the cancer patients had fecal nuclear-dehydrogenating *clostridia* (NDC), while only 43% of the controls had NDC. Seventy percent of the cancer patients had a combination of NDC and high FBA levels, compared with only 9% of the control patients. Nuclear-dehydrogenating *clostridia* are of interest because of their capacity to dehydrogenate the steroid nucleus of bile acids and

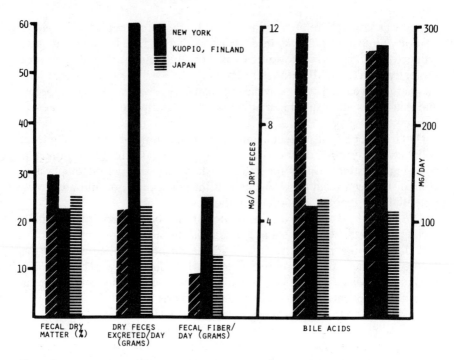

Figure 1-3. Fecal constituents of high- and low-risk population for colon cancer. *(From S. Winawer, D. Schottenfeld, and P. Sherlock, eds. Colorectal Cancer: Prevention, Epidemiology, and Screening. Raven Press, New York, 1980, p. 30. Copyright © 1980 by Raven Press.)*

cholesterol metabolites, a process necessary for the conversion of these compounds to polycyclic, aromatic carcinogens.

Murray and associates attempted to replicate Hill's work in a population known to have a high incidence of colorectal cancer.[45] Thirty-seven patients with colorectal cancer in Glasgow, Scotland were compared with 36 controls without gastrointestinal disease. Biochemical analyses of the total FBA, lithocholic, deoxycholic, and cholic acids, and NDC were isolated in stool specimens. The main FBA concentration in the controls was significantly *higher* ($P < 0.001$). Bacteria capable of metabolizing steroids were thus implicated in the etiology of colorectal cancer; however, the relationship between FBA and colorectal cancer was considered to require further evaluation.

Based upon the review of animal and human studies, Weisburger et al. postulate that bile acids can serve as *promoters* of colon cancer.[35, 36] Furthermore, they suggested that secondary (bacterially produced) bile acids

Table 1-1. Current Concepts on Colon-Cancer Causation and Development

Risk factors: Diets high in fat, cholesterol, and fried foods and low in fiber

Established mechanisms:

High fat ⟶ High cholesterol biosynthesis ⟶ High gut-bile-acid levels
    High dietary cholesterol ⟋

Low fiber ⟶ High concentration of gut bile acids
    (low dilution through lack of bulk)

High bile-acid concentration ⟶ Promoting effect in colon carcinogenesis

Mechanisms under study:

Fried food ⟶ Mutagens ⟶ Colon carcinogens?

Role of micronutrients (vitamins and minerals) and different types of fiber in production and metabolism of carcinogens, bile acids, promoters?

Mechanisms of promotion?

Source: From S. Winawer, D. Schottenfeld, and P. Sherlock, eds., *Colorectal Cancer: Prevention, Epidemiology, and Screening.* Raven Press, New York, 1980, p. 37. Copyright © 1980 by Raven Press.

are more potent than primary bile acids in colon carcinogenesis. Importantly, these same compounds are present in human stools in relatively high concentrations. In certain circumstances, (e.g., a low dose of or brief exposure to cocarcinogens), colon cancer failed to appear when the promotional stimulus from the luminal contents was removed. Studies at the infrahuman level have shown that removal of the gut contents, including bile-acid flow by colostomy, strongly suppressed colon carcinogenesis. Weisburger et al. emphasized that fat, rather than protein, appears to be the dietary ingredient more closely associated etiologically with colon cancer.[35, 36] Figure 1-3 reveals fecal bulk, fiber content, and bile-acid excretion in three geographies with markedly contrasting values for colorectal cancer (see also Fig. 1-1 and Fig. 1-2). Table 1-1 incorporates findings into a model for colorectal cancer causation.

Qualitative studies of the intestinal flora have not consistently demonstrated a difference in the *number* of species between high-risk colon cancer subjects and low-risk controls.[44, 45, 49-51] It was, therefore, suggested that the relation between colon cancer incidence and fecal bacteria cannot be attributed to a single species or group of related species and depends, instead, on the rate of metabolic activity of the bacteria. Such metabolic activity includes the conversion of primary bile acids to secondary bile acids (7-alpha-dehydroxylase), conversion of cholesterol to coprostanol and coprostanone (cholesterol dehydrogenase), introduction of double bonds into the steroid nucleus (nuclear dehydrogenase), and release of toxic products from conjugated compounds (beta-glucuronidase).[52]

Reddy and Wynder found concentrations of deoxycholic and lithocholic acid, cholesterol, coprostanol, and cholestan-3-alpha, 5-alpha, 6-alpha-triol in colon cancer patients and patients with adenomatous polyps to be higher than controls.[38] Consequently, 7-alpha-dehydroxylase and cholesterol-dehydrogenase activity were elevated. Further study of endogenous breakdown products was recommended.

GENETIC-ENVIRONMENTAL INTERACTION

Reddy found that patients with colon cancer precursors such as familial polyposis coli (FPC), ulcerative colitis, and adenomatous polyps, fall into three distinct groups relevant to fecal-bile-acid and metabolite profiles.[38, 39]

Patients with FPC excrete higher amounts of undegraded cholesterol than controls. Those with adenomatous polyps excrete more cholesterol-metabolite bile acids than normal controls.[53-55] Those with ulcerative colitis yield relatively greater concentrations of neutral sterols but no excess of bile acids. The central focus—cholesterol metabolites—was therefore believed to be genetic.

Genetic control is also apparent in other syndromes characterized by colon cancer (discussed at length in other sections of this book). These include the cancer family syndrome (CFS), Peutz-Jeghers syndrome, and juvenile polyposis coli, all of which follow an autosomal-dominant mode of inheritance and are characterized by multiple primary malignancies and an early age of onset.

Chemical carcinogenesis occurs in two stages: initiation and promotion.[56] Knudson's model of malignant transformation in hereditary cancer syndromes based on a two-stage process presupposes that the two stages of malignant transformation in hereditary cancer are germinal mutation and somatic mutation.[57] In hereditary forms of cancer, a germinal mutation predisposes malignant transformation by a single mutagenic event. Multiple primary malignancies and early age of onset, both characteristics of hereditary forms of cancer, are easily explained by this model. A germinal mutation may affect all cells in a cell line, resulting in multiple opportunities for primary tumor development. A germinal mutation is present at birth, and the time span required for a single somatic mutation is genetically significantly less than that required for two somatic mutations in patients lacking in inborn traits. Supportive examples of this "two-hit" hypothesis include xeroderma pigmentosum (XP), retinoblastoma, and adenomatosis of the colon and rectum.

Following an autosomal-recessive mode of inheritance, XP is characterized by sensitivity to sunlight and multiple cutaneous cancers. The primary defect is in the genetically determined enzyme system necessary for deoxyribonucleic acid (DNA) repair of ultraviolet light-induced damage. Mutations occurring as a result of exposure to sunlight constitute the second hit or promoting phase and result in development of skin cancers.[58]

Adenomatosis of the colon and rectum is a familial polyposis syndrome in which the entire intestine may be carpeted with polyps. If untreated, colon cancer develops in nearly 100% of these patients.[57] The disorder is inherited as an autosomal-dominant trait, and Purtilo et al. suggest that a prezygotic germinal mutation represents the primary defect.[59] Somatic mutations are then necessary for the development of polyps and adenocarcinomas.

Evidence for a similar two-hit process in familial forms of colon cancer is found in work by Kopelovich et al. who induced neoplastic transformation in skin fibroblasts from patients with hereditary adenomatosis of the colon and rectum by treating the cells with tumor-promoting agents only.[60] Fibroblasts from patients without the syndrome were not transformed by this treatment. The promoting activity associated with the secondary bile acids may provide the second hit in familial forms of colon cancer.

In a preliminary study, we examined the enzyme 7-alpha-dehydroxylase and its proposed role in colon cancer.[61] The enzyme converts primary bile acids to secondary bile acids. Subjects for the study consisted of members of families who fulfilled the criteria of the CFS and were divided as follows:

Group I: five people previously diagnosed with colon cancer and treated by local resection
Group II: six people previously diagnosed with endometrial cancer, but free of colon cancer
Group III: eight spouses of subjects in Groups I and II

Fecal samples were collected from each person and assayed for 7-alpha-dehydroxylase activity. The results of these analyses (Table 1-2)

TABLE 1-2. Mean Values of 7-*a*-Dehydroxylase Activity in Groups I, II, and III

GROUP I	GROUP II	GROUP III
35.4 ± 10.1	49.7 ± 10.7	42.1 ± 10.4

Source: After J. D. Keathley and C. A. Needham, Analysis of the fecal microflora and its enzymatic activity in individuals genetically predisposed to colon cancer, *Cancer Res.* **42:**4284-4288, 1982.
Note: Mean value of 7-alpha dehydroxylase activity expressed as % conversion to deoxycholic acid per 100 mg dry feces ± standard error.

showed no significant differences among CFS family members who had developed colon cancer, CFS family members who had not developed colon cancer, and persons with very similar dietary and environmental exposure who lacked a family history of colon cancer.

In a similar study by Mastromarino et al.[62] fecal 7-alpha-dehydroxylase activity was measured in colon cancer subjects with no known familial history and compared to levels of activity in nonhereditary, adenomatous polyp patients and healthy controls.[61] A significant increase in activity was found in patients with colon cancer and adenomatous polyp vis-à-vis healthy controls.

The results from these two studies indicate possible differences in familial and environmentally induced forms of colon cancer. If bile acids do play a role in colon tumorigenesis, that role appears to be less important cumulatively in familial colon cancer. In other words, the increased activity of 7-alpha-dehydroxylase seen by Mastromarino in presumptive environmentally induced cases is not necessary for tumorigenesis in genetically predisposed subjects.

Based on Knudson's hypothesis, the inherited trait characteristic of CFS may result in a state of increased susceptibility of these persons to levels of promoting agents, such as secondary bile acids, that would not affect nonfamily members. Therefore, levels of enzymatic activity associated with production of promoting agents would be expected to fall into an average range in familial syndrome subjects, even in those who develop colon tumors. People from the general population, with no familial history, may instead require increased levels of promoting agents, and thus increased associated enzymatic activity, before tumorigenesis will occur. The extent of the inherited susceptibility may vary among familial syndromes as well as all people, thereby accounting for a broad range of susceptibility–resistance to colon cancer in the entire population.

ADDENDUM

Since this chapter was submitted for publication, the first report of our epidemiologic-family study of colorectal cancer in Nebraska has been published.[63] This case/control interview study was conducted in two rural counties (Butler and Colfax) in eastern Nebraska in order to determine reasons for the elevated colon cancer mortality rates from 1950-1969.[64] The investigation involved 86 residents of these counties who were diagnosed with colorectal cancer from 1970-1977. For each case identified, two controls were selected from hospital admissions lists and matched to the case by hospital, year of hospitalization, county of residence, age (±5 years), race, and sex. The mean age of study subjects was 74 years and the mean length of residence in the respective counties was 45 years.

Findings disclosed an increased risk of colorectal cancer among persons of Czech background, with persons of Bohemian and Moravian extraction predominating in this region of the United States. The findings suggested an interaction between Bohemian ancestry and certain dietary patterns that may have contributed to colorectal cancer pathogenesis in this particular region. Of interest was the finding of elevated colon cancer risk among commercial beer drinkers regardless of their ethnic background, although Bohemians reportedly were heavy consumers. The results also suggested an influence of obesity on the area's high colon cancer rates, since the mean heights and weights of the control group approximate the United States average seen in a recent nationwide study. In addition, an excess risk was associated with intestinal polyps—a finding more often present among Moravians—and with familial occurrence of gastrointestinal and other cancers. A threefold excess of cancer was found among patients with a history of colon cancer in a close relative, a finding that was consistent with previous surveys of familial risk of colon cancer.[65]

REFERENCES

1. Armstrong, B., and Doll, R.: Environmental factors, cancer incidence and mortality in different countries, with special reference to dietary practices. *Intern. J. Cancer* **15:**617-631, 1975.
2. Drasar, B.S., and Irving, D.: Environmental factors and cancer of the colon and breast. *Br. J. Cancer* **27:**167-172, 1973.
3. Haenszel, W.: Cancer mortality among the foreign-born in the U.S. *JNCI* **26:**37-132, 1961.
4. Doll, R.: General epidemiologic considerations in etiology of colorectal cancer. In: *Colorectal Cancer: Prevention, Epidemiology, and Screening* (Winawer, S.; Schottenfeld, D.; and Sherlock, P., eds.). New York, NY: Raven Press, 1980, pp. 3-12.
5. Eisenberg, H., Sullivan, P.D.; and Connelly, R.R.: *Cancer in Connecticut, 1935-1962.* Hartford, CT: Connecticut State Department of Health, 1966.
6. Correa, P., and Haenszel, W.: Comparative international incidence and prevention. In: *Cancer Epidemiology and Prevention* (Stewart, S.T., ed.). Springfield, MA: Charles C. Thomas Co., 1975, p. 386.
7. Lee, J.A.H.: Recent trends of large bowel cancer in Japan compared to United States and England and Wales. *Intern. J. Epid.* **5:**187-194, 1976.
8. Cook, P.; Doll, R.; and Fellingham, S.A.: A mathematical model for the age distribution of cancer in man. *Intern. J. Cancer* **4:**93-112, 1969.
9. Rosato, F.E., and Marks, G.: Changing site distribution patterns of colorectal cancer at Thomas Jefferson University Hospital. *Dis. Colon Rect.* **24:**93-95, 1981.
10. Morgenstern, L., and Lee, S.E.: Spatial distribution of colonic carcinoma. *Arch. Surg.* **113:**1142-1143, 1978.

11. Abrams, J.S., and Reines, H.D.: Increasing incidence of right-sided lesions in colorectal cancer. *Am. J. Surg.* **137:**522-526, 1979.
12. Selikoff, I.J., and Hammond, E.C.: Asbestos associated disease in United States shipyards. *Cancer* **28:** 87-99, 1978.
13. Peto, J.; Doll, R.; Howard, S.V.; Kinlen, L.J.; and Lewinsohn, H.C.: A mortality study among workers in an English asbestos factory. *Br. J. Ind. Med.* **34:**169-173, 1977.
14. Broghamer, W.L.; McConnell, K.P.; and Blotchy, A.L.: Relationship between serum selenium levels and patients with carcinoma. *Cancer* **37:**1384-1388, 1976.
15. Shamberger, R.J.; Rukovena, E.; Longfield, A.K.; Tytko, S.A.; Deodhar, S.; and Willis, C.E.: Antioxidants and cancer. I. Selenium in the blood of normals and cancer patients. *JNCI* **50:**863-870, 1973.
16. Shamberger, R.J.; Tytko, S.A.; and Willis, C.E.: Antioxidants and cancer. VI. Selenium and age adjusted human cancer mortality. *Arch. Env. Health* **31:**231-235, 1976.
17. Enstrom, J.E.: Colorectal cancer and beer drinking. *Br. J. Cancer* **35:**674-683, 1977.
18. Dean, G.; MacLennan, R.; McLoughlin, H.; and Shelley, E.: Causes of death of blue-collar workers at a Dublin brewery. *Br. J. Cancer* **40:**581-589, 1979.
19. Bjelke, E.: Epidemiologic studies of cancer of the stomach, colon, and rectum, with special emphasis on the role of diet. Vols. III and IV. Ann Arbor, MI: University Microfilm, 1963.
20. Graham, S.; Dayal, H.; Swanson, M.; Mittelman, A.; and Wilkinson, G.: Diet in the epidemiology of cancer of the colon and rectum. *JNCI* **61:**709-714, 1978.
21. Burkitt, D.P.: Fiber in the etiology of colorectal cancer. In: *Colorectal Cancer: Prevention, Epidemiology, and Screening* (Winawer, S.; Schottenfeld, D.; and Sherlock, P., eds.). New York, NY: Raven Press, 1980, pp. 13-18.
22. Wynder, E.L., and Shigematsu, T.: Environmental factors of cancer of the colon and rectum. *Cancer* **20:** 1520-1561, 1967.
23. MacLennan, R.; Jensen, O.M.; Mosbech, J.; and Vuori, H.: Diet, transit time, stool weight, and colon cancer in two Scandanavian populations. *Am. J. Clin. Nutr.* **31:** S.239-242, 1978.
24. Reddy, B.C.; Hedges, A.R.; Laakso, K.; and Wynder, E.L.: Metabolic epidemiology of large bowel cancer: fecal bulk and constituents of high-risk North American and low-risk Finnish population. *Cancer* **42:**2832-2838, 1978.
25. Chen, W.; Patchefsky, A.H.; and Goldsmith, H.: Colonic protection from dimethylhydrazine by a high fiber diet. *Surgery* **147:**503-506, 1978.
26. Fleiszer, D.; Murray, D.; MacFarlane, J.; and Brown, R.A.: Protective effect of dietary fibre against chemically induced bowel tumors in rats. *Lancet* **2:**552-553, 1978.
27. Cruse, J.P.; Lewin, M.R.; and Clarke, G.C.: Failure of bran to protect against experimental colon cancer in rats. *Lancet* **2:**1278-1279, 1979.
28. Newcombe, R.R.Q.: Bran and experimental colon cancer. *Lancet* **1:**108, 1979.
29. Macdonald, I.A.; Sinsh, G.; Mahony, D.E.; and Meier, C.E.: Effect of pH on bile salt degradation by mixed fecal cultures. *Steroids* **32:**245-256, 1978.
30. Macdonald, I.A.; Webb, G.R.; and Mahony, D.E.: Fecal hydroxysteroid

dehydrogenase activities in vegetarian Seventh-Day Adventists, control subjects, and bowel cancer patients. *Am. J. Clin. Nutr.* **31:**5233-5238, 1978.

31. Walker, A.R.; Walker, B.F.; and Segal, I.: Faecal pH value and its modification by dietary means in South African black and white school children. *S. Afr. Med. J.* **55:**495-498, 1979.

32. Antonis, A., and Bersohn, I.: The influence of diet on faecal lipids in South African white and Bantu prisoners. *Am. J. Clin. Nutr.* **11:**142-155, 1962.

33. Land, P.C., and Bruce, W.R.: *Origins of Human Cancer.* Cold Spring Harbor, NY: Cold Spring Harbor Laboratory, 1976.

34. Ershoff, B.A.: Antitoxic effects of plant fibre. *Am. J. Clin. Nutr.* **27:**1395-1398, 1974.

35. Weisburger, J.H.; Reddy, B.S.; and Joftes, D. (eds.): Colorectal cancer. *UICC Tech. Rpt. Ser.* **19:**1-143, 1975.

36. Weisburger, J.H.; Reddy, B.S.; Springarn, N.E.; and Wynder, E.L.: Current views on the mechanisms involved in the etiology of colorectal cancer. In: *Colorectal Cancer: Prevention, Epidemiology, and Screening,* Winawer, S.; Schottenfeld, D.; and Sherlock, P., eds. New York, NY: Raven Press, 1980, pp. 19-41.

37. Hill, M.J.; Drasar, B.S.; William, R.E.O.; Meade, T.W.; Cox, A.G.; Simpson, J.E.P.; and Morson, B.C.: Faecal bile acids and clostridia in patients with cancer of the large bowel, *Lancet* **1:**535-538, 1975.

38. Reddy, B.S., and Wynder, E.L.: Metabolic epidemiology of colon cancer: fecal bile acids and neutral sterols in colon cancer patients and patients with adenomatous polyps. *Cancer* **39:**2533-2539, 1977.

39. Reddy, B.S.: Nutrition and colon cancer. *Adv. Nutr. Res.* **2:**199-218, 1979.

40. Burkitt, D.P.: Epidemiology of cancer of the colon and rectum. *Cancer* **28:**3, 1971.

41. Armstrong, B., and Doll, R.: Environmental factors, cancer incidence, and mortality in different countries, with special reference to dietary practices. *Int. J. Ca.* **14:** 617-631, 1975.

42. Miller, J.A., and Miller, E.C.: Carcinogens occurring naturally in foods. *Fed. Proceedings* **35:**1316-1321, 1976.

43. Nagao, M.; Honda, M.; Seino, T.; Yahazi, R.; and Sugimura, R.: Mutagenicities of smoke condensates and the charred surface of fish and meat. *Cancer Lett.* **2:**221-226, 1977.

44. Hill, M.J.; Drasar, B.S.; Aries, V.C.; Crowther, J.S.; Hawkesworth, G.; and Williams, R.E.O.: Bacteria and aetiology of cancer of the large bowel. *Lancet* **1:**95, 1971.

45. Murray, W.R.; Blackwood, A.; Trotter, J.M.; Calman, K.C.; and MacKay, C.: Faecal bile acids and clostridia in the aetiology of colorectal cancer. *Br. J. Cancer* **41:** 923-928, 1980.

46. Goldin, B.R., and Gorbach, S.L.: The relationship between diet and rat fecal bacterial enzymes implicated in colon cancer. *JNCI* **57:**371-375, 1976.

47. Wattenberg, L.W.: Studies of polycyclic hydrocarbon hydroxylases of the intestine possibly related to cancer. *Cancer* **28:**99-102, 1971.

48. Jacobs, M.M.; Jansson, B.; and Griffin, A.C.: Inhibitory effects of 1, 2-

dimethylhydrazine and methylazoxymethanol acetate induction of colon tumors. *Cancer Lett.* **2:**133-138, 1977.

49. Peach, S.; Fernandez, F.; Johnson, F.; and Drasar, B.S.: The nonsporing anaerobic bacteria in human feces. *J. Med. Microbiol.* **7:**213-221, 1974.

50. Cummings, J.H.; Wiggans, H.S.; Jenkins, D.J.A.; Houston, H.; Jivraj, T.; Drasar, B.S.; and Hill, M.J.: Influence of diets high and low in animal fat on bowel habit, gastrointestinal transit time, fecal microflora, bile acid, and fat excretion. *J. Clin. Inv.* **61:**953-963, 1978.

51. Finegold, S.M., and Sutter, V.L.: Fecal flora in different populations, with special reference to diet. *Am. J. Clin. Nutr.* **31:**5116-5122, 1978.

52. Mastromarino, A.J.; Reddy, B.S.; and Wynder, E.L.: Fecal profiles of anaerobic microflora of large bowel cancer patients and patients with nonhereditary large bowel polyps. *Cancer Res.* **38:**4458-4462, 1978.

53. Reddy, B.S.; Mastromarino, A.; Gustafson, C.; Lipkin, M.; and Wynder, E.L.: Fecal bile acids and neutral sterols in patients with familial polyposis. *Cancer* **38:** 1694-1698, 1976.

54. Drasar, B.S.; Bone, E.S.; Hill, M.F.; and Marks, C.G.: Colon cancer and bacterial metabolism in familial polyposis. *Gut* **16:**824-825, 1975.

55. Watne, P.L.; Lai, H.L.; Mance, T.; and Core, S.: Fecal steroids and bacterial flora in polyposis coli patients. *Am. J. Surgery* **131:**42-46, 1976.

56. Miller, E.E.: Some current perspectives on chemical carcinogenesis in humans and experimental animals: Presidential address. *Cancer Res.* **38:**1479-1496, 1978.

57. Knudson, A.G.; Strong, L.C.; and Anderson, D.E.: Heredity and cancer in man. *Prog. Med. Genet.* **9:**113-152, 1973.

58. Cleaver, J.E.: Defective repair replication of DNA in xeroderma pigmentosum. *Nature* **218:**652-656, 1968.

59. Purtilo, D.T.; Paquin, L.; and Gindhart, T.: Genetics of neoplasia-impact of ecogenetics in oncogenesis. *Am. J. Path.* **91:**609-688, 1978.

60. Kopelovich, L.; Bias, N.E.; and Helson, L.: Tumor promoter alone induces neoplastic transformation of fibroblasts from humans genetically predisposed to cancer. *Nature* **282:**619-621, 1979.

61. Keathley, J.D., and Needham, C.A.: Analysis of the fecal microflora and its enzymatic activity in individuals genetically predisposed to colon cancer. *Cancer Res.* **42:**4284-4288, 1982.

62. Mastromarino, A.; Reddy, B.S.; and Wynder, E.L.: Metabolic epidemiology of colon cancer: enzyme activity of fecal flora. *Am. J. Clin. Nutr.* **29:**1455-1460, 1976.

63. Pickle, L.W.; Green, M.H.; Ziegler, R.G.; Toledo, A.; Hoover, R.; Lynch, H.T.; and Fraumeni, J.F.: Colorectal cancer in rural Nebraska. *Cancer Res.* **44:**363-369, 1984.

64. Blot, W.J.; Fraumeni, J.F.; Stone, B.J.; and McKay, F.W.: Geographic patterns of large bowel cancer in the United States, *JNCI* **57:**1225-1231, 1976.

65. Correa, P., and Haenszel, W.: The epidemiology of large bowel cancer, *Adv. Cancer Res.* **26:**1-141, 1976.

2
Investigation of a Genetic Model

A.M.O. Veale, M.B., Ch.B., Ph.D.

The possibility that hereditary factors might be important in the causation of colorectal cancer has been highlighted ever since it was recognized that some rare, hereditary, large bowel syndromes led to the development of malignancy. Handford drew attention to the occurrence of malignancy complicating what we now call familial polyposis coli (FPC),[2] and other writers of the time[2-4] all described cases occurring in relatives. Lockhart-Mummery, in a paper entitled "Cancer and Heredity," presented data from three polyposis families and placed the association of this condition with large bowel cancer beyond all reasonable doubt.[5] Speculation about the role (if any) of genetic factors in the causation of most, if not all, cases of bowel and other cancers has continued ever since.

The investigation of the incidence of large bowel cancer among index cases with the condition has been a favorite method of attack. Findings such as those of Macklin,[6] Woolf,[7] Lynch et al,[8] Bjelke,[9] and Lovett[10] have established that the frequency among relatives is undoubtedly increased over that of the general population. Unfortunately, whether this increase is due to genetic or environmental factors has not been resolved because of the tendency of investigators to regard such causative agents as mutually exlcusive and also because of the lack of a suitable model that might make some kind of genetic analysis possible.

The evidence for environmental factors in the causation of large bowel cancer is considerable, but we should bear in mind that such factors may exert their influence on populations in which there exist persons who, by virtue of their genotype, may have a greater or lesser susceptibility to environmental stresses. In the discussion that follows, the genetic argument in no way conflicts with variations in the incidence of bowel cancer that have been shown to be associated with defined epidemiological variables. Just as the increased frequency of large bowel cancer among relatives of index cases is confirmed finding, so is the association of incidence with such factors as diet, social class, fiber intake and country of residence and origin. Perhaps the isolation of a genetic component with respect to susceptibility to colorectal cancer will clarify other epidemiological findings.

A GENETIC MODEL

The purpose of this section is to examine in some detail how appropriate data might be analyzed genetically in the light of a model first suggested by Veale.[11] The hypothesis was formulated to explain the absence of parent-child correlations in various age parameters associated with FPC. Although sibling to sibling correlations for age of appearance of polypi, age of onset of cancer, and age at death from cancer were all statistically equal to the expected value of +0.5, the parent to child correlations were all 0. In addition, the data suggested that among the patients there were two overlapping age distributions with one group having an earlier onset and more severe clinical course than the other. These findings were to be expected if an allelic series of genes existed at the polyposis locus. Such series was proposed consisting of the polyposis gene for FPC designated P, a polyp gene designated p, and a normal (wild type) designated gene +. The genotype Pp represented a more severe form of FPC with earlier onset of polypi, cancer, and death than the alternative genotype $P+$. As all FPC patients would receive the modifying allele from their *unaffected* parent, no correlation between the affected parents and their affected offspring was expected. In contrast, the sibling to sibling correlation would be +0.5 for any frequency of the p and + genes in the general population.

The next question to be resolved was the effect (if any) of the variant genotypes pp, $p+$, and $++$ on nonpolyposis patients. It was proposed that there was no effect except for persons of the pp genotype. Here it was suggested that such patients would inevitably produce a few adenomata of the colon and rectum.

It has long been known that a significant proportion of the population over age 40 harbors one or more adenomatous lesions of the large bowel. At one time there was much debate over the relationship between isolated adenomas and cancer, but it is now accepted that the presence of an adenoma increases one's risk of colorectal cancer.[12] Morson has shown that at least half the cases of colorectal cancer may develop in a preexisting adenoma, and that remnants of adenomas are frequently found in malignant lesions.[13] Hill and Hill et al. have formalized the operation of environmental factors at three levels on the postulated susceptible genotype pp, suggesting that all cases of colorectal cancer arise in such patients, and that racial and other epidemiological differences in cancer incidence reflect variation in the magnitude of the factors operating at the three stages necessary for the production of a carcinoma.[14, 15]

Formal consequences of such a mechanism are

1. That there should be an increased incidence of colorectal cancer among index cases. (This has already been established.)
2. That there should be "polyp prone" people in the population. This has been claimed on a number of occasions.[12, 16, 17]
3. That, occasionally, we could expect to see families in which the incidence of bowel cancer was notably high but who did not have multiple polyps as in FPC. Such "cancer families" have been reported by Warthin,[18, 19] Macklin,[6] and Lynch et al.,[8, 20] among others.
4. That if the "cancer proneness" bestowed on a patient by virtue of his genotype (pp) should manifest itself in other organs as well as the colon, we could expect to see associated cancer occurring in cancer families with a frequency not explainable by chance alone. Such an association in colon-cancer families with endometrial cancer and multiple, primary malignancies has been reported by Lynch et al.[21] and others.
5. That if cancer proneness has a genetic basis, there might be some manifestation of this in a tissue-culture system.

Apparently, if a formal genetic model of carcinogenesis in the large bowel is to be based on the presence of a susceptible genotype (pp) in the population then we must not only estimate the frequency of pp persons and, hence, the gene frequency of p, but also ascertain the risk of a pp person developing carcinoma. Veale[11] noted that the most frequent estimate of the prevalence of adenomas in adults was around 10%, although the range was from 2 to 20%. Basing his estimate mainly on the work of Andren and Frieberg,[22] Veale took the prevalence of pp persons as 9% corresponding to a gene frequency for the gene p of $u = 0.3$ and + of $v = (1 - u) = 0.7$. These gene frequencies correspond to an equilibrium in the population of 9% pp, 42% $p+$, and 49% $++$.

The various types of mating that will exist in the population can now be calculated and if, in addition, we postulate that the risk of a pp person developing cancer is 1/3, then we could expect 9% $\times$ 1/3 = 3% of all persons dying to have died from or to have had and been cured of colorectal cancer. The figure of 3% is the approximate proportion of all deaths from colorectal cancer in England and Wales in the period 1930 to 1974. However, in order to explore the genetic model more formally, it is necessary to estimate the gene frequency of p (u) and the risk of developing cancer (x, given that the patient is pp) from actual family and population data. For this purpose, the analysis is based on the data of Lovett[10] but a different technique was used and two families now known to have FPC were omitted. The amended series now consists of 207 index cases with colorectal cancer, their parents, and 672 siblings. The patients consisted of consecutive admissions to St. Mark's Hospital, London, during the period of December, 1969 to March, 1973.

ANALYSIS BASED ON THE PARENTS

We will now examine this series of patients and their relatives in terms of the Veale hypothesis and obtain estimates of u (the gene frequency of p) and x (the risk of a pp person developing colorectal cancer). Note that $v =$ gene frequency of the $+$ gene and $u + v = 1$. The genotypes pp, $p+$, and $++$ will be in the proportions u^2, $2uv$, and v^2 respectively. A proportion x of the pp population will develop colorectal cancer, so that the population incidence will be u^2x. In England and Wales this value of u^2x is approximately 0.03. If colorectal cancer is a random event with a probability of 0.03, then the frequency of cases among both, one, or neither parent of our index cases can be calculated. This has been done in Table 2-1 for the 207 cases in the series. Included among the 414 parents are 53 who are still alive, which, unfortunately, artificially increases the proportion of unaffected parents and diminishes the actual observed difference from expectation, making the result less statistically significant than it actually is. Table 1-2 clearly shows that there are too many affected parents when the expectation is based on the population incidence (probability $p < 0.001$).

In terms of our hypothesis, we know that since each index case is of genotype pp, each parent must have passed at least one p gene on to his offspring. The frequency of the companion gene (allele) can be expressed in terms of gene frequencies. The allele to the p gene we know to be present in each parent will be another p gene with frequency $= u$ (the gene frequency

Table 2-1. Expected and Observed Cases of Colorectal Cancer Among Parents of Index Cases, Assuming a Random Incidence of 0.03

	BOTH PARENTS AFFECTED	1 PARENT AFFECTED	0 PARENTS AFFECTED	TOTAL
Observed	1	34	172	207
Expected	0.19	12.05	194.76	207

Note: Combining the first 2 columns x^2 (1 df) = 44.98 (probability = $p < 0.001$).

of p) and $a +$ gene with frequency $= v$ (the gene frequency of $+$). In other words, each parent of an index case will be pp with frequency u and $p+$ with frequency v. Hence, the risk of actually having colorectal cancer in a parent of an index case is ux ($=$ risk of being pp $\times$ risk of developing cancer). The chance of a parent not developing cancer either because he is $p+$ or because, although he is pp, cancer does not develop, is $1 - ux$. The expected proportions of parents with both affected, one affected, or neither affected are given by $(ux)^2$, $2ux (1 - ux)$, and $(1 - ux)^2$ respectively.

The value for ux is given by the proportion of parents with cancer $=$ $36/414 = 0.087$. Using this value, we can calculate the expected proportions of parental types (0, 1, or both affected) and compare this with what was actually observed. The comparison is made in Table 2-2 where it is clear that the agreement between the observed and expected matings is very good. Parenthetically, we can observe that even if there had been no families with both parents affected and 36 sets of parents with only 1 affected ($ux = 0.087$) the value of x^2 would have been only 1.87, which is still in good agreement. However, 4 or more sets of parents with both affected, and 28 or less with 1 affected so as to maintain $ux = 0.087$ would give highly significant departures from expectation.

As we now have estimates of $u^2x = 0.03$ and $ux = 0.087$, it is easy to see that $u = u^2x/ux = 0.03/0.087 = 0.34$ and $x = 0.25$. These estimates of the gene frequency of the p gene (u) and the chance of a pp person developing cancer (x) are derived from all the parents including some who are still alive and may develop cancer. Hence, our estimate of ux (0.087) may be a little too small. If more parents should develop cancer, ux will increase, and since u is obtained by dividing ux into $u^2 x$ (a constant), the value for u may diminish and the value for x increase. The value of u corresponds to a proportion u^2 of the population being of the polyp-prone-at-risk-for-cancer genotype ($= 11.56\%$), and if x of these (0.25) should develop cancer, the value for u^2x is 0.0289 ($= 0.03$).

Table 2-2. Expected and Observed Cases of Colorectal Cancer Among Parents of Index Cases Assuming $ux = 36/414 = 0.087$

	BOTH PARENTS AFFECTED	1 PARENT AFFECTED	0 PARENTS AFFECTED	TOTAL
Observed	1	34	172	207
Expected	1.57	32.88	172.55	207

Note: x^2 (1 df) $= 0.25$ (0.7 $>$ probability > 0.5).

INCIDENCE OF CANCER IN SIBLINGS

Independent estimates of u and x can be made from sibling data, but this is more complicated than simply measuring the proportion of affected siblings observed. Lovett's[10] analysis compared the death certifications of deceased siblings with the expectation of death being from colorectal cancer for persons of the appropriate age, sex, and time of death. (These expectations were derived from population figures for England and Wales from 1930–1970.) Among 104 siblings dying in this period, the number of deaths from colorectal cancer was 5.34 times the expectation. The actual number of cancer deaths was 18, or 17.31%. In spite of this, Lovett made the observation that "the incidence of large bowel cancer is too low to be consistent with a simple, single locus determination, either heterozygous or homozygous, in all the families" (p.15). We will see that, far from being too low, it is too high— probably a reflection of a bias towards over-representation of deaths from colorectal cancer in the deceased siblings when so many others are still alive and thought to be cancer-free.

In the more up-to-date series, there are 207 siblings containing 166 deceased and 506 live siblings, some of the latter being of advanced age (the oldest is 101). In order to achieve a worthwhile analysis, all such sibships should be followed to extinction, and hopefully, future studies based on index cases will try to do this.

We have already seen that the parents of an index case (known to be of genotype pp) will be pp with frequency u and $p+$ with frequency v. Each parent will generate gametes carrying p with frequency $[u + (\frac{1}{2}) v]$, and so the frequency of children with genotype pp among the siblings of an index case will be $[u + (\frac{1}{2})v]^2$. Since the risk of developing cancer is x, the chance that a sibling of an index case will develop colorectal cancer is $[u + (\frac{1}{2})v]^2 x$, and this is the quantity we wish to estimate when observing the incidence of colorectal cancer among siblings of index cases. Using the values for u and x already derived, the average risk is 11.22%. Unfortunately, the risk to siblings does not correspond to the observed incidence in siblings due to inherent biases in the method of ascertaining sibships.

For example, albinism is a rare, autosomal-recessive condition where, except under exceptional circumstances, all cases arise from the mating of two heterozygous but otherwise normal carriers. The chance of an affected offspring is 1 in 4 for each pregnancy arising from an appropriate mating; in all other matings, the chance is 0. So, in a large number of families at risk, if each had two children (size=two sibship)

9/16 $[= (\frac{3}{4})^2]$ will have two normal children
3/16 $(= \frac{3}{4} \times \frac{1}{4})$ will have the first child normal and the second affected
3/16 $(= \frac{1}{4} \times \frac{3}{4})$ will have the first child affected and the second normal
1/16 $(= \frac{1}{4} \times \frac{1}{4})$ will have both children affected

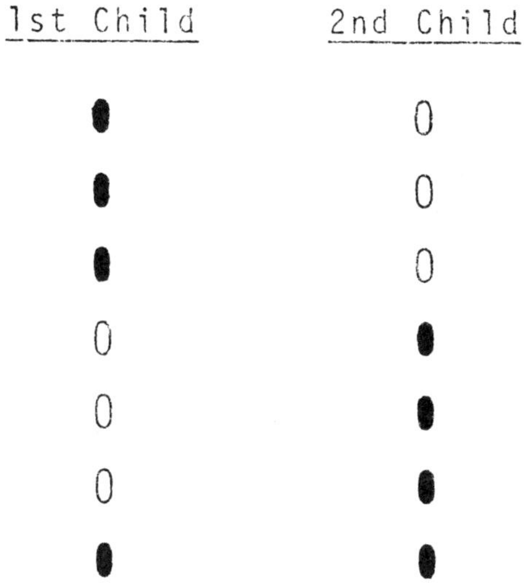

Figure 2-1.   The relative frequencies of 2 child families containing an albino detected by complete ascertainment of all families containing affected children. That the risk of an affected child is ¼ is not immediately apparent. Solid circles = affected. Open circles = normal. (Not shown and not detected are 9 sibships where both children are normal.)

If now we set out to demonstrate that the chance of an affected child is indeed 1 in 4, a peculiar difficulty arises. Since we ascertain appropriate matings by the occurrence of an affected child, we have no way of detecting and counting those matings where both children were normal. Thus, if we found every sibship of size two containing an albino, the relative frequencies would be as in Figure 2-1. If we now omit the case by which we first ascertained the family, we find in the remainder that the observed incidence is 1 in 7, even though we know that the risk is actually 1 in 4. For exactly the same reason (not detecting families where all the children are unaffected), the incidence of cancer among the siblings of index cases will be less than the risk $[u + (\frac{1}{2}) v]^2 x$, and the amount depends not only on the magnitude of the risk that we are trying to estimate, but also on the sibship size.

ASCERTAINMENT BIAS

This method of selecting appropriate matings by means of an affected child is said to be truncated because of the omission of families where the offspring are all normal. Having selected our sibships by the presence of at least one affected member, we refer to sibship where all the other siblings are unaffected as "simplex." If one or more of the siblings of the index case are affected, the sibship is said to be "multiplex." This is the nomenclature of Morton.[23]

Ascertainment is "complete" when the relative proportions of various multiplex sibships to each other and to simplex sibships are consistent with the truncated binomial distribution determined by the sibship size *(N)* and the segregation ratio (risk) being estimated. In Figure 2-1, the ratio of simplex to multiplex is 6 to 1 corresponding to $N = 2$ and a segregation ratio of 1 in 4. Special methods of analysis such as those of Hogben[24] or the "sib" method of Weinberg[25] can be used to give the correct segregation ratio when we are sure that ascertainment is complete. Note that complete ascertainment does not depend on finding all cases in the population (although that would do it) but rather on determining whether the various types of sibships exist in the correct proportions.

More commonly, multiplex sibships tend to be over-represented with respect to simplex sibships and do not bear the same relationships to each other and the simplex sibships as they would if ascertainment was complete. In extreme cases, multiplex sibships are present in proportions dependent on the truncated binomial distribution and the number of affected persons in the sibship. Under these conditions, ascertainment is "incomplete," and the "propositus" method of Weinberg[25] or the sib method of Fisher[26] must be used.

Usually, however, ascertainment is neither complete nor incomplete, lying somewhere between the two. Consequently, yet another genetic parameter must be introduced: the ascertainment probability, defined as the chance that an affected person will become an index case. Under conditions of complete ascertainment this quantity is tending to 1 (certainty), and under incomplete ascertainment it is tending to 0, making multiplex sibships more likely to be ascertained because they contain more affected members. In this situation, methods such as Morton's[23] should be used, but a body of data for colorectal cancer suitable for these powerful analytic techniques has probably never been collected.

If ascertainment was known to be incomplete, the estimation of the segregation ratio ($[u + (\frac{1}{2}) v]^2$) would be obtained by omitting the index case and finding the proportion affected in the remainder. However, the assumption about incomplete ascertainment implies that sibships with two affected members will be detected with twice their appropriate frequency in the population, and sibships with three affected members will have three times their frequency. But this situation is known to occur in human genetics only rarely when affected siblings coexist in their affected state. As the cases of colorectal cancer in sibships are observed *not* to coexist, except in rare instances, it is difficult to imagine that anything approaching incomplete ascertainment is actually present. If anything, the bias should favor complete ascertainment, necessitating the use of the more complex analytic techniques.

ANALYSIS OF SIBLING DATA

The disposition of siblings of index cases from the amended Lovett[10] series is shown in Table 2-3. All the sibships with an affected member in them are indicated, and in two instances there are two affected siblings. In three cases, the affected sibling is still alive, but he is counted as dead for the purposes of this analysis. If an estimate of the segregation ratio is obtained by confining the analysis to estimating the proportion of affected siblings to all deceased siblings, the answer is approximately 14%. We have already seen that this method of estimating the risk corresponds to an implicit assumption of incomplete ascertainment, which is intrinsically unlikely and rendered more so when we consider that 503 siblings have been excluded because they are still alive. Furthermore, our example showed that the proportion so estimated is actually less (by an arbitrary amount) than the actual risk. Assuming complete ascertainment and applying the appropriate method of analysis, the estimate of the risk—$(u + (\frac{1}{2}) v)^2x$ in terms of our model— is close to 25%, over twice our expected value of 11.22%. The model may be wrong, but it would be premature to assume this while 503 surviving and unaffected siblings remain unassessed.

In brief, the straight proportion of affected siblings is $24/672 = 3.57\%$ (already greater than the population incidence), and 503 unaffected siblings are still alive. Some of these will surely develop colorectal cancer. We must also remember that this figure is an underestimate because it assumes

Table 2-3. Siblings of 207 Index Cases with Colorectal Cancer

		Alive Siblings											
		0	1	2	3	4	5	6	7	8	9	10	11	TOTAL
	0	16	29	27	15	5	8	6				1	1	108
	1	6	8	**21	***9	*5	*2	***5	*2					58
	2	2	*†6	*6	*2	**4	*1	†1	1					23
Deceased 3		1	1	1	5	2		*2						12
Siblings 4		*1			1	*1	1							4
	5		2											2
TOTAL		26	46	55	32	17	12	14	3			1	1	207

* = sibship with 1 affected sibling
† = sibship with 2 affected siblings
Deceased siblings = 166
Alive siblings = 506
Number affected = 24

incomplete ascertainment. The analysis based on the existence of complete ascertainment gives an estimate of the risk to siblings of 6.42%, which will also be an underestimate because of the large number of surviving siblings.

FUTURE INVESTIGATIONS

It is apparent that the exploration of a genetic model alleging a predisposition to colorectal cancer demands a body of data that has not yet been collected and analyzed appropriately. To undertake any kind of dependable segregation analysis to estimate gene frequencies and the risk to siblings, all sibships should be followed to extinction. Confining the analysis to a single point in time while a significant proportion of siblings are still alive is bound to introduce the error of having affected patients over-represented among the deceased group.

An additional problem is that following sibships until all are deceased would probably occupy a working lifetime for the investigators. During this time, no great change in gene frequency need be anticipated, but almost certainly the value of x (risk of developing colorectal cancer) may alter, introducing further complications of analysis. Nevertheless, in areas with cancer registration centers, extending the registration to include unaffected siblings and subsequent comparison of this list with new registrations and death certifications for the area, would do much towards gathering more meaningful data. The demonstration of an increased incidence of cancer among relatives or the documentation of cancer-prone families will not advance our knowledge of possible genetic factors unless a model is proposed and the formal consequences explored.

The difficulties in gathering data are obviously considerable, but a new method of attack may soon present itself. Danes[27, 28] reported an increased frequency of cells showing tetraploidy in tissue culture preparations from split skin biopsies of patients with Gardner's syndrome. It is now known that the presence of this cytogenetic marker depends on the culture containing a proportion of growing epithelial cells; the marker will not be shown if the culture consists of fibroblasts alone. The marker has been followed through several generations of patients with Gardner's syndrome and is also found in some patients at risk for developing the condition.

More recently, Danes et al. have shown that occasionally this marker is not present in patients with Gardner's syndrome or FPC, but it is present in their siblings and affected parents.[29] The researchers have suggested that the marker may be recognizing not the main gene for the heritable colorectal cancer syndrome but rather the postulated unfavorable modifying allele p. If this is correct, it then follows that, occasionally, apparently normal persons— not members of Gardner or FPC families—who have been found to show the marker may be of genotype pp. Confirmation of this theory may soon be obtained by investigating sibships where the index case is known to be positive for the marker and no question of Gardner's syndrome or FPC arises.

It is also known that some tissue culture preparations show an increased tendency to undergo partial *in vitro* transformations indicative of increased sensitivity to genetic change resulting in the observed change in cellular behavior. Such changes include alterations in cellular morphology and plating efficiency, loss of density-dependent growth regulation, lowering of serum requirements for growth, ability to grow in agar or methocel. Danes has demonstrated that a preexisting variant genotype may predispose a cell-culture preparation to undergo transformation.[30] A transformed cell population growing in suspension arose in single monolayer sublines obtained from five biopsies from four patients with FPC. These sublines showed altered cellular morphology, ability to grow in suspension, and an apparently indefinite life span.

These findings indicate that there is every hope of being able to isolate a tissue-culture property present in index cases with colorectal cancer. The use of such an *in vitro* cellular abnormality will greatly simplify the process of deciding whether a genetic predisposition exists as postulated. All siblings studied could enter the analysis, since there is no need to wait for them to develop cancer before assigning a genotype. The increased and complete body of data will allow measurements of any bias in ascertainment to be made. The method used by Morton[23] will allow not only estimates of segregation ratios (leading to gene-frequency estimates) and the ascertainment probability but also measurements of whether there exists a significant number of environmentally induced cancer cases independent of the hypothesized cancer-prone genotype. Isolating these cases from the remainder for more detailed study is bound to be rewarding.

The data presented here show that methods of analysis that try to implicate genetic factors as significant influences on the occurrence of colorectal cancer have been unsatisfactory. We have also seen that the observed frequency of cancer among parents of index cases is consistent with a simple genetic model. In the case of siblings, analysis is more difficult, but results indicate that the frequency is not too small and may, in fact, be too great. This latter finding could well be a reflection of strong intrafamilial, environment factors that are not excluded by any genetic model but make interpretation of family data more difficult. The next step must be a combined approach by cancer epidemiologists, geneticists, and all the armamentarium of the tissue-culture laboratory.

Acknowledgments.   The writer wishes to thank Dr. B. C. Morson and Dr. H. J. R. Bussey for access to the St. Mark's Hospital polyposis and colorectal cancer family registers.

REFERENCES

1. Handford, H.: Disseminated polypi of the large intestine becoming malignant. *Trans. Path. Soc. Lond.* **41:**133, 1890.
2. Cripps, H.: Two cases of disseminated polypus of rectum. *Trans. Path. Soc. Lond.* **33:**165, 1882.
3. Smith, T.: Three cases of multiple polypi of the lower bowel occurring in one family. *St. Bartholomew's Hospital Report* **32:**225, 1887.
4. Bickersteth, R.A.: Multiple polypi of the rectum occurring in a mother and child. *St. Bartholomew's Hospital Report* **26:**299, 1890.
5. Lockhart-Mummery, J.P.: Cancer and heredity. *Lancet* **1:**427, 1925.
6. Macklin, M.T.: Inheritance of cancer of the stomach and large intestine in man. *JNCI* **24:**551-557, 1960.
7. Woolf, C.M.: A genetic study of carcinoma of the large intestine. *Am. J. Hum. Genet.* **10:**42-47, 1958.
8. Lynch, H.T.; Guirgis, H.; Swartz, M.; Lynch, J.; Krush, A.J.; and Kaplan, A.R.: Genetics and colon cancer. *Arch. Surg.* **106:**669-675, 1973.
9. Bjelke, E.: *Epidemiologic Studies of Cancer of the Stomach, Colon and Rectum: With Special Emphasis on the Role of Diet.* Ann Arbor, MI: University Microfilms, 1973, 5p. Cited by Correa, P., and Haenszel, W., In: *Adv. Cancer Res.* **26:**93, 1978.
10. Lovett, E.: Family studies in cancer of the colon and rectum. *Br. J. Surg.* **63:**13-18, 1976.
11. Veale, A.M.O.: Intestinal polyposis. In: Eugenics Laboratory Memoir Series No. 40. London, England: Cambridge University Press, 1965, pp. 1-104.
12. Brahme, F.; Ekelund, G.R.; Norden, J.G.; and Wenckert, A.: Metachronous colorectal polyps: comparison of development of colorectal polyps and carcinomas in persons with and without histories of polyps. *Dis. Colon. Rect.* **17:**166-171, 1974.
13. Morson, B.C.: Precancerous and early malignant lesions of the large intestine. *Br. J. Surg.* **55:**725-731, 1968.
14. Hill, M.J.: Carcinogenesis and gastrointestinal cancer. *Frontiers Gastrointest. Res.* **4:**1-16, Karger, Basel, 1979.
15. Hill, M.J.; Morson, B.C.; and Bussey, H.J.: Aetiology of adenoma-carcinoma sequence in large bowel. *Lancet* **1:**245-247, 1978.
16. Woolf, C.M.; Richards, R.C.; and Gardner, E.J.: Occasional discrete polyps of the colon and rectum showing an inherited tendency. *Cancer* **8:**403, 1955.
17. Rider, J.A.; Kirsner, J.B.; Moeller, H.C.; and Palmer, W.L.: Polyps of colon and rectum: Four year to nine year follow up study of 537 patients. *JAMA* **170:**633, 1959.
18. Warthin, A.S.: Heredity with reference to carcinoma. *Arch. Int. Med.* **12:**546-555, 1913.
19. Warthin, A.S.: The further study of a cancer family. *J. Cancer Res.* **9:**279-286, 1925.
20. Lynch, H.T., and Krush, A.J.: Heredity and adenocarcinoma of the colon. *Gastroenterology* **53:**517-527, 1967.

21. Lynch, H.T.; Shaw, M.W.; Magnuson, C.W.; Larsen, A.L.; and Krush, A.J.: Heredity factors in cancer: study of two large mid-western kindreds. *Arch. Intern. Med.* **117**:206-212, 1966.

22. Andren, L., and Frieberg, S.: Frequency of polyps of rectum and colon, according to age, and relation to cancer. *Gastroenterology* **36**:631, 1959.

23. Morton, N.E.: Genetic tests under incomplete ascertainment. *Am. J. Hum. Genet.* **11**:1-16, 1959.

24. Hogben, L.: *Nature and Nurture,* rev. ed., London, England: George Allen & Unwin, 1945.

25. Weinberg, W.: Weitere Beitrage zur Theorie der Vererbung, 4. Uber Methode und Fehlerquellen der Untersuchung auf Mendelsche Zahlen beim Menschen. *Arch. Rass. u. Ges. Biol.* **9**:165, 1912.

26. Fisher, R.A.: The effect of methods of ascertainment upon the estimation of frequencies. *Ann. Eugen. Lond.* **6**:13-25, 1934.

27. Danes, B.S.: The Gardner Syndrome: A study in cell culture. *Cancer* **36**:2337 (suppl.), 1975.

28. Danes, B.S.: Increased tetraploidy in cultured skin fibroblasts. *J. Med. Genet.* **13**:52, 1976.

29. Danes, B.S. Alm, T.; and Veale, A.M.O.: Hypothesis: Modifying alleles in in vitro expression of mutant genes of the heritable colorectal cancer syndromes with polyps. *Med. Hypotheses* **5**:1057-1064, 1979.

30. Danes, B.S.: In vitro evidence for adenoma-carcinoma sequence in large bowel. *Lancet* **2**:44-45, 1979.

3
Hereditary Adenomatosis of the Colon and Rectum

Thor Alm, M.D.

For about 100 years, adenomatosis of the colon and rectum (ACR), also called familial polyposis coli (FPC), has been recognized as a disease entity. In 1890, Handford was the first to call attention to the enormous risk of malignancy even in young patients.[1] During the early decades of the twentieth century, an increasing number of family investigations confirmed that heredity played a role, but no hypothesis concerning the mode of inheritance was suggested until 1927 when Coccayne postulated that the disease was inherited as a Mendelian dominant character.[2] The pioneer investigations at St. Mark's Hospital in London were initiated by Lockhart-Mummery who, in the *Lancet* under the heading "Cancer and Heredity," presented families.[3] In 1952, Dukes[4, 5] reported 33 fully investigated families— 22 of these had two or more affected members and 11 had only one affected member. Since no difference existed in the clinical picture in patients with and without a family history, Duke postulated that the solitary cases were manifestations of gene mutation and would eventually transmit the disease to their offspring.

In the early 1950s, ACR was generally considered a fairly simple disease with autosomal dominant inheritance and associated with benign extracolonic tumors in a minority of families. The adenomatous polyposis was believed to be restricted to the colon and rectum, and only a few observations of gastric and small bowel involvement had been published. In a few instances, association with malignant tumors outside the colon had also been reported.

During the last 25 years, the topic has become more complex. A large number of malformations and extracolonic tumors, benign as well as malignant, have been reported in association with ACR. In the 1950s, Gardner and co-workers[6-9] reported an association with sebaceous or epidermoid cysts, osteomas, and desmoid tumors. The eponym *Gardner's syndrome* for this association seems now to be generally accepted in the literature, and is often used even if the syndrome is far from fully developed. A number of reports have appeared of adenomatous polyposis involving the stomach or parts of the small bowel, mainly the duodenum and distal ileum, in a high percentage of ACR patients.[10-14] Site-specific malignancies outside the colon, for example, pancreatico-duodenal, thyroid, or kidney tumors, have also been reported in ACR families.[15] Turcot et al. reported two cases of association with malignant tumors of the central nervous system.[16] This might indicate an inherited tendency in ACR families to develop neoplastic activity involving all three embryonic layers.

Reed and Neel investigated 23 families in Michigan.[17] They found it reasonable to assume the ACR was "determined by a single gene whose penetrance is of the order of 90% in persons of age 50" (p. 250). Veale made a most comprehensive study of the subject, analyzing the reported data from a total of 102 families.[18] Based on analysis of the different age parameters (age at onset of symptoms, at diagnosis of ACR, and at death from cancer, he proposed a genetic model involving the main ACR gene called P and two recessive, modifying alleles called p and $+$. If p was carried in conjunction with P, it was supposed to cause the unfavorable form of ACR with an early age of manifestation. The normal allele $+$ together with P, would cause a later age of manifestation and death.

Smilow et al.[19] and Veale et al.[20] presented families in which diffuse juvenile polyposis had occurred in two or more members and in two or three generations; congenital anomalies were also present in some members. During the last 15 years, studies of a number of similar families and associations have also been published. Veale et al. introduced a further modifying allele, labelled j,[20] to Veale's previously proposed genetic model. The researchers hypothesized that since mutation to the P form of the gene occurred, this would from time to time take place in a person carrying one or two j genes, so that the genotype would be Pj and juvenile polyposis would develop. Mixed forms of juvenile and adenomatous polyposis that this model well have also been reported in a number of cases,[21] occurring either in the same person or within a family where one person was affected with ACR and another with juvenile polyposis.

Irrespective of the great variation in extracolonic manifestations, adenomatous polyposis of the colon and rectum and the inevitable malignant degeneration are the same in all the varieties of ACR. This is the main reason for including ACR in a textbook entitled *Colon Cancer Genetics.* Furthermore, ACR has served, and in the future will probably also serve, as a model disease for studying different aspects of colorectal cancer.

THE ST. ERIK'S HOSPITAL ACR REGISTER

The accumulated experience from more than 20 years' work with a national register of Swedish ACR families is presented in this chapter. The building up of this register started in 1959. Most of the affected persons diagnosed after the investigation started, and their first degree relatives, still alive, were examined by me. The results up to the end of 1972 were published previously.[22, 23]

During the last 10 years, the treatment and regular follow-up of affected persons and their relatives, from new families and from some of the earlier ones, has been taken over by doctors at their local hospitals. As a consequence, some variation in the treatment principles was unavoidable. The results presented are based on my observations during the continuous surveillance of "older" families. As a number of "new" families reported to the registry are far from fully investigated, supplementary information has been added only to the extent that I have verified it.

Classification of Families

The investigated families were divided into two main groups: those with only one affected member, labeled S (solitary cases) and those with at least two affected members, labeled F. Families in which extracolonic manifestations were present, either in members with ACR or their first degree relatives, had the suffix e added, giving a total of four family types: F, F_e, S, and S_e. Non-affected family members, regardless of age, were classified as *quasi-normals* (QN) to indicate the possibility that they, despite a negative examination or lack of symptoms, might carry the gene and manifest ACR at a later date.

The total number of families investigated was 106 (Table 3-1), comprising

Table 3-1. Classification of Families: Number of Family Members and Affected Members in Each Family Type

TYPE OF FAMILY	NO. OF FAMILIES	AFFECTED			
		NO. OF FAMILY MEMBERS	ACR/ACR + ca	DEDUCED	TOTAL
F	43 (24 + 19)	607	208	36	244
F_e	35 (32 + 3)	558	214	22	236
$F + F_e$	78 (56 + 22)	1.165	422	58	480
S	23 (21 + 2)	129	23		23
S_e	5 (3 + 2)	23	5		5
Total	106	1.317	450	58	508

1317 members (i.e., affected persons, their siblings, and children). Deduced cases, mainly from earlier generations, are those for whom no definite information on ACR is available. Most of these cases have died, usually at a young age, from "bowel trouble" or nonspecified malignancies, and the majority of them were ascertained by at least two lines of affected offspring. Since the end of 1972, the number of families has increased from 80 to 106. In Table 3-1, the 1972 numbers and the increase for the different family types are given within brackets. In 28 families—roughly one-fourth of the total—there is presently only 1 affected member. This statistic is similar to findings in other investigations and is the expected figure. In the present series, this figure has not changed appreciably between 1972 and 1981 (0.3-0.25).

In 2 of the 1972 S families, children of the propositus have developed ACR, and in a third S family, 2 elder siblings of the propositus have done the same. In another S family, extracolonic manifestations, but so far no ACR, were found in 2 first degree relatives of the proband, altering the family from S to S_e. Thus, the 1972 number of S families has been reduced by 4, and the real increase of S families is, therefore, 6 (2 + 4), while 2 S_e families have been added (1 + 1). As the table shows, the relation of F to F_e families has switched from 24/32 to 43/35. Now, there are 19 new F families, 3 of which were converted to F from the old S families.

The majority of affected members and first-degree relatives in 16 previously uninvestigated families were not examined by the author. As extracolonic manifestations are not easily detected when not specially sought for, it may well be that they have been missed in some persons, falsely reducing the number of F_e families. During future surveillance of these families, some members of F as well as S families will be further affected, and probably one or more members will exhibit some extracolonic manifestation. At present, in about 40% of the families, one or more members have been found to have such manifestations.

Pathology

The macro- and microscopic pathology of ACR has been described in detail by Morson and Dawson,[24] Bussey,[25] and Bussey and Morson.[26] Other types of intestinal polyposis and the importance of elaborate microscopic examination for differential diagnosis are also discussed by the same authors and by Welch[27] and Alm and Licznerski.[22]

The clinical expression "polyposis" indicates the presence of multiple polyps. *But how many polyps make polyposis*—or, in the case of ACR, adenomatosis? According to current literature, most authors seem to agree on a number of at least 100 although 200 or 50 have also been mentioned. No doubt, in the ordinary case of fully developed ACR, there are hundreds or

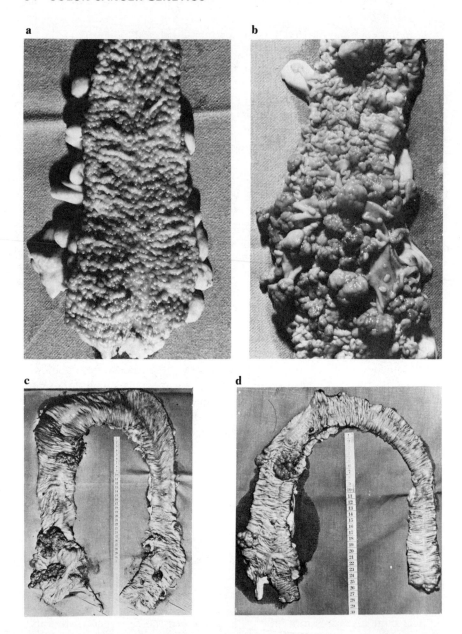

Figure 3-1.   ACR: (a) Common variant: densely packed, small sessile adenomas of fairly uniform size; (b) Another common variant: variable size of sessile and pedunculated adenomas; (c) and (d) Uncommon variant: a few minor tabular adenomas and 3-5 large, sessile, pedunculated villous adenomas. Brother and sister, 45 and 42 years of age, respectively. *(c: From T. Alm and G. Licznerski, The intestinal polyposes. Clin. Gastroenterol. 2:586, 1973. Copyright © 1973 by W. B. Saunders Company.)*

thousands of adenomas present in varying stages of development (see Fig. 3-1a and 3-1b). But, just as obvious, there are exceptions to this rule as illustrated in Figures 3-1c and 3-1d, the operation specimens from a brother and sister, 45 and 42 years of age, respectively. Furthermore, by repeated examination of a number of children of affected parents, I had the opportunity to notice the first appearance of a few, tiny, sessile adenomas already in children between age 5 and 10 and the later, successive increase in number and size of adenomas up to the time for surgical intervention, usually in the late teens or early twenties. Of course, this has been true for ACR from the beginning.

The real problem, most certainly met with by all investigators, emerges when an adult appears carrying a limited number of adenomas, say 30 to 40, distributed throughout the entire large bowel. As long as no kind of marker that specifically identifies ACR is known, the question of whether such a person suffers from ACR cannot be immediately answered. In such a situation, a thorough family history must be taken, and the siblings and children of the patient must be recommended for examination of the colon and rectum and, depending on age, regular follow-ups for a defined period of time.

Although the distribution of adenomas in the present series of patients was, as a rule, very similar between members of the same family, a relatively large variation existed between families. In general, the tumors were fairly evenly distributed throughout the entire large bowel, but the highest density areas were usually the rectosigmoid and descending colon. Adenomas of the left side of the large bowel also tended to be larger than those of the right side. A most important feature is that adenomas were present in the rectum of all the patients I observed. The density varied considerably, from patients in whom no normal mucosa was visible between the densely packed polyps to those with only a few polyps (as in Fig. 3-1c and Fig. 3-1d).

The consequence in clinical practice of this observation is that proctosigmoidoscopy, with biopsies for microscopic examination, is sufficient for diagnosis. This leaves colonoscopy or x-ray examination with the double-contrast method to provide complementary information about the extent of the lesions or the presence of cancer beyond the reach of the ordinary stiff sigmoidoscope—information that might influence the planning of surgery.

Polypoid Lesions Outside the Colon and Rectum. We particularily looked for lesions outside the colon and rectum from the start of the investigation. X-ray examination of the stomach, usually using a double-contrast technique, and of the small bowel, preferably using the intubation technique according to Sellink,[28] was performed in all ACR patients. (Of course, during the last 5 years, the routine x-ray examination was replaced by fiberoptic gastroduodenoscopy.) Multiple gastric or duodenal adenomas were found in only three patients; in a fourth patient, a hamartomatous polyp the size of a hazel nut was removed from the pyloric region. However, gastroduodenoscopy, which is a much better method than x-ray for diagnosing gastroduodenal adenomatosis, has been performed in only a limited number of patients. Furthermore, repeated examinations as performed by Ranzi et al.[14] have not been done in symptom-free persons without polypoid lesions at the original examination. The observed very low frequency of gastroduodenal adenomatosis might, therefore, be somewhat too low, but it is certainly far from that reported by the Japanese investigators. In a number of patients, usually in younger age groups, polypoid lesions in the terminal ileum were found when during colectomy, but histologic examination invariably disclosed only lymphoid hyperplasia.

Cancer of the Colon and Rectum.   In the St. Erik's Hospital ACR register, cancer and carcinoma always mean invasiveness. Terms such as "carcinoma *in situ*," and "focal carcinoma" are not used. Severe epithelial dysplasia or atypia indicates cytological changes that are, beyond doubt, of malignant nature but are still restricted to the mucosa (i.e., no invasion across the lamina propria). Among the propositi group of patients operated on, including those who turned out to be inoperable or who only had segmental resections, cancer was found in around 65% of the cases. In the symptom-free patients, the call-up group, cancer was present in 7.4%. The corresponding figures for the St. Mark's material were, according to Bussey, 66.2% and 9.4% respectively.[25] In other words, when a person with adenomatous polyposis seeks medical help, usually because of bleeding or altered bowel habits, he runs a 2 to 3 risk of having malignant degeneration, fairly often multicentric and already metastasizing.

In the call-up group, there is also a substantial risk of malignancy. In the stage of development when the investigator strives to collect all affected families in a defined population, the sample of persons at risk will represent a wide age range. Although symptom free, one in ten of these people will already have cancer. Not until every person at risk is put under continuous surveillance from childhood and operated on with colectomy as soon as ACR is confirmed, will the frequency of malignancy approach the zero level. However, cancer in ACR patients will never, even under the most favorable conditions, reach the absolute zero level because a number of persons, representing fresh mutations, will not be identified until they seek medical help, and at that time, they already run the above-mentioned 2 to 3 risk of malignancy. At present, the only way to find these people is by regular proctosigmoidosocopic examinations of the total population, too formidable a task for any health organization.

Distribution of Colorectal Carcinoma

The percentage distribution of the tumors within the large bowel in the St. Erik's Hospital series of patients is presented in Table 3-2. Comparison is made with two unselected series of patients with large bowel cancer and with a series of patients with an inherited type of colorectal cancer without adenomas. The figures for ACR and the unselected patients are identical with 75 to 80% of the carcinomas situated within the distal part of the colon and rectum and less than one-fourth to the right of the splenic flexure. In the 220 patients with the inherited type, the situation is the reverse.

Additional Neoplastic Activity

All additional neoplastic activity, benign as well as malignant, and some congenital anomalies encountered from the pedigree charts are summarized in Table 3-3.

Three male patients from three different families died from brain tumors at age 6, 7, and 25. None of the patients was examined with respect to ACR, but all of them had an affected parent; the 7-year-old boy also had an affected brother. The histological type of the brain tumor—a cerebellar medulloblastoma—is known only for this boy. A fourth patient with brain tumor, a woman aged 42, had an affected daughter and affected grandchildren, but no affected siblings or parents. It is possible that these four persons represent another four cases of Turcot's syndrome, although this cannot be proven.

Table 3-2. Percentage Distribution of Colorectal Carcinomas

SITE	INHERITED TYPES WITHOUT ADENOMAS[a]	ACR[b]	UNSELECTED PATIENTS	
			SERIES A[a]	SERIES B[c]
Cecum	20,5 ⎫	7 ⎫	11,3 ⎫	7 ⎫
Ascending	18, 6 ⎬ 65	4 ⎬ 21	4,9 ⎬ 23, 7	4 ⎬ 20
Hepatic flexure	⎬	2 ⎬	⎬	2 ⎬
Transverse	25,9 ⎭	6 ⎭	7, 5 ⎭	4 ⎭
Splenic flexure		2		3
Descending	8, 6	5	5, 6	4
Sigmoid	16, 8 ⎬ 26,4	26 ⎬ 74	37, 3 ⎬ 70,7	20 ⎬ 76
Rectum	9, 6 ⎭	48 ⎭	33,4 ⎭	56 ⎭

Source: From S. Winawer, D. Schottenfeld, and P. Sherlock, eds. *Colorectal Cancer: Prevention, Epidemiology, and Screening.* Raven Press, New York, 1980, p. 111; Copyright © by Raven Press.
[a] No. of patients: inherited types 220, unselected patients 1,599[29]
[b] St. Erik's Hospital register, 229 tumors
[c] Three large series, 9,811 tumors

Table 3-3. Additional Neoplastic Activity and Anomalies in ACR families

KIND OF TUMOR OR ANOMALY	F				F_e				S				S_e			
	AFFECTED		QN		AFFECTED		QN		AFFECTED		QN		AFFECTED		QN	
	M	F	M	F	M	F	M	F	M	F	M	F	M	F	M	F
Sebaceous/epidermoid cysts					25	20	3	4						1	1	
Osteomas					6	7										
Desmoid tumors					7	17		1					2			
Excessive intra-abdominal adhesions		1			3											
Impacted supernumerary teeth					1											
Epipharyngeal angiofibroma					2											
Gastroduodenal polyps	1				2	1										
Gastric cancer	1	1	4	2							5	1				
Pancreatic cancer	2	1						2								
Hepatic cancer			1	1			1	2								
Thyroid cancer						2	2	2								
Urinary tract cancer	2						2					1				
Prostatic cancer	1		2				1								1	
Ovarian/uterine cancer				3				5								
Brain tumor	1		1				2	1								
Leukemia	1		1				1	1								
Miscellaneous tumors			3	3	2		3	6			1	3				
Congenital heart disease								1								
Situs inversus														1	1	

Thyroid cancer appeared in two female ACR patients, a mother and daughter, and in two other females without known ACR and belonging to other families. Four of the five patients who died from hepatic carcinoma were young—24 to 35 years of age. The fifth was a female of 65. All of them had an ACR-affected parent and affected siblings but no children of their own to help ascertain the diagnosis of ACR. Nevertheless, it seems probable that these patients did, in fact, have colorectal cancer on the basis of ACR and liver metastases.

Gastric cancer was encountered in 20 patients, 18 of whom were first degree relatives. In some of these patients who died before age 40, the diagnosis was not confirmed during surgery or by autopsy. So they may well have died from metastasizing colorectal cancer related to ACR. With the exception of thyroid cancer, which occurred only in F_e families, and pancreatic cancer, which occurred only in F families, the malignancies outside the large bowel were almost equally distributed in the two family types. A young boy with a brain tumor, a young woman with "excessive intra-abdominal adhesions," and two elderly women dying from urinary tract cancer, were the only members of the largest pedigree (125 numbers, 56 affected) who presented any additional neoplastic activity or abnormality. Taken together, these observations indicate that there is no absolute demarcation line between the two family types in regard to extracolonic malignancies.

Extracolonic lesions of the original Gardner type were sought by physical examination and x-ray of parts of the skeleton (cranium and long bones) from the beginning of the investigation in every ACR patient and in a number of their relatives. To determine how often such lesions precede or appear dissociated from ACR, it would have been of interest to perform these examinations on every family member. However, since family members were spread throughout the country, this was impossible. Interestingly, in the present series, there is not a single person with full-blown Gardner's syndrome and no family had a combination of more than two extracolonic manifestations of this kind.

Cysts and osteomas were found in equal numbers in males and females, while desmoid tumors were twice as common in females. Altogether, there were 27 patients with desmoids, about one-fourth of them occurring many years before diagnosis of ACR and the rest after surgery in the mesentery or abdominal incisional scar. One woman had surgery for an intestinal obstruction on the basis of a mesenteric desmoid tumor diagnosed 20 years before ACR was revealed. One of her daughters had a colectomy and an ileorectal anastomosis at age 29 and 3 years later developed a rapidly growing desmoid tumor. Although, within a few months, the tumor occupied a large part of the abdominal cavity, it has remained unchanged for 4 years. According to Dahn, desmoid tumors appear in the general population with "an incidence of about two cases per year per million persons" (p. 312).[30] They are obviously at least 100 times more common in ACR patients.

GENETICS

Incidence

The incidence of ACR in the general population of different countries is presented in Table 3-4. In this context, incidence means the frequency at birth of persons with the gene for ACR. Postulating a population in equilibrium, the incidence has been calculated according to Reed and Neel by the formula $f = P/D$, where $P =$ all persons with the gene dying in a specified time interval and $D =$ all deaths in the same time.[17] There is good agreement between the figures from the United States, Japan, and Sweden, while the figures from the United Kingdom differ appreciably. Although the number of families recorded at the St. Mark's Hospital Polyposis Register in London has increased considerably during the last 10 to 15 years, the statement of Bussey and Morson,[26] cited as a note to the table, is the most probable explanation of the difference. If the incidence in the United Kingdom is of the same order as in the other countries referred to, the number of families registered would be at least three times greater.

A bias to overestimation of the incidence exists in the decreased life expectancy of people with the gene. On the other hand, a bias to underestimation lies in the fact that some people fail to die from, or are not recognized as having died from, cancer secondary to ACR. This latter bias is probably the more important one, giving an overall tendency to underestimation of the real frequency at birth of the ACR gene.

Table 3-4. Incidence of ACR in the General Population.

REFERENCE	COUNTRY	INCIDENCE
Reed and Neel[17] (1955)	United States	1:8.300
Veale[18] (1965)	England	1:23.790
Komatsu[31] (1968)	Japan	1:9.467
Pierce[32] (1968)	United States	1:6.850
Alm and Licznerski[22] (1973)	Sweden	1:7.646
Bussey and Morson[26] (1978)	England	at least 1:40.000[a]
Bülow[b] (1981)	Denmark	1:13.491

[a] "The St. Mark's Hospital Polyposis Register does not as yet include all cases occurring in the United Kingdom and the actual proportion is not known, so a direct incidence rate cannot be calculated from this source, except that it is at least 1 in 40,000" (p. 281).
[b] personal communication

Penetrance

The regularity with which a gene produces its effect is usually expressed as the percentage of all persons possessing the gene who show the traits. This can be estimated by more or less sophisticated methods. Alm and Licznerski made estimations for F and F_e families separately.[22] The found values, 94% to 95% for both family types, were in good agreement with Reed and Neel who found that the manifestation of the ACR gene in persons aged 50 was on the order of 90% and would be still higher in older persons.[17] The practical/clinical consequence of this high penetration rate is an almost negligible risk of "skipped generations."

Inheritance, Sex Ratio

Since ACR is inherited as a Mendelian dominant character of such rarity that homozygosity has never been encountered, the ratio of affected to unaffected children is expected to be 1 to 1. The calculations made by Alm and Licznerski revealed no significant deviation from this ratio in either family type or in the total material.[22] Both sexes were equally affected in the F as well as the F_e families. In the total material, the proportion of males was 53.5%, which did not significantly differ from the sex ratio for births in Sweden, which was 51.5%.

When calculations were made with respect to the sex of the parent, a slight tendency was found for affected mothers of the F_e families to have an excess of affected sons. In the other groups, there was no significant deviation from the 1 to 1 ratio. This was in contrast to Pierce who found a stronger, yet not significant, tendency of affected parents to produce an excess of affected children of like sex.[32] Chance variation seems to be the most probable explanation for the divergent tendencies in relatively small numbers.

Biological Fitness

When a crude estimation was made by comparing the sibship sizes of propositi, of affected cases except propositi, and of QNs for the F and F_e families, the means for the sibship sizes of the two groups of affected persons were larger than the mean for the QN cases. With respect to the many sources of error, no definite conclusions were justified, but the general impression was that fertility was not reduced by the action of the ACR gene. Elaborate studies on genetic fitness (mean fecundity) and evolutionary fitness (probability that a single mutant line will not become extinct) were recently published by Murphy[33] and applied to ACR by Murphy and Krush.[34]

Age Variation

Age of first appearance of adenomas obviously varies within rather wide limits between as well as within families. I have regularly examined a number of children at risk from age 5 to 10 when no pathologic changes were present up to fully developed ACR, usually in the late teens or early twenties. These patients represent those with an early age of manifestation, the youngest was a 2-year-old girl who had to have a proctocolectomy at age 4 because of serious symptoms.

The routine at St. Erik's hospital is to call persons at risk for scheduled proctosigmoidoscopies every third year until age 45, and also offer check-ups on their own initiative after age 45—an offer accepted by many. Very rarely has the diagnosis of ACR in this category of patients been made after age 30 and never after age 45. However, finding those with an eventual very late age of manifestation would require another 25 years of observation of a sufficiently large number of persons.

Age at Onset of Symptoms

Most of the patients with symptoms were able to relate almost exactly when they appeared, and the most homogeneous group were the propositi. The analysis showed a statistically younger age at onset for males of the F_e families than for males of the F families. Male propositi of the F_e families also differed significantly from female propositi of the same family. No significant differences were found between the other subgroups. The average age at onset of symptoms was 33.7 years.

Age at Diagnosis of Cancer

This was the age parameter most uniformly determined. The average was 4.5 years later than the age at diagnosis and 7 to 8 years later than onset of symptoms. As surgery interfered with the natural course of the disease in the majority of patients, the exact age at death from cancer was available only for a limited number of persons. An "adjusted age at death" was set to 1 year later than the diagnosis. Further analyses of the age parameters, by adopting the methods of Veale,[18] to estimate the parent-child and sibling-sibling correlations gave indecisive results that neither proved nor disproved Veale's allelic hypothesis. For details, see Alm and Licznerski.[22]

Treatment

Because of the numerous adenomas disseminated over the colorectal mucosa, radical surgery is the only possible treatment. This can be achieved either as total proctocolectomy with ileostomy (PCI) or a colectomy and ileorectal anastomosis (IRA). The ileostomy can be performed either as a conventional one *ad modum* Brooke[35] or as a continent ileal pouch *ad modum* Kock,[36] or maybe, when further experience is gained, as an ileal reservoir and anal anastomosis according to Parks et al.[37] During the last three years increased experience and favorable outcome with the latter type of operation has resulted in the recommendation from many centers that this should be the method of choice (see, for example, Pemberton et al.[50] and Motson et al.[51]). If IRA is considered, the following conditions must be fulfilled:

1. The number of adenomas in the rectum must be limited to give a fair chance of removing them without permanent damage to anorectal function.
2. The rectum or lower sigmoid must be free of signs of malignancy.
3. The patient must be cooperative and prepared to come for regular check-ups every third to twelfth month.
4. The patient must be informed that a second operation, abdominoperineal resection of the rectum and ileostomy (Sec. I), might be necessary if malignancy is revealed or strongly suspected at a control examination.
5. The out-patient surveillance program must be well organized to guarantee that the patients really turn up for regular check-ups.

The operations performed with the aim of cure on the patients of the St. Erik's Hospital Register, as well as the outcome, are summarized in Table 3-5. The overall surgical mortality was 3.5%; it was 4.2% in the propositi group and 3% in the call-up group. All surgical deaths occurred before 1962, and during the last 20 years when 142 of the operations were performed, there were no surgical deaths or other serious postoperative complications.

In the propositi group, 50% of the cases had cancer at the time of operation, and 14 of the 34 patients later died from metastases. In the call-up group, around 7% had malignancies at the time of colectomy, and so far there has been only one late death from metastases. This patient and two in the propositi group who all had Sec. Is in the mid-1960s and within 5 years died from metastases, would never have had an IRA according to the prerequisites just outlined. The three other malignancies were primary tumors of pancreas, lung, and kidney.

Among the 89 call-up patients operated on initially with IRA, 4 had Sec. I performed 1, 3, 11, and 14 years later. Biopsies revealed severe dysplasia, and one patient had invasive cancer when the entire removed rectum was examined. In another of these patients, a segmental resection was made because of cancer 3 years before diagnosis of ACR.

Table 3-5. Number of Patients Operated on, Types of Operation, and Outcome

GROUP OF PATIENTS	TYPE OF OPERATION	NO. OF PATIENTS				LATE DEATHS FROM OTHER MALIGNANCIES	OTHER CAUSES	ALIVE 31.10.1981
		OPERATED ON	WITH CANCER	SURGICAL DEATHS	METASTASES			
Propositi	PCI	44	24	1	9	2	5	27
	IRA	21	10	2	5	–	–	14
	Sec. I	7	5	–	2	–	–	5
Total		72	39	3	16	2	5	46
Call-up Group	PCI	11	3	1	–	–	–	10
	IRA	85	4	2	–	1	2	80
	Sec. I	4	1	–	1	–	–	3
Total		100	8	3	–	1	2	93
Grand total		172	47	6	17	3	7	139

PCI = proctocolectomy with ileostomy
IRA = colectomy and ileorectal anastomosis
Sec. I = abdominoperineal resection of the rectum and ileostomy

44

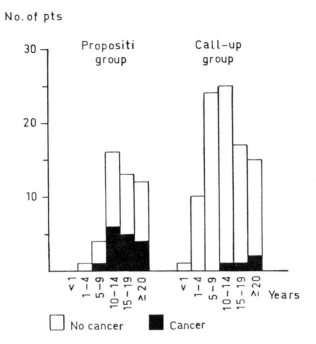

Figure 3-2.   Number of patients operated on and postoperative observation time in years. PCI *n* 37, IRA *n* 102 *(8 had Sec. I).*

The postoperative observation time for the total material is illustrated in Figure 3-2. In the propositi group, 89% have been followed for more than 10 years, and in the call-up group the corresponding figure is 62%. Thirty-five patients in the call-up group were followed for less than 10 years. In none of them was cancer present at colectomy.

In accordance with the conditions listed above, IRA was practiced in 90% of the call-up patients. Moertel et al. condemned this method because of a surprisingly large number of deaths due to cancer of the rectal stump, an accumulated risk of 59% after 23 years of observation.[38] This is in sharp contrast to Bussey and Morson who calculated a 7% risk over a 20-year period.[26] Schaupp and Volpe recorded one, single case of rectal carcinoma in 48 patients.[39] In the present series, there has been so far only the above-mentioned patient with invasive cancer of the rectal stump in the 89 patients operated on. The period of observation for the other 88 patients is illustrated in Figure 3-2.

Malignant degeneration may occur not only in adenomas but also directly from the intervening mucosa. During the continuous follow-up of the IRA

No. of pts

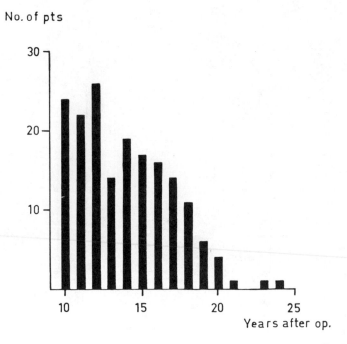

Figure 3-3. Postoperative follow-up. 3-5 biopsies from macroscopically normal rectal mucosa once yearly from tenth postoperative year.

patients, the procedure I applied was to remove the polyps with a biopsy forceps for microscopic examination. Furthermore, from 10 years after IRA, three to five biopsies from macroscopically normal mucosa were regularly made once yearly. In 38 patients, biopsies were taken on 172 occasions up to 24 years postoperatively (see Fig. 3-3). In none of the biopsies was epithelial dysplasia noted by the pathologist.

SUMMARY AND CONCLUSIONS

More than 20 years' surveillance of a number of families (at present, 106) with ACR has confirmed that the disease is inherited as a Mendelian, autosomal-dominant character with a very high rate of penetrance, 95% or more. The frequency at birth of the ACR gene is at least 1 in 7,600. Fertility does not seem to be substantially reduced by the action of the gene. Age at onset of symptoms preceded diagnosis of ACR by about 3 years and diagnosis of cancer by 7 to 8 years. Death from cancer occurred 1.5 years after diagnosis; the mean age was 43.8 years.

The first appearance of adenomas was in the younger age groups, and with appropriate examination, the diagnosis of ACR should be able to be made before age 45 or even earlier. The wide variation in age at onset of symptoms and manifestation of cancer might reflect only a large variation in the speed of development—either genetically or environmentally determined or both—rather than commencement of adenoma appearance.

Radical surgery—PCI or IRA—is the only possible treatment. Provided that some clearly defined conditions are fulfilled and strictly followed, IRA seems to be a safe method in most of the call-up patients, while PCI is usually recommended for patients who present with symptoms.

In almost half of the investigated families, extracolonic manifestations of the original Gardner type were found in one or more affected persons and also in some first degree relatives without obvious ACR. The full-blown Gardner's syndrome is obviously a rare occurrence running in a small number of families. In the present series, no person had all the components and no family had a combination of more than two of them. The lesions are of special interest because they sometimes appear before the large bowel adenomatosis is manifested. In the general population, multiple sebaceous cysts at sites other than the scalp, epidermoid cysts, osteomas, and especially, desmoid tumors are rare. A person presenting with one of the anomalies or a combination of them should, therefore, have the colon examined, regardless whether he is a member of an ACR family. Mesenteric desmoid tumors, although lacking classical malignant patterns, run a fatal course in a few patients because of their tendency to local invasive growth, intestinal obstruction, and the impossibility of radical excision.

In the discussion concerning phenotypic expression and genetic background, a second main mutant gene labelled G was introduced for Gardner's syndrome. The confusion sometimes characterizing this debate is at the moment probably best answered by McConnell's statement that

the genetic theory which would best explain the family data so far collected is that there is one major pleotropic gene underlying the inheritance of all these syndromes. Without this gene, neither the polyposis nor the extracolonic lesions will develop . . . other genes will determine whether or not extracolonic manifestations develop and also their type. (pp. 69-70)[40]

However, McConnell adds a reservation: "The implications of cell culture studies are difficult to assess at present, but if they establish that there is increased tetraploidy in some families and not in others, a revision of the single major gene theory would have to be considered" (p. 70). Studies along these lines are in progress,[41-47] but at present, no definite conclusions are justified (see Chapter 8). Also, the genetic model and its application to families with impressive aggregations of colon cancer but without adenomatosis is elaborated by Veale in Chapter 2. He includes a discussion of the future possibilities opened up by marker studies like those just mentioned.

The clinician's hope for the future is that the search for a genetic marker, with some not-too-complicated or too-expensive assay capable of identifying the carriers of the ACR gene, will be successful. In addition to the cell culture studies, a great deal of research along different lines has been initiated at many centers. Blood groups were studied by Veale,[18] the human leucocyte antigen (HLA) genes by Vargish et al.,[48] and carcinoembryonic antigen (CEA) by Alm and Wahren,[49] among others (without success, however). For the future surveillance of affected persons and families and in order to keep the pedigrees up to date, a central register is essential, preferably run by a main gastroenterologic unit. National registers, or in countries with very large populations, local registers for a well-defined subpopulation, would enable international cooperation for comparison and further studies of this fascinating, heritable condition.

ADDENDUM

In volume 26 of *Diseases of the Colon and Rectum* (1983, issue nos. 6-9), a number of articles have been published presenting current information on various aspects of the hereditary intestinal polyposes. See also in volume 26 the article by S. Schröder, D. Moehrs, J. von Weltzien, R. Winkler, and H. Otto entitled "The Turcot Syndrome. Report of an Additional Case and Review of the Literature."

REFERENCES

1. Handford, H.: Disseminated polypi of the large intestine becoming malignant; strictures (malignant adenoma) of the rectum and splenic flexure of the colon; secondary growths in the liver. *Trans. Path. Soc. Lond.* **41:**133-137, 1890.
2. Coccayne, E.A.: Heredity in relation to cancer. *Cancer Rev.* **2:**337-347, 1927.
3. Lockhart-Mummery, J.P.: Cancer and heredity. *Lancet* **1:**427-429, 1925.
4. Dukes, C.E.: Familial intestinal polyposis. *Ann. Eugen. Lond.* **17:**1-29, 1952.
5. Dukes, C.E.: Familial intestinal polyposis. *Ann. Roy. Coll. Surg. Eng.* **10:**293-304, 1952.
6. Gardner, E.J., and Stephens, F.E.: Cancer of the lower digestive tract in one family group. *Am. J. Hum. Genet.* **2:**41-48, 1950.
7. Gardner, E.J.: Genetic and clinical study of intestinal polyposis, predisposing factor for carcinoma of the colon and rectum. *Am. J. Hum. Genet.* **3:**167-176, 1951.
8. Gardner, E.J., and Richards, R.C.: Multiple cutaneous and subcutaneous

lesions occurring simultaneously with hereditary polyposis and osteomatosis. *Am. J. Hum. Genet.* **5:**139-148, 1953.

9. Gardner, E.J.: Follow-up study of a family group exhibiting dominant inheritance for a syndrome including intestinal polyposis, osteomas, fibromas, and epidermoid cysts. *Am. J. Hum. Genet.* **14:**376-390, 1962.

10. Yonemoto, R.H.; Slayback, J.B.; Byron, R.L.; and Rosen, R.B.: Familial polyposis of the entire gastrointestinal tract. *Arch. Surg.* **99:**427-434, 1969.

11. Hoffman, D.C., and Goligher, J.C.: Polyposis of the stomach and small intestine in association with familial polyposis coli. *Br. J. Surg.* **58:**126-128, 1971.

12. Utsunomiya, J.; Maki, T.; Iwama, T.; et al.: Gastric lesions of familial polyposis coli. *Cancer* **34:**745-754, 1974.

13. Watanabe, H.; Enjoji, M.; Yao, T.; and Ohsato, K.: Gastric lesions in familial adenomatosis coli: their incidence and histologic analysis. *Hum. Pathol.* **9:**269-283, 1978.

14. Ranzi, T.; Castagnone, D.; Velio, P.; Bianchi, P.; and Polli, E.E.: Gastric and duodenal polyps in familial polyposis coli. *Gut* **22:**363-367, 1981.

15. Pauli, R.M.; Pauli, M.E.; and Hall, J.G.: Gardner syndrome and periampullary malignancy. *Am. J. Med. Genet.* **6:**205-219, 1980.

16. Turcot, J.; Despres, J.P.; and St. Pierre, F.: Malignant tumours of the central nervous system associated with familial polyposis of the colon: report of two cases. *Dis. Colon Rect.* **2:**465-468, 1959.

17. Reed, T.E., and Neel, J.V.: A genetic study of multiple polyposis of the colon (with an appendix deriving a method of estimating relative fitness). *Am. J. Hum. Genet.* **7:** 236-263, 1955.

18. Veale, A.M.O.: Intestinal polyposis. In: *Eugenics Laboratory Memoirs,* Vol. XL. London, England: Cambridge University Press, 1965, 104p.

19. Smilow, P.C.; Pryor, C.A.; and Swinton, N.W.: Juvenile polyposis coli. *Dis. Colon Rect.* **9:**248-254, 1966.

20. Veale, A.M.O.; McColl, I.; Bussey, H.J.R.; and Morson, B.C.: Juvenile polyposis coli. *J. Med. Genet.* **3:** 5-16, 1966.

21. Sandler, R.S., and Lipper, S.: Multiple adenomas in juvenile polyposis. *Am. J. Gastroenterol.* **75:** 361-366, 1981.

22. Alm, T., and Licznerski, G.: The intestinal polyposes. *Clin. Gastroenterol.* **2:**577-602, 1973.

23. Alm, T.: Hereditary Adenomatosis of the Colon and Rectum in Sweden. M. D. thesis, Karolineka Institutet, Stockholm, Sweden.

24. Morson, B.C., and Dawson, I.M.P.: *Gastrointestinal Pathology.* Oxford, England: Blackwell Scientific Pub., 1972, 676 p.

25. Bussey, H.J.R.: *Familial Polyposis Coli: Family Studies, Histopathology, Differential Diagnosis, and Results of Treatment.* Baltimore, MD: Johns Hopkins University Press, 1975, 104p.

26. Bussey, H.J.R., and Morson, B.C.: Familial polyposis coli. In: *Gastrointestinal Tract Cancer* (Lipkin, M., and Good, R.A., eds.) New York, NY: Plenum Medical Book Co., 1978, pp. 275-294.

27. Welch, C.E.: Polypoid lesions of the gastrointestinal tract. In: *Major Problems*

in Clinical Surgery, Vol. 2 (Dunphy, J.E., ed.). Philadelphia, PA: W.B. Saunders Co., p. 148.

28. Sellink, J.L.: Radiologic examination of the small intestine by means of duodenal intubation. *Acta. Radiol. (Diagn.)* **15:**318-332, 1974.

29. Anderson, D.E.: Risk in families of patients with colon cancer. In: *Colorectal Cancer: Prevention, Epidemiology, and Screening* (Winawer, S.; Schottenfeld, D.; and Sherlock, P., eds.) New York, NY: Raven Press, 1980, pp. 109-115.

30. Dahn, I.; Johnson, N.; and Lundh, G.: Desmoid tumours: a series of 33 cases. *Acta. Chir. Scan.* **126:**305- 314, 1963.

31. Komatsu, I.: A clinical genetic study of multiple polyposis and allied conditions. *Jpn. J. Hum. Genet.* **12:** 246-297, 1968.

32. Pierce, E.R.: Some genetic aspects of familial multiple polyposis of the colon in a large kindred of 1422 members. *Dis. Colon. Rect.* **11:**321-329, 1968.

33. Murphy, E.A.: Genetic and evolutionary fitness. *Am. J. Hum. Genet.* **2:**51-79, 1978.

34. Murphy, E.A., and Krush, A.J.: Familial polyposis coli. *Prog. Med. Genet.* **4:**59-101, 1980.

35. Brooke, B.N.: The management of an ileostomy. *Lancet* **2:**102, 1952.

36. Kock, N.G.: Intra-abdominal "reservoir" in patients with permanent ileostomy. *Arch. Surg.* **99:**223-231, 1966.

37. Parks, A.G.; Nicholls, R.J.; and Belliveau, P.: Protocolectomy with ileal reservoir and anal anastomosis. *Br. J. Surg.* **67:**533-538, 1980.

38. Moertel, C.G.; Hill, J.R.; and Adson, M.A.: Surgical management of multiple polyposis: the problem of cancer in the retained bowel segment. *Arch. Surg.* **100:**521-526, 1970.

39. Schaupp, W.C., and Volpe, P.A.: Management of diffuse colonic polyposis. *Am. J. Surg.* **124:**218-222, 1972.

40. McConnell, R.B.: Genetics of familial polyposis. In: *Colorectal Cancer: Prevention, Epidemiology, and Screening* (Winawer, S., Schottenfeld, D., and Sherlock, P., eds.). New York, NY: Raven Press, 1980, pp. 69-71.

41. Danes, B.S.: Increased *in vitro* tetraploidy: tissue specific within the heritable colorectal cancer syndromes with polyposis coli. *Cancer* **41:**2330-2334, 1978.

42. Danes, B.S.; Alm, T.; and Veale, A.M.O.: Role of modifying alleles in the heritable colorectal cancer syndromes with polyps. *Med. Hypotheses* **5:**1057-1064, 1979.

43. Danes, B.S., and Alm, T.: *In vitro* studies on adenomatosis of the colon and rectum. *J. Med. Genet.* **16:**417-422, 1979.

44. Danes, B.S.; Alm, T.; and Veale, A.M.O.: Modifying alleles in heritable colorectal cancer syndromes with polyps. *In: Colorectal Cancer: Prevention, Epidemiology, and Screening* (Winawer, S.; Schottenfeld, D.; and Sherlock, P., eds.). New York, NY: Raven Press, 1980, pp. 73-81.

45. Danes, B.S., and Alm, T.: *In vitro* evidence of genetic heterogeneity within the heritable colon cancer syndromes with polyposis coli. *Scan. J. Gastroenterol.* **16:**421-427, 1981.

46. Kopelovich, L.: Phenotypic markers in human skin fibroblasts as possible diag-

nostic indices of hereditary adenomatosis of the colon and rectum. *Cancer* **40**:2534-2541, 1977.

47. Kopelovich, L.: Hereditary adenomatosis of the colon and rectum: recent studies on the nature of cancer promotion and cancer prognosis *in vitro.* In: *Colorectal Cancer: Prevention, Epidemiology, and Screening* (Winawer, S.; Schottenfeld, D.; and Sherlock, P., eds.). New York, NY: Raven Press, 1980, pp. 97-108.

48. Vargish, T.; Dawkin, H.G.; Heise, E.; and Myers, R.T.: Serologic detection of persons at risk in familial polyposis coli. In: *Surgical Forum,* Vol. 26, 61st Annual Congress, American College of Surgeons, 1975.

49. Alm, T., and Wahren, B.: Carcinogembryonic antigen in hereditary adenomatosis of the colon and rectum. *Scan. J. Gastroenterol.* **10**:875-879, 1975.

50. Pemberton, J.H.; Heppel, J.; Beart, R.W., Jr.; Dozois, R.R.; and Telander, R.L.: Endorectal ileoanal anastomosis. *Surg. Gynecol. Obstet.* **155**:417-424, 1982.

51. Motson, R.W.; Pescatori, M.; Nicholls, R.J.; and Parks, A.G.: Restorative proctocolectomy with ileal reservoir for ulcerative colitis and familial adenomatosis: clinical results in 62 patients followed for up to six years. *Gut* **24**:A476, 1983.

4
Hereditary Nonpolyposis Colon Cancer: Epidemiologic and Clinical-Genetic Features

Patrick M. Lynch, J.D., M.D., Henry T. Lynch, M.D.,
and Jane F. Lynch, B.S.N.

In this chapter heritable colon cancer (HCC) will be operationally defined as any familial aggregation of colon cancer showing apparent Mendelian segregation and requisite clinical features but not including any of the familial *Adenomatosis coli* syndromes. It will include those families whose members are also prone to cancer of *other* anatomic sites (namely, the cancer family syndrome [CFS]) as well as heritable cancer limited to the colorectum (hereditary, site-specific colon cancer).

HISTORICAL DEVELOPMENT: CASE REPORTS

Historically, early case reports of remarkable family clusters of colon cancer yield to more quantitative studies that attempted to characterize the familial component in colon cancer generally. The first description of the familial tumor spectrum that is now known as CFS is attributed to a 1913 report by Warthin.[1] This kindred (Family G) was ascertained in the course of a chart review of family histories of cancer patients treated at the University of Michigan Hospitals between 1895 and 1913. Family G, updated by several authors in more recent years,[2-4] was at that time characterized by a susceptibility to carcinoma of the uterus (histology unspecified) and stomach (Fig. 4-1). Later, colon cancer came to be regarded as the primary gastrointestinal site,[4] paralleling a similar temporal shift in the general population.[5] In his initial report, Warthin cited studies by Levin and Williams of modest familial clusters of carcinoma of the uterus and gastrointestinal tract.[6, 7] More recent surveys of Family G document the prospectively occurring lesions in the descendents of the patients described originally by Warthin (Fig. 4-2). As will be discussed in further detail, the rare opportunity to longitudinally follow a family with CFS for many generations provides some of the strongest evi-

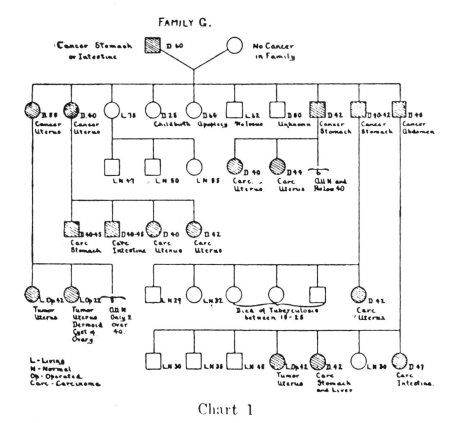

Chart 1

Figure 4-1. Family G of Warthin, as originally published in 1913. *(From A.S. Warthin. Heredity with reference to carcinoma. Arch. Int. Med. 12:549, 1913.)*

dence for both the existence of nonpolypotic, heritable colon cancer and for inferences as to the mode of inheritance.

In both the 1913 report[1] and a 1925 follow-up,[2] Warthin suggested that the pattern of familial tumor expression was consistent with the existence of a *recessively* inherited cancer susceptibility. This erroneous impression of the mode of genetic transmission of cancer in Family G was based on the total cancer experience in the adult membership of the family, involving both cancer-affected and cancer-free branches. Obviously, total cancer incidence in an extended kindred, without regard to whether a given adult had an affected parent, sibling, or progeny, is not informative as to genetic mechanisms. If one were to perform a similar evaluation on a large kindred with familial, multiple, adenomatous polyposis coli (FPC), known to be a classically inherited autosomal-dominant disorder, one might easily arrive at a total

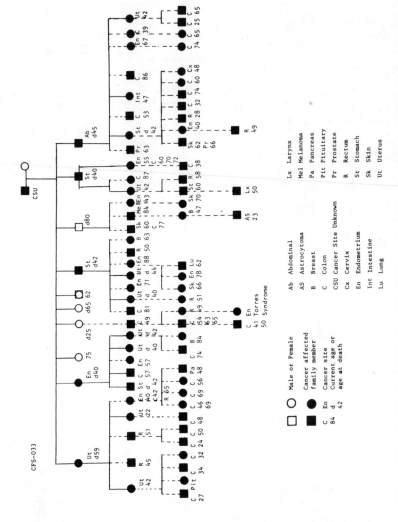

Figure 4-2. Family G. Abridged pedigree illustrating cancer occurrences over the past seven decades. *(From H.T. Lynch, P.M. Lynch, W.A. Albano, and J.F. Lynch. The cancer family syndrome: A status report. Dis. Col. Rect. 24(4):312, 1981.)*

54

incidence of 25% or less in a given family because of the inclusion of the preponderant, low-incidence, nonsegregating lineages.

Aside from Warthin's studies, nearly all investigations of cancer familiality in the early part of this century were conducted at European centers.[8-10] As had been the case with Warthin's evaluation of cancer familiality in a consecutive patient series, these investigations pursued the still elusive goal of specifying the frequency and nature of cancer heritability, employing methods that in certain instances have not been greatly improved on in more recent years.

In 1908, Bashford reported a small kindred in which four brothers died of carcinoma of the cecum and a sister of carcinoma of the uterus (four other siblings were unaffected).[8] The mother and a maternal uncle also died of cancer, sites unspecified. A nephew of the affected siblings died of colonic cancer at age 28. Bashford stressed the infrequency of such occurrences. Focusing on an issue that has long bedeviled efforts to sort out hereditary influences in cancer, Bashford stated that "the great frequency of cancer as a cause of death in adult life discounts very largely any value which might otherwise attach to a succession of cases or to its mere appearance and reappearance in a family as evidence of heredity" (p. 1509).

In 1932, Cholewa reported the case of a 70-year-old woman dying of carcinoma of the uterus and breast. Five of her 12 children expressed carcinomas; three involving the uterus, one, the breast, and one, the ovary. These affected offspring, in turn, had 3 children with carcinoma of the breast, uterus, and rectum. Six of the nine total affected relatives were diagnosed before age 50. The progenitor also had a sister with uterine cancer who, in turn, had a daughter similarly affected; further details were not provided. Unfortunately, as in so many early reports, the critical distinction between endometrial and cervical carcinoma was not made.

In 1941, Bargen et al. reported on the familiality of cancer in a series of patients with colorectal cancer and compared these patients to control groups consisting of patients with hypertrophic arthritis and kidney tumors.[11] Cancer-affected relatives were classified as having gastrointestinal, specified other, or unspecified other cancer and were documented by patient and family recall, supposedly using the same diligence in all three groups. The frequency of unspecified cancer was similar for all groups, while the frequency of gastrointestinal tract cancer in families with colorectal cases was 1.5 times that of the two control groups. The authors reported three specific "cancer families," one of which is worthy of particular note. Of 9 siblings, 6 had gastrointestinal cancer and 1 had ovarian cancer. Seven of the 11 offspring manifested carcinoma of various sites (4, in the gastrointestinal tract), at a substantially earlier age of onset than their parents.

Other than the anecdotal case reports just noted, few examples of HCC families were published between 1913 and the early 1960s. This was, perhaps, partly because of the attention being devoted to the study of adenomatosis coli, particularly by the investigators at St. Mark's Hospital in London, beginning in the 1920s.[12, 13] Notwithstanding a preoccupation with the polyposes and the disappointing findings from case-control studies of cancer familiality (discussed next), the past several decades have witnessed a rapid increase in published accounts of nonpolyposis colon cancer prone families, a development that began to accelerate as criteria for CFS were refined. While a majority of such reports have been of American families,[14-18] informative CFS kindreds have been reported by authors from Denmark,[19] England,[20, 21] Germany,[22] Switzerland,[23, 24] Norway,[25] Finland,[26] Yugoslavia,[27] Uruguay,[28] and New Zealand,[29] a listing that is by no means exhaustive. While all of these reports have been of caucasian families, we are aware of the occurrence of HCC in a black kindred from the United States (D. Purtillo, M.D., personal communication), in several Japanese families (J. Utsunomiya, M.D., personal communication), and in one American-Indian family (Family C-251) currently under study. Further details and accompanying pedigrees regarding this particular kindred and other CFS families from our resource are provided in the Appendix.

HISTORICAL DEVELOPMENT: CASE-CONTROL STUDIES OF FAMILIALITY

In 1924, Samter reviewed the earlier work of C. C. Little in which an increased cancer risk was seen in families of cases, relative to controls.[30] However, in noting Little's failure to ascertain inheritance mechanisms, Samter suggested that the study of individual family genealogies would be the only means of elucidating inheritance patterns. It is of more than historical interest that a distinction was drawn between the knowledge to be gained through the study of familial cancer frequency in large patient series and genealogic investigation of individual "informative" kindreds. Yet, while the usefulness of case-control studies of cancer familiality has long been limited by their inability to elucidate mechanisms of inheritance, genealogic workups of individual families have been criticized on the somewhat justifiable grounds that any given cancer cluster, when ascertained on the basis of aggregation itself, might well simply represent a chance aggregation of such lesions.

By 1908, if not earlier, there existed calculations of expected chance aggregation of lesions from family units of arbitrary size, based on derivations from prevailing mortality rates.[8] While the predictable frequency of such chance aggregations has been used as an argument against the genetic basis for any given familial cluster down to more recent times, it should be noted that such projections dealt with the possibility of familial clustering of cancer of any anatomic site, while most reported cancer families have involved the occurrence of lesions affecting a narrow range of anatomic sites, carrying with them a correspondingly lesser, but still predictable, probability of chance occurrence.

In one of the more oft-quoted studies done since 1960, Macklin considered a series of 145 patients with cancer of the large intestine and 167 patients with gastric carcinoma.[31] Cancer of the large intestine was found significantly more often in relatives of probands with cancer of the large intestine than in the general population, but no excess of gastric cancer was found in the families of colon cancer patients. Conversely, a significant excess of gastric cancer was found in the families of gastric cancer probands, but no excess of colon cancer was observed. Patterns of simple inheritance were not found in the families of colon cancer probands who lacked diffuse adenomatous polyposis of the colon, and the conclusion was that the excess of site-specific cancers in these families was attributable to polygenic inheritance, an opinion shared by many investigators to this day. The methodology employed in this study merits careful scrutiny since the study purports to identify an element of familiality and imputes a hereditary basis to it, yet identifies no simple pattern of inheritance.

Age-specific proportionate death rates (ASPDR) for the state of Ohio were used for decades beginning in 1910, with deaths classified in quinquennial age groups from 40 to 90+ (males) and 30 to 90+ (females). Deceased relatives were arranged in quinquennial age groups and by the decades in which they died; these observed numbers were compared with respective values from the ASPDR for Ohio.

Macklin found that family history information was largely unavailable or could not be substantiated on several classes of more-or-less-remote relatives—grandparents, parents, aunts, and uncles.[31] Most died before the advent of modern mortality record keeping, and many diagnoses were unreliable even when death records were available. Children of many patients were too young to have expressed cancer. Although it was noted that the same difficulties existed for the state of Ohio as a whole, the availability of information on family members (if limited to parents, siblings, and children) tended to preclude the identification of simple patterns of inheritance, even if such patterns existed.

The well-known limitations of reliance on mortality data were particularly critical in this study and may have led to systematic underreporting of familial cancers vis-a-vis the matched control sample. For example, studies by our Creighton group have shown that in families known to be prone to colon cancer, 5- to 10-year survival rates may be higher than in the general population.[32] Regardless of whether this is due to earlier onset alone or to biological differences in the behavior of the tumors themselves, increased survival would be negatively correlated with the likelihood of cancer being listed as a cause of death on death certificates. The survival data similarly suggest that a greater fraction of such patients might still have been living at the time of the study. Consequently, exclusive reliance on death certificates could conceivably lead to a systematic underreporting of colon and other associated cancers in families that are, in fact, cancer prone. This is particularly characteristic of kindreds in which the disease is single gene determined and, therefore, typified by *earlier* onset. In addition, death certificates of relatives from earlier generations (except those who died at advanced ages) could not have been obtained. This would also bias the reporting against cancers occurring at the early ages that are now considered to be characteristic of hereditary colon cancer.

In 1958, Woolf conducted a similar study in which the frequency of deaths due to carcinoma of the large intestine (and other sites) in families of colon cancer probands was compared with the frequency in a control sample.[33] Probands were selected from death certificates in Utah between 1931 and 1951. Family history data from the Archives of the Latter Day Saints (Mormon) Genealogic Society in Salt Lake City were available on approximately one-fourth of the colon cancer probands. Death certificates were then obtained for all parents and siblings of the probands when such relatives died later than 1905, the first year of population mortality record keeping. Controls consisted of persons whose sex, year of death, place of death (county) and approximate age of death matched the deceased relatives of the probands. The tabulated data involved death certificates for 145 fathers of probands, 142 mothers, 309 brothers, and 167 sisters (with corresponding numbers of death certificates for the matched controls). From the total of 763 patients, 26 had carcinoma of the large bowel, as compared with 8 of 763 controls ($P < 0.01$). As in Macklin's study, the significant excess was limited to colon cancer.

Recent Series Assessing Colon Cancer Familiality

More recently, Lovett conducted a study of a series of 209 colorectal cancer patients according to a protocol much like that of Woolf.[34] All patients admitted to St. Mark's Hospital between the end of 1969 and mid-1973 were included in the series. All patients referred to the center because of a known positive family history of colon cancer were excluded. Others were excluded because of diagnoses of multiple polyposis, inability to provide family history, or lack of traceable family members. Although death certificates were relied on to a large extent (they were more available than medical records), morbidity data were traced whenever possible. Of 430 deaths, 47 were attributable to large bowel cancer (nine *living* relatives had a cancer diagnosis; see also discussion of prolonged survival). These death rates were compared with mortality statistics in which colorectal-cancer mortality rates were arranged in quinquennia for each sex; deaths from all causes were similarly tabulated. In each category of first degree relatives, there was a significant excess of deaths from large bowel cancer compared to the mortality expected from similar age groups in the general population. Although the increase over the general population was statistically significant, Lovett concluded (as had Macklin and Woolf) that the incidence was still too low to be consistent with a simple, single, gene-determined pattern of inheritance. Lovett concluded that when all case-control variables could not be attributed to simple inheritance patterns, one must consider the possibility of genetic heterogeneity—that is, sex linked, recessive, autosomal dominance with incomplete penetrance, polygenic inheritance, shared environmental experience, and chance aggregation—all coexisting within the pool of cancer families. In short, it must be considered unrealistic to expect a unifactorial etiology for a disease that is known to otherwise be so obviously heterogeneous.

Lovett was apparently quite aware of the occasional presence of families who did have single-gene-determined, colon-cancer susceptibility within the larger, herterogeneous category of elevated-empiric-risk families, since she provided a case report of a large family in an article from the same volume.[35] Because of the pattern of tumor expression, autosomal-dominant inheritance was inferred in the particular kindred.

One of the most interesting observations in Lovett's series was the correlation between age of onset in probands and the likelihood of having affected relatives. Five of the eight index cases diagnosed before age 40 reported a positive family history of colonic cancer; of the probands diagnosed over age 40, only 25% reported one or more affected relatives. The inference is that any patient diagnosed before age 40 has an increased likelihood of having other members of his family affected. Moreover, based on findings from this series, a patient with colon cancer at any age is fairly likely to have another family member affected, and this likelihood is higher than would be expected by chance alone. The significance of early onset in suggesting a familial susceptibility is underscored if we consider that the older proband will probably have a larger family at an older average age and, consequently, be more apt to express cancer of a nongenetic etiology.

Our own group reviewed the familiality of cancer among 4,515 consecutive patients in a multiphasic, mobile, cancer detection unit.[36] Although the self-referral of community volunteers could certainly have constituted a selection bias, the population screened was not selected for any particular risk factor. The work-up of family history was akin to that reported in the previous studies, but it also incorporated a diligent search for histologic verification of all reported cancers among the probands and their relatives. In plotting the incidence of cancer in the people screened (i.e., by having a carcinoma detected in the screening unit or by history) against the number of first degree relatives with cancer, we discovered a linear increase in risk from 10% of patients with one first degree relative with cancer to 27% of patients with three or more first degree relatives with cancer. Average family size was seen to increase with mean age of relatives. Not surprisingly, then, the mean number of relatives and their mean ages increased as the number of family members affected with cancer increased, consistent with the known age distribution of most cancers in the population.

These data support the notion that elevated cancer risk exists in probands with a family history of cancer, but that such probands themselves may be older.

Cardinal Features of Heritable Colon Cancer Without Polyposis

As the number of CFS reports increased and detailed clinical and pathologic evaluations of large, informative families became more commonplace, the following criteria for the syndrome were established: a high frequency of adenocarcinoma of the colon, endometrium, and ovary[37-39] (other adenocarcinomas including breast, stomach, and, possibly, mesodermal tumors[14-40] may be additional components of the tumor spectrum); a lack of multiple adenomatous polyposis in any affected family members; an excess of proximal colonic involvement in members with colon cancer;[41] an early age of cancer onset (mean of approximately 45 years)[42] when compared to sporadically occurring counterparts in the general population (mean onset, approximately 62 years); an excess of multiple primary cancer in affected patients;[43] a pedigree expression consistent with an autosomal-dominant mode of genetic transmissions;[44] an occasional occurrence of sebaceous adenomas, epitheliomas, and carcinomas in patients with the syndrome cancers (Torre's syndrome);[45, 46] and an increased frequency of prolonged survival in affected patients.[32, 47] Thus the "idealized" patient would be a woman who presents at age 40 with anemia and weight loss and is diagnosed as having two distinct adenocarcinomas of the cecum and ascending colon but who has no other evidence of adenoma formation. Her history might include an adenocarcinoma of the endometrium at age 33. She might also report a family history of similarly affected relatives on one side of her family. On long-term follow-up, the patient would be expected to have a better longevity, stage for stage. But she might develop additional malignancies, perhaps in the remaining colonic segments, in the ovaries, or, possibly, in other anatomic sites.

In hereditary, site-specific colon cancer, the criteria are essentially the same except for the lack of extracolonic tumors.

SELECTED CLINICAL FEATURES

Proximal Colonic Excess

In a large family (C-198) from our registry showing hereditary, site-specific colon cancer (without multiple adenomatous polyps of the colon and also lacking endometrial and ovarian cancer), it was noted that most cases of colorectal cancer involved the right colon (see Appendix for pedigree). Twenty-one of 26 initial diagnoses of colon cancer in this family were proximal to the splenic flexure.[48] This striking contrast to the site distribution seen in the general population (where only 25-35% are proximal)[49] stimulated a review of the other families in our registry. Published findings pertaining to ten CFS families revealed that 65% of *all* cases involved the proximal colon.[41] Updated figures on these and nine additional families[38] are summarized in Table 4-1. Available data on colon cancer subsites in nonpoly-

Table 4-1. Proximal Colonic-Cancer Incidence Among 19 Families

	TOTAL COLONIC-CANCER OCCURRENCE[a] (INITIAL DIAGNOSIS ONLY)	FIRST OCCURRENCE AT PROXIMAL COLON[a]	PERCENT
Family 1	7	7	100
Family 33	27	11	41
Family 51	6	3	50
Family 120	7	5	71
Family 196	11	4	36
Family 200	7	6	86
Family 30	4	4	100
Family 35	3	2	67
Family 115	7	6	86
Family 113	5	4	80
Family 164	6	4	67
Family 199	4	4	100
Family 250	6	2	33
Family 007	2	2	100
Family 198	26	21	81
Family 069	4	4	100
Family 194	3	1	33
Family 010	2	1	50
Family 203	2	1	50
	139	92	66

[a]Only tumors verified as to subsite are included; all families include additional cases in which colonic cancers could not be verified or could not be verified as to subsite.

posis-colon-cancer-prone families reported by other American and foreign authors strongly support the site distribution just quoted.

This site distribution in CFS is patently inconsistent with theories of environmental colon carcinogenesis, which have been offered as an explanation for, among other things, the distal colonic predominance observed in western, high-risk countries.[50] In conjunction with early onset and other syndrome features, proximal colonic involvement serves as a useful criterion for distinguishing hereditary cancer clusters from random aggregations.[41]

Of geographic–epidemiologic interest in the well-documented excess of proximal colonic lesions in developing countries, relative to the left-sided predominance seen in western countries.[50] Conceding that increasing rates in western immigrants may be due to the adopted environment or life-style, the converse also ought to be true—namely, that occurrences in endemically low-risk areas (presumably with low carcinogenic exposures) are reflective of a baseline host susceptibility. Logically, a number of colon cancers occurring in high-risk countries arise through the same mechanism, which accounts for the bulk of cases in low-risk geographies, but are simply submerged within the larger mass of "environmental" cases that occur in high-risk areas.

Prognostic (Survival) Considerations

Anecdotal reports suggest that survival characteristics of certain hereditary forms of cancer may differ from their sporadic counterparts.[51-53] A review of disease-free survival was conducted on the hereditary-colon-and breast-cancer families from our registry, prompted by several observations of prolonged survival in individual patients with invasive disease.[52]

The 20 most well-documented families with hereditary colon cancer (exclusive of polyposis) were evaluated. Primary medical-document review included medical records, pathology reports, and autopsy or death records. Each family medical history was traced over multiple generations, and treatment had been administered in differing geographic locations. Hence, the specific documentation varied considerably from person to person. Staging at initial presentation followed the criteria of the American College of Surgeons (ACS) tumor registries[54] when sufficient documentation was available. Age at onset, tumor characteristics, and disease-free survival were compared with the published, ACS long-term audits for colon cancer. There were 117 patients available for analysis.

The colon cancer patients were significantly younger ($P < 0.05$) than those reported in the ACS audit. The mean age at diagnosis in the 117 HCC patients was 46 years with 36.5% diagnosed under the age of 40. Only 6% of patients from the ACS colon audit were diagnosed under the age of 40.

Adequate documentation for accurate clinical-pathological staging was available in 70% of the hereditary cancer patients. Among these patients, no appreciable differences were noted in staging as compared to the ACS audit studies.

A significant excess of right-sided colon lesions (ascending–transverse colon; $P < 0.05$) was found among patients with HCC compared to the ACS colon audit, which demonstrated the rectum and sigmoid as the favored cancer sites.

Disease-free survival intervals for the 117 patients with HCC yielded a follow-up period ranging from 6 months to over 20 years. The overall 5-year survival was 52%, significantly better ($P < 0.05$) than the 35.3%, 5-year disease-free survival reported in the ACS audit.

These preliminary data are compatible with the existence of a substantial biological difference in the natural history of sporadic and hereditary forms of nonpolyposis colon cancer. Caution must obviously be exercised pending evaluation of a much larger series. The clinical stages in our small series were similar for both the hereditary and ACS patients. Possible biases occasioned by early detection in high-risk patients are, thus, unlikely. None of the 30% of patients lacking enough information for adequate staging had been participants in any formal surveillance programs for cancer at the time of diagnosis.

Another possible explanation for improved survival in hereditary cases (aside from true biological variations or subtle staging differences) is their younger age per se and, consequently, their better ability to withstand major surgery and to fight infections, regardless of stage of disease. However, reported series of young patients with colon cancer have demonstrated a markedly *poorer* survival than that reported in the ACS audits.[55] While small sample sizes have hampered efforts to classify young patients by stage of disease, higher clinical stage at time of diagnosis has been considered to be a critical finding in several series in which poor survival was observed.[56, 57]

If actually present, differences in survival in the hereditary forms of cancer could have a bearing on the evaluation of therapeutic trials. Typically, therapeutic trials comprise a heterogeneous pool of patients, including both unrecognized and unspecified hereditary and nonhereditary cases. But such subgroups are rarely, if ever, classified and assessed separately. Varying survival between the two groups could affect estimates of treatment efficacy, particularly if the therapeutic advantage were marginal. Therefore, stratification in clinical trials, classifying for family history, might be important in evaluating differences in treatment response.

THE TORRE'S SYNDROME AS A CUTANEOUS SIGN OF HERITABLE COLON CANCER

In 1967, Torre described the first patient who would subsequently be recognized as having Torre's syndrome (TS).[58] In the same year, Muir and associates published a case that also seems to represent TS.[59] It is of considerable interest that a review of these original cases as well as the more recent descriptions of TS show them to share certain common features with the CFS.[60-71] These features include multiple visceral adenocarcinoma with early age at onset and, on occasion, a remarkably benign clinical course. However, these disorders have been thought to differ by virtue of an association of multiple sebaceous neoplasms in the TS and their alleged absence in the CFS and a well-defined autosomal-dominant pattern of cancer transmission in the CFS,[44] with a lack of information supportive of familial clustering in TS.

Although our protocol for the study of CFS included a meticulous search for cancer of all anatomic sites as well as all major causes of morbidity and mortality in probands and their available relatives, only modest attention was given to examination of the skin. Prompted by a recent observation of sebaceous neoplasms and unusually long survival from multiple primary cancer in one of our CFS patients (features that were remarkably similar to case reports of the TS),[58-71] we reevaluated records of patients from our extensive CFS resource for evidence of cutaneous findings.[45] Positive cases were found in four CFS kindreds (C-113, C-197,[72] and C-200[73]) and Family G of Warthin.[1-4] Pathology slides and tissue blocks were retrieved for independent microscopic review of biopsied lesions from these patients.

Family C-113. Patient III-3 is a member of a family that fulfills the criteria of the CFS. At age 30, because of a Grade-3 adenocarcinoma of the cecum, she had a right hemicolectomy with ileotransverse anastomosis. At age 51, an adenocarcinoma of the endometrium necessitated total abdominal hysterectomy with bilateral salpingo-oophorectomy and postoperative radiation therapy. Six months later, she underwent a segmental colonic resection for carcinoma of the remaining distal transverse colon. The lesion did not penetrate the muscular layers of the colon. At age 67, she had a fourth primary tumor, an invasive carcinoma of the rectum. During the same · hospitalization, a sebaceous epithelioma was excised from the patient's right flank (Fig. 4-3). She died 6 months later of metastatic rectal cancer. Further family cancer history, including corresponding pedigree, are found in the Appendix.

Family C-197. The proband from this CFS kindred, at age 40, 50, and 51, had a carcinoma of the endometrium, a primary invasive carcinoma of the proximal transverse colon, and a sebaceous epithelioma of the skin of the neck (see Appendix for pedigree).

The patient's identical twin sister had a carcinoma of the endometrium diagnosed three months before the same diagnosis was established in her twin. This patient has not had colon cancer, and she does not admit to having

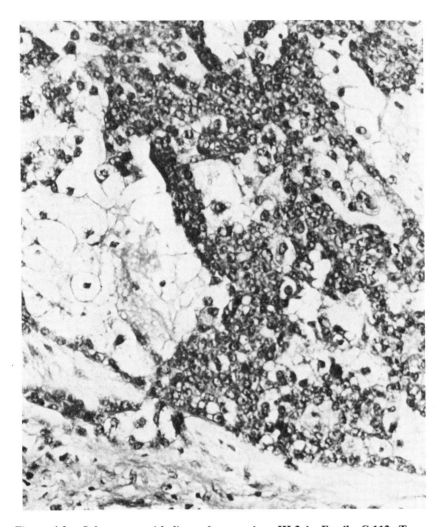

Figure 4-3. Sebaceous epithelioma from patient III-3 in Family C-113. Tumor consists of germinative cells with evidence of sebaceous maturation (hematoxylin-eosin, origin magnification × 160). *(From H.T. Lynch, P.M. Lynch, R. Fusaro, and J. Pester. The cancer family syndrome: Rare cutaneous pheontypic linkage of Torre's syndrome. Arch. Int. Med. 141:609, 1981. Copyright © 1981 by the American Medical Association.)*

cutaneous lesions. However, she has not been examined by a physician for evidence of this. The brother of these sisters had a malignant rectal polyp at age 46 and an invasive adenocarcinoma of the splenic flexure at age 51. Previously, at age 50, he was reported to have had a squamous cell carcinoma

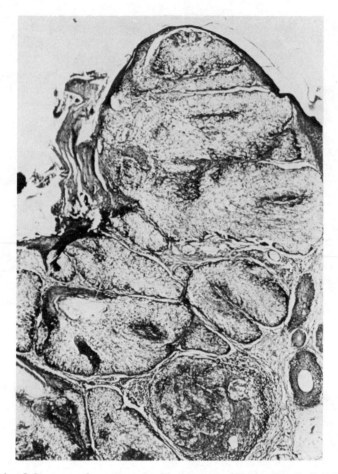

Figure 4-4. Sebaceous adenoma excised from patient III-11 in Family C-113. Tumor consists of several lobules of mature sebaceous cells (hematoxylin-eosin, original magnification × 19). *(From H.T. Lynch, P.M. Lynch, R. Fusaro, and J. Pester. The cancer family syndrome: Rare cutaneous pheontypic linkage of Torre's syndrome. Arch. Int. Med. 141:609, 1981. Copyright © 1981 by the American Medical Association.)*

and a sebaceous carcinoma removed from the eyebrow and the temple. At independent dermatopathologic evaluation, the lesions were interpreted as a keratoacanthoma and a sebaceous adenoma. Finally, the mother of these siblings was diagnosed as having carcinoma of the endometrium at age 60 and carcinoma of the rectum at age 77. She is alive and well at age 90.

Family C-200.   This family includes a 48-year-old woman who had cutaneous stigmata of the TS, but who to date has not manifested visceral carcinoma.

At age 43, a sebaceous adenoma on the face was removed (Fig. 4-4). Five months later, a well-differentiated squamous cell carcinoma of the skin of the nose was excised. While it was stated that the patient has had no evidence of visceral cancer to date, a mucinous cystadenoma of the left ovary was removed at age 42. This patient is a candidate for visceral cancers of the CFS and will require meticulous surveillance. Additional family cancer history, including pedigree, are found in the Appendix.

Family G.[1-4]   In 1974, Bitran and Pellettiere described a 57-year-old woman who was treated at age 33 for an epidermoid carcinoma of the vulva.[62] At age 43 she had an adenocarcinoma of the endometrium treated with intracavity radiotherapy. Concurrently, a pneumonectomy for a left hilar mass confirmed a metastatic adenocarcinoma consistent with the endometrial primary tumor. She subsequently underwent a hysterectomy and bilateral salpingo-oophorectomy. At age 42, before the diagnosis of endometrial carcinoma, she had had a waxy, papular, sebaceous adenoma and a sebaceous epithelioma excised. No mention of family history was given in the 1974 report.[62] From Dr. Pellettiere, who made additional contact with this patient, we learned that she was a member of the direct genetic line of descent of Family G of Warthin (the original CFS kindred). It is of further interest that this patient, although extremely knowledgeable about her family history, had not disclosed any of these facts to her husband—nor had she told her four children, who are at 50% risk for the CFS.

Review of Torre's Syndrome

In 1967, Torre reported the case of a 57-year-old man with asymptomatic, papular, waxy lesions of the face, trunk, and scalp, variously documented as "sebaceous adenomas," "sebaceous carcinomas," and "basal cell epitheliomata with sebaceous differentiation."[58] Almost incidentally, the patient was reported to have had a primary carcinoma of the ampulla of Vater at age 48 and a primary carcinoma of the colon at age 51; no mention was made of presence or absence of a family history of either the unusual skin lesions or of the internal cancer.

Earlier in 1967, Muir et al. reported the rather striking case of a patient with at least seven internal carcinomas associated with multiple molluscum sebaceum (keratoacanthoma).[59] Specifically, the patient was diagnosed with a moderately differentiated squamous cell carcinoma of the larynx (Broder's Grade III) at age 37 followed by diagnosis of four, apparently primary, carcinomata located predominantly in the proximal colon, as well as three benign colonic polyps. At age 41, two primary malignancies of the duodenum, including a periampullary carcinoma that obscured the ampulla itself, were noted. Muir et al. suggested that the lesions must have been of low-grade malignancy, although their histologic appearance did not support such a contention. In other words, the authors found it remarkable that none of the rather invasive tumors had metastasized. During the 6-year period before and all during this previously described sequence of events, the patient had been diagnosed with recurrent, multiple molluscum sebaceum of the face, none described as cancerous. The lesions ranged

from hyperplasia of a group of follicles with hyperkeratosis of the lining epithelium . . . to that of the fully developed keratoacanthoma in which numerous hyperkeratotic follicles had merged into a crater-like mass. . . . The base of the lesion showed regular downgrowths of squamous epithelium forming keratin and associated with a heavy infiltrate of chronic inflammatory cells in the adjacent dermis . . . a highly differentiated sebaceous gland tumour composed of irregular lobules consisting of a peripheral layer of generative basal cells with a central mass of mature sebaceous cells. (Muir et al.,[59] p. 192)

In 1971, Bakker and Tjon-A-Joe reported the first case of Torre's syndrome in which a family history was reported (the patient's father died of colon cancer).[63] At age 43, the reported patient manifested a well-differentiated squamous cell carcinoma of the cheek which, on independent evaluation, appeared more like a benign keratoacanthoma. The following year, at age 44, a large, ulcerating carcinoma of the ascending colon was diagnosed, invading the fatty mesocolon but with no nodes involved. Nine years later, a sebaceous gland carcinoma of the back was excised followed by 18 similar lesions in the ensuing years, appearing on the back, breast, face, and extremities. At age 63, a carcinoma of the transverse colon was diagnosed and at age 65, an anaplastic carcinoma of the stomach. In discussing etiology, Bakker and Tjon-A-Joe state:

The factor responsible for this predisposition to tumor formation in this special place (sebaceous cells) remains uncertain. Extrinsic physical and chemical agents cannot perhaps be totally excluded but seem improbable; a chronic disease of the sebaceous gland and hair sheath cells that could have given rise to a precancerous state can be reasonably excluded. Therefore, a hereditary predisposition seems to be the most important factor and becomes, in our view, quite acceptable because the only cases of multiple tumors of sebaceous glands described in the literature were seen in patients with multiple tumors in widely different organs. (p. 56)

They conclude that their case, as well as those of Torre[58] and Muir et al.[59] "are examples of a rare syndrome, characterized by the occurrence of multiple lesions of the skin, partly sebaceous gland tumors and partly keratoacanathoma, in patients with multiple tumors of the internal organs, mostly of a low grade malignancy"(p. 56).

In 1973, Rulon and Helwig reviewed 105 cases of sebaceous neoplasia from the Armed Forces Institute of Pathology charts and found 5 patients who also had had internal cancer.[60] The 5 cases were similar in that each involved cutaneous lesions of widely varying histologic appearance, each having multiple visceral carcinomas, typically of the proximal colon, and each showing prolonged survival.

In 1974, Jakobiec reported a patient who, in addition to the characteristic sebaceous adenomas and keratoacanthomas, exhibited a fungating carcinoma of the rectosigmoid at age 49.[64] This patient's family history was the most striking reported up to that time, in that the father had a benign "fibrous" growth of the colon at age 36, and also had skin lesions described as squamous cell carcinoma, basal cell epithelioma, and pseudoepitheliomatous hyperplasia in his sixties. At age 65, a right hemicolectomy was performed on the father for carcinoma followed at age 69 by a left hemicolectomy for a second colonic carcinoma.

In 1974, Sciallis and Winkelmann reported two cases of Torre's syndrome.[65] The first patient, a white male, presented with sebaceous adenoma of the temple at age 42, followed by sebaceous adenoma of the upper back at age 55, basal cell carcinoma at age 56, sebaceous adenoma of the chest at age 56, and two sebaceous adenomas of the forehead at age 57. Sebaceous hyperplasia of the nasolabial fold was also reported to have occurred at age 57. At age 53, a Grade III adenocarcinoma of the cecum was diagnosed. No polyposis was evident. No recurrence of the tumor was reported. The father of this patient was reported to have had an adenocarcinoma of the colon at age 40 and lived to age 77. The patient could not recall whether or not the father had cutaneous lesions.

The second case was a white female who, at age 57, manifested a Grade III adenocarcinoma of the hepatic flexure, without invasion. At age 60, a sebaceous adenoma was removed from the occipital region of the scalp. No recurrence of either the colonic or cutaneous lesions was reported. The family history was not known.

Also in 1974, Leonard and Deaton reported the case of a white female who, at age 47, was diagnosed with carcinoma of the descending colon, invading the muscularis but without evidence of lymph node metastases.[66] At age 52, squamous cell carcinoma of the vocal cord was diagnosed, and at age 56, a noninvasive adenocarcinoma of the endometrium was treated. None of the lesions recurred. Between the ages of 55 and 63, six sebaceous adenomas and squamous cell carcinomas of the skin were removed from the left breast, anterior chest wall, neck, left arm, and back. The family history was quite significant in that the mother was reported to have had carcinoma, as were six out of ten siblings. The lesions included two carcinomas of the cervix, one of the colon, three that were "other gastrointestinal," and one whose primary site was unknown.

In 1976, Reiffers et al. reported a case of a 45-year-old Swiss male diagnosed with multiple sebaceous hyperplasia, benign adenoacanthoma, keratoacanthoma, and squamous cell epitheliomas, primarily of the face.[61] Previously, at age 34, an adenocarcinoma of the sigmoid colon with a second primary located more proximally in the colon were diagnosed. At age 43, an epidermoid cancer of the external auditory meatus was detected. A micropolyp of the rectosigmoid was removed at this time. A villous adenoma of the colon was removed at age 45 at approximately the same time that the multiple skin lesions appeared. This patient presented with a most remarkable and informative family history, describing for the first time in the literature of Torre's syndrome the degree of variable expressivity that can occur. The patient's brother died at age 33 of intestinal cancer and was reported to have had none of the cutaneous lesions observed in the proband. Conversely, the father manifested cutaneous lesions, reported to have been quite similar to those observed in the proband, yet did not manifest intestinal cancer.

Also in 1976, Tschang et al. reported the following case: a 40-year-old white female who underwent a hysterectomy for endometrial carcinoma followed at age 46 by a Duke's A adenocarcinoma of the rectum and a Duke's B adenocarcinoma of the sigmoid colon.[67] One of the resected colonic lesions involved the periureteral soft tissue and ileal wall. Between ages 48 and 50, two sebaceous adenomas and two keratoacanthomas were removed from her face. At age 54, lesions described as keratoacanthoma (left cheek) and basal cell carcinoma (infraorbital) were excised. Her family history was also significant in that her father and seven of his ten siblings were reported to have died of abdominal malignancies. Of the patient's four siblings, one had endometrial carcinoma and skin lesions of undetermined type. Multiple adenomas of the colorectum have been encountered rarely in patients otherwise appearing to express Torre's syndrome.[74, 75] Sebaceous adenomas and keratoacanthomas have also been observed in at least one patient with malignant lymphoma in the absence of polyposis coli.[76]

One patient with multiple sebaceous gland tumors and evidence of polyposis coli was reported by Lynn-Davies et al. in 1974.[74] At age 48, a white male was diagnosed by sigmoidoscopy as having "many sessile and pedunculated polypoid tumors, varying in size between 1 cm and 2 cm, beginning at the anal verge" (p. 1378). Radiography and subsequent laparotomy demonstrated "multiple polyposis of the large bowel" (p. 1378). A 6 cm × 5 cm, well-differentiated papillary adenocarcinoma was detected in the cecum. Several regional lymph nodes were extensively replaced with secondary adenocarcinoma. During the 25 years before this time, multiple asymptomatic tumors of the forehead, face, and upper trunk had gradually increased in size and number. Skin biopsies performed at approximately the same time as the colon surgery showed the lesions to be sebaceous adenomata. Two years later, a 1 cm osteoma of the right tibia was shown on skeletal survey. The patient died at age 52, and at autopsy was found to have massive metastatic adenocarcinoma of the liver. Additional findings included exostosis of the right calcaneus and right tibia, neural hamartoma of the right adrenal medulla, and solitary chromophobe adenoma of the pituitary.

The patient's sister had had a carcinoma of the large bowel removed 20 years previously, at age 26. Although no further details were provided, there had apparently been no recurrence. Another sister had multiple cutaneous lesions of the forehead, face, and upper trunk. While small and less numerous than those observed in her brother, they had the same microscopic appearance. Evaluation of the colon showed only a small (4 mm), sessile, adenomatous polyp of the rectum. Although the patients in this report bear a superficial resemblance to the expression seen in Gardner's syndrome, the noncystic nature of the sebaceous lesions and the lack of polyposis in the sister with cutaneous lesions may partially serve to distinguish these cases from the typical expression of Gardner's syndrome.

In 1980, Schwartz et al. described a 75-year-old man in whom isolated rectal and multiple colonic polyps respectively had been removed at age 36 and 60, the latter involving at least one focus of microinvasive adenocarcinoma and necessitating resection of 90 cm of bowel.[75] Isolated polyps were removed over the ensuing 15 years. From age 73 to 75, numerous asymptomatic papules (sebaceous epitheliomas, keratoacanthomas, and sebaceous adenomas) were removed from his face and head. Family history was negative except for cancer (site unknown) in the patient's mother at age 52 and prostatic cancer in a fraternal half brother at age 86. No information regarding collateral maternal relatives was available.

In an excellent review of differential diagnosis of sebaceous tumors, Sciallis and Winkelmann[65] differentiated the sebaceous adenoma–sebaceous gland carcinomas that occur in the Torre's syndrome from several other disorders (see also Table 4-2).[77-84] The "Nevus Sebaceous of Jadassohn" is distinguished on the basis of its congenital onset. Senile sebaceous hyperplasia lacks stromal reaction or atypical keratinization; moreover, Sciallis and Winkelmann found no relationship to gastrointestinal malignancy in a review of 50 cases from the Mayo Clinic with a ten-year follow up. A review by Nickel and Reed, cited by Sciallis and Winkelmann, deleted adenoma sebaceum from classification as a sebaceous gland disorder.[65] Nevertheless, for completeness, the disorder has been listed in Table 4-2.

Recently, Anderson reported a family in which 4 of 5 patients with colonic

TABLE 4-2. Differential Diagnosis [a]

DISORDER	DESCRIPTION
Torre's syndrome[58-71]	Single or multiple sebaceous neoplasia associated with early onset and multiple, primary, visceral cancer (typically gastrointestinal) in absence of polyposis; prolonged survival common; familiality suggested but not rigorously evaluated
Cancer family[1-4, 14-24] syndrome	Early onset, multiple, primary, visceral cancer (predominantly proximal colon and endometrial) in absence of polyposis; prolonged survival common; in some patients, evidence of sebaceous neoplasia; familial clustering repeatedly documented as consistent with autosomal-dominant genetic transmission
Signs of Leser-trelat[77-78]	"Sudden appearance and rapid increase in size and number of seborrheic keratosis" secondary to internal cancer (usually adenocarcinoma of the stomach); as in acanthosis nigricans, skin changes postulated to be result of latent genetic abnormality that is only expressed in the presence of a highly malignant carcinoma
Gardner's[79] syndrome	Colonic polyposis as of FPC (hereditary basis well established); sebaceous cyst as leading skin sign; also osteomas (mandible, maxilla, skull are common sites), abnormal dentition, abdominal fibrosis, desmoid tumors (less frequently), periampullary malignancy

72

Disorder	Description
Perifollicular [80, 81] dermal fibroma with colon polyps	Multiple dermal perifollicular fibromas appearing as skin tags (one family report); associated isolated adenomatous colon polyps
Tuberous [82] sclerosis (epiloia, Bourneville's disease)	Autosomal-dominant inheritance; cerebral-cortical nodules (neural deficiency, epilepsy, death before age 20 common); angiofibromas (adenoma sebaceum) at nasoLabial folds; shagreen patches; "ash leaf" depigmentation; retinal tumor; rhabdomyosarcoma; skeletal abnormality; kidney and heart tumors
Nevoid basal-cell [83] carcinoma syndrome	Multiple, nevoid, basal-cell cancers; frontal bossing; hypertelorism; bone cysts; bifid ribs; agenesis of corpus callosum; brachymetacarpalism; palmar pits; endocrine anomalies; medulloblastoma; jaw fibrosarcoma; ameloblastoma, ovarian fibroma; autosomal dominance well established; no significant gastrointestinal or other adenocarcinoma association
Generalized [84] keratoacanthoma	Diffuse eruptive keratoacanthomas with prurific and mucous-membrane involvement but without internal malignancy; multiple or solitary keratoacanthoma with squamous carcinoma of larynx, rectum, and anus; may in fact be related to Torre's syndrome except that sebaceous lesions and adenocarcinomas are not expressed.

[a] Several of the disorders listed are clearly not examples of sebaceous-gland activity, hereditary disease, or gastrointestinal-tract cancer associations but have been listed in the interest of providing a broader background.

or small bowel cancer supposedly had skin tumors consistent with Torre's syndrome.[85] One patient, a male, was diagnosed at age 49 with duodenal carcinoma, and three basal cell carcinomas were treated between ages 48 and 59. A second member of this family was diagnosed with carcinoma of the sigmoid colon at age 70. Between ages 73 and 91, he had multiple skin lesions classified as basal cell carcinoma, sebaceous hyperplasia, keratoacanthoma, actinic, and seborrheic keratoses. A third male relative was diagnosed with carcinoma of the rectosigmoid colon at age 43 and was found at age 51 to have "multiple hyperkeratotic lesions." The status of the fourth patient was not discussed in Anderson's text.

In no case did there appear to be histopathologic verification of the more unusual lesions associated with Torre's syndrome (i.e., sebaceous adenoma, epithelioma, and carcinoma) that characterized the earlier case reports. It is entirely possible that independent, dermatopathologic review of existing slides and tissue sections, coupled with intensive screening of affected and high-risk patients, might have disclosed such cases in the family reported by Anderson. This issue is stressed because it is apparent that a consensus is lacking as to precisely what cutaneous lesions are actually associated with visceral neoplasms in the Torre's syndrome. Because lesions such as basal and squamous cell carcinomas and actinic and seborrheic keratoses are so common in older age groups, they cannot (and should not) serve as evidence that the syndrome exists in any given patient.

One of the most insightful case reports of the Torre's syndrome was that of Householder and Zeligman,[70] who reported the following cases:

Case 1. The patient was diagnosed at age 59 with a keratoacanthoma and sebaceous adenoma and, later, with a sebaceous carcinoma and another sebaceous adenoma. At age 64, a second keratoacanthoma was removed and in the following 3 years, two sebaceous epitheliomas were removed. At age 39, the cecum was removed due to cancer, and at age 53, cancer of the transverse colon was resected. In later years, several isolated adenomatous polyps were removed.

Case 2. A 71-year-old woman had a 20-year history of a lesion ultimately diagnosed as a sebaceous adenoma. At age 45, carcinoma of the uterus was diagnosed, and at age 59, the colon was resected for adenocarcinoma.

Both patients were reported to have had positive family histories of colon cancer, though no information was available regarding the status of relevant skin lesions in close relatives. Householder and Zeligman suggested that the key feature of Torre's syndrome was the occurrence of sebaceous neoplasia with visceral cancer and that keratoacanthoma was frequent, though not invariably, present. Thus, Householder and Zeligman suggested that the patient could not be classified as having Torre's syndrome on the basis of visceral neoplasm and keratoacanthoma alone, but that the presence of sebaceous neoplasia are essential. The authors disagreed with several earlier commentaries suggesting that the skin lesions were in some way a consequence of visceral malignancy. Householder and Zeligman's review indicated that roughly one-third of the reported patients had had sebaceous neoplasia before the onset of colonic and other visceral cancer and that, in this respect, there was some predictive value in the lesions themselves. These authors suggested, then, that any patient presenting with such a skin lesion should be evaluated for possible presence of visceral cancer. Finally, noting the frequent suggestion of positive, though loosely documented, family histories, the presence of Torre's syndrome in a given patient was considered adequate indication for evaluation and screening of close relatives. However, the report did not specify the need for stool guaiac and barium enema or colonoscopy as means of achieving early detection of colorectal cancer, the most frequently occurring visceral malignancy.

Two reports in the recent literature have conflicting findings as to familiality. Namia et al. describe a 64-year-old Japanese male with a history of carcinoma of the stomach (age 36), the sigmoid colon (age 45), the cecum (age 47), the sigmoid colon (age 50), the stomach (age 54), the ileum (age 54), the transverse colon (age 57, two lesions), the nasal vestibule (a sebaceous carcinoma, age 62), and the stomach and descending colon (age 64, at autopsy).[71] Obviously, the gastrointestinal lesions had only been locally resected, contributing in large part to the great multiplicity of primary lesions that occurred. Widespread metastases were apparent at autopsy. Notably, the family history was reported to be unremarkable.

Fahmy et al. recently described a patient with eight primary visceral malignancies, sebaceous neoplasia, keratoacanthoma, and a family history that is positive for gastrointestinal cancer but with apparently no further examples of sebaceous lesions.[46] The pedigree of this kindred summarizes these findings (Fig. 4-5).

Fahmy et al. also considered at some length the basis for a possible relationship between true sebaceous neoplasia and keratoacanthomas. The perifollicular location of each was considered a unifying histologic feature with an emphasis on the occasional "overlap between subaceous and epidermoid proliferation" called "squamoproliferative (with) foci of sebaceous cells" (Rulon and Helwig,[86] p. 90) or "squamous cell epithelioma with sebaceous differentiation" (Urban and Winkelman,[87] p. 66). Of significance to the differential diagnosis of sebaceous lesions is the conclusion by Fahmy et al. in concordance with the current consensus of dermatopathologic opinion, that senile sebaceous hyperplasia are not helpful in diagnosis because of the high frequency of these lesions in older patients.

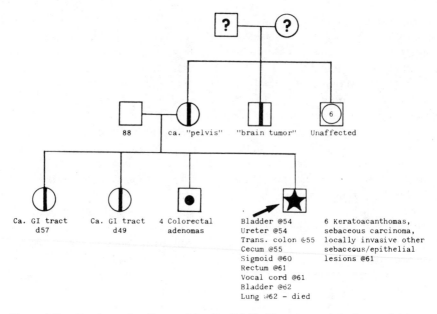

Figure 4-5. Condensed pedigree of family C-010. *(Based on original material from Fahmy et al.*[46] *and personal communication from W. Burgdorf, 1981.)*

Summary and Classification of Skin Lesions

Previous case reports of Torre's syndrome (Table 4-3) described a range of cutaneous lesions including sebaceous adenoma, sebaceous epithelioma, sebaceous carcinoma, keratoacanthomas, and a variety of lesions encountered frequently in older persons, such as seborrheic, actinic, and other keratoses, as well as typical basal and squamous cell carcinomas. The sebaceous lesions, and to a lesser extent, keratoacanthomas, when coupled with visceral malignancy, form the core criteria for Torre's syndrome. The remaining skin lesions appear to have been catalogued mainly for purposes of completeness. It seems unlikely that one would classify a patient as having Torre's syndrome if that patient had, in addition to visceral malignancy, only the more commonly encountered skin lesions just described.

The coexistence of sebaceous skin lesions, early-onset visceral carcinoma, and prolonged survival in patients from families with CFS clearly integrates the Torre's syndrome as a phenotypic component of CFS. For this reason, CFS may now be considered a cancer-associated genodermatosis, albeit one in which the cutaneous signs are not always fully penetrant.

Table 4-3. Case Reports—Cutaneous Manifestations and Visceral Carcinomas

SOURCE	SEBACEOUS ADENOMAS	OTHER SKIN LESIONS[a]	VISCERAL MALIGNANCY	FAMILY HISTORY OF TUMORS
Muir, et al.[59]	Multiple	Keratoacanthomas	Larynx, colon, duodenum	
Torre[58]	Multiple	Sebaceous carcinoma, sebaceous BCC, SCC	Ampulla of Vater, colon	
Rulon and Helwig[60]				
Case 1	10	Keratoacanthoma, sebaceous hyperplasia, SCC	Colon	
Case 2	2	Sebaceous BCC	Renal pelvis, urinary bladder	Father: carcinoma of colon and prostate
Case 3	11	Benign keratosis, dermatofibroma	Colon, ureter	
Case 4	8	Epidermal cyst	Colon, stomach	Sister: carcinoma of breast; Brother: carcinoma of colon, colon polyps, carcinoma of bladder; Brother: carcinoma of liver
Case 5	2	Sebaceous BCC	Colon	
Bitran and Pellettiere[62]	8	Sebaceous epithelioma, SCC of vulva	Endometrium	

[a]Sebaceous BCC indicates basal-cell carcinoma with sebaceous differentiation; BCC indicates basal-cell carcinoma; SCC indicates squamous-cell carcinoma

(continued)

Table 4-3. *(continued)*

SOURCE	SEBACEOUS ADENOMAS	OTHER SKIN LESIONS[a]	VISCERAL MALIGNANCY	FAMILY HISTORY OF TUMORS
Bakker and Tjon-A-Joe[63]	19	Keratoacanthomas	Colon, stomach	Father: carcinoma of colon
Sciallis and Winkelmann[65]				
Case 1	5	BCC; sebaceous hyperplasia	Ileoceal valve	Father: carcinoma of colon
Case 2	1	None	Colon	Negative
Jakobiec[64]	17	Keratoacanthoma; sebaceous hyperplasia, sebaceous BCC	Rectosigmoid	Father: carcinoma of colon
Leonard and Deaton[66]	6	SCC	Colon, larynx, endometrium	Carcinoma of colon, cervix, gastrointestinal tract
Tschang et al.[67]	5	Keratoacanthomas, BCC	Endometrium, rectum, sigmoid colon	Father: carcinoma; Sister: carcinoma of endometrium
Reiffers et al.[61]	5	Keratoacanthoma; sebaceous epitheliomas, sebaceous hyperplasias, SCC	Rectosigmoid, colon	Brother: carcinoma of colon
Householder and Zeligman[70]				
Case 1	2	Keratoacanthoma, sebaceous epitheliomas, sebaceous carcinoma; carcinoma of adnexal origin	Colon, duodenum	Father: carcinoma of colon; Mother: carcinoma of uterus; Brother: carcinoma

Case 2	1	None	Colon, uterus	Mother: carcinoma of liver; Son: carcinoma of rectum
Poleksic[68]	None	Keratoacanthoma, SCC	Colon, prostate, esophagus	
Lynn-Davies and Brown[74]				
Case 1	Multiple	None	Colon	Sister: carcinoma of colon
Case 2	Multiple	None	Colon	
Anderson[85]				
Case 1	None	BCC	Duodenal	All three patients from same kindred
Case 2	None	BCC, sebaceous hyperplasia, keratoacanthoma	Colon	
Case 3	None	SCC	Colon	
Lynch et al.[17]				
(C-113, III-3)	None	Sebaceous epithelioma	Distal colon, proximal colon, rectum	Numerous collateral relatives with cancer of CFS type[22]
(C-197, III-2)	None	Sebaceous epithelioma	Endometrium, proximal colon	
(C-197, III-1)	1	Keratoacanthoma	Rectum, distal colon	
(C-200, III-11)	1	SCC	None	

[a]Sebaceous BCC indicates basal-cell carcinoma with sebaceous differentiation: BCC indicates basal-cell carcinoma: SCC indicates squamous-cell carcinoma

(continued)

Table 4-3. *(continued)*

SOURCE	SEBACEOUS ADENOMAS	OTHER SKIN LESIONS[a]	VISCERAL MALIGNANCY	FAMILY HISTORY OF TUMORS
(C-033)[1-4] (from Family G of Warthin—same as Bitran and Pellettiere)[62]	8	SCC of vulva, sebaceous epithelioma	Endometrium	Numerous collateral relatives with cancers of CFS type
Schwartz et al.[75]	Numerous	Keratoacanthomas	Microinvasive cancer, adenocarcinoma of colon multiple colonic polyps	Mother with carcinoma, site unknown
Namia[71]		Sebaceous carcinoma	Stomach, sigmoid, cecum, ileum, transverse colon	Unremarkable
Fahmy et al.[46]		Keratoacanthomas, sebaceous carcinoma	Bladder, ureter, cecum, transverse sigmoid colon, rectum: lung	Two sisters with cancer of gastrointentinal tract at 49, 57; Brother with isolated colonic adenomas; Mother: cancer of pelvis; Maternal uncle: brain tumor

[a]Sebaceous BCC indicates basal-cell carcinoma with sebaceous differentiation; BCC indicates basal-cell carcinoma; SCC indicates squamous-cell carcinoma

In light of this linkage with Torre's syndrome, all CFS kindreds should be reevaluated, with particular attention to the integument, in order to learn what fraction of patients with the syndrome actually manifest the subject cutaneous stigmata. Conversely, meticulous attention to family history should be devoted to any patient with Torre's syndrome. Any patient with the cutaneous lesions, with or without a known family history of cancer, should be screened for visceral cancer. In their paper on the topic, Fahmy et al. concur with this view.[46]

The natural history of the cutaneous signs must be critically scrutinized in an effort to isolate the factors that elicit the cutaneous signs (i.e., primary vs. secondary manifestations of underlying cancer.

EVIDENCE OF AUTOSOMAL DOMINANCE

In the absence of distinguishing physical signs (e.g., adenomatosis) or closely associated biomarkers (chemical-cytogenetic findings) or gene linkage, it is impossible to unequivocally prove that the CFS is caused by a single, deleterious, autosomal-dominant gene. This point is emphasized even though casual pedigree inspection is consistent with this assumption of the mode of inheritance. Nevertheless, in spite of our limitations from the biomarker standpoint, there are now several strong descriptive lines of support for an autosomal-dominant mode of genetic transmission in CFS.

The first line of support is the high lifetime incidence of colorectal-endometrial cancer to progeny of matings that involve an affected direct-line parent, using pooled data from many families. Figure 4-6 contrasts the cumulative, age-specific incidence curve for 581 progeny (307 males and 274 females) of CFS-affected patients with that of the general population. Notably, the lifetime risk for tumors of the two primary anatomic sits (colon and endometrium) is approximately 55% compared to only 6 to 7% in the general population. The excess lifetime risk to progeny of affected parents is, therefore, approximately 50%, consistent with the notion that one-half of these persons received a deleterious, cancer-predisposing gene from a heterozygous direct-line parent.

The second line of support is that findings from segregation analysis of one of our pedigrees (C-196; see Appendix for pedigree), using maximum likelihood techniques, are consistent with an autosomal-dominant inheritance pattern with gene carriers showing a lifetime susceptibility (penetrance) of 89% and a mean age of cancer onset of 42.5.[88]

The final line of support, and perhaps the most compelling to the clinician lacking highly technical genetic and mathematical sophistication, is

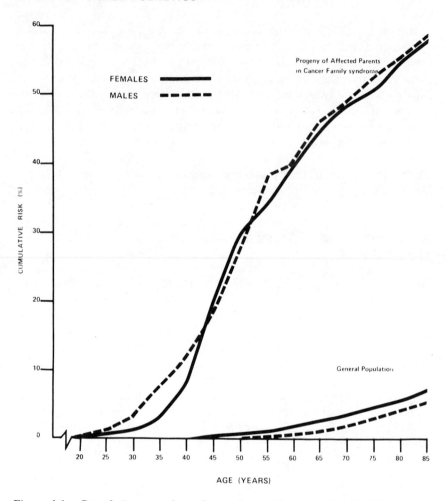

Figure 4-6.   Cumulative rates for colon-endometrial cancer in high-risk patients from pooled families contrasted with expected population incidence. Colorectal cancer in males; colorectal-endometrial cancer in females. Rates for the general population are based on the Third National Cancer Survey. *(From H.T. Lynch, P.M. Lynch, and R.E. Harris. Minimal genetic findings and their cancer control implications: A family with the cancer family syndrome. JAMA 240:537, 1978. Copyright © 1978 by the American Medical Association.)*

our long-term prospective follow-up of a number of kindreds with a simple segregating pattern of vertical cancer expression and equal sex distribution. However, before such observations can have any value in distinguishing dominant from recessive, sex-linked, maternal, polygenic, cytoplasmic, or "other" putative inheritance mechanisms, one must first establish that a given familial cancer cluster shows *any* etiology consistent with primary genetic factors.

By way of analogy, the search for infectious agents in Hodgkin's disease has been slowed and to some extent discredited by the persistent inability to conclusively prove that reported time–space clusters of the disease could not have been mere chance aggregations. Because cancer, particularly colorectal cancer, is such a common disease, it did not take long for early investigators to recognize the possibility of random clustering in families, as alluded to in the previous reference to Bashford's 1908 report. Certainly, in a sufficiently large population with a common disease, striking clusters are inevitable on the basis of chance alone. And while the features already cited (early onset, tumor multiplicity, proximal cancer predominance) tend to decrease the random probability of a given observed event, they cannot completely rule out random occurrence, at least not if the events are considered from an entirely retrospective time frame. However, prospective occurrence of such events in a small predefined sample, if showing a segregation pattern fulfilling one's *a priori* hypothesis, would provide near conclusive evidence of inheritance. Even here, the rigid requirement of segregation must be imposed to rule out the rather vague suggestion of "shared environmental influences," or a perpetuated infection.

SIGNIFICANCE OF EXTRA-COLONIC LESIONS

For years, descriptions of CFS have supposed that anatomic sites in addition to the colon comprise part of the heritable tumor spectrum. These inferences have been predicted on many, often anecdotal, observations that a limited range of tumors is found at an early age in patients who also manifest colon cancer at an early age. In certain cases, demonstration of vertical transmission in a family required that a given patient having only extracolonic cancer be regarded as a presumptive gene carrier given the "typical" expression in his descendents.

In an attempt to more reliably assess the significance, if any, of extracolonic lesions, previously coded information pertaining to all of the largest families in our registry were subjected to life-risk analysis. All family members had been classified as high (50%) risk, low (less than 25%) risk, and indeterminate (25-50%) risk. In the respective groups, direct-line parents were (1) affected with colonic or specific other cancer; (2) cancer-free; or (3) of unknown cancer status. The so-called high-risk group was comprised of subjects whose immediate parents had colon cancer as well as those whose parents may have had cancer of some other site but who could reasonably be regarded as gene carriers by virtue of having an affected parent, siblings/or child. Such parents had typically died early enough to have been unlikely to show clinical disease, regardless of their gene-carrier status (see also Chap. 10). Assignment to low-risk categories was also somewhat arbitrary inasmuch as the status of cancer-free parents was determined in relation to their age or age at death and by accuracy of medical history. Indeterminate risk, as the name implies, occurs when the carrier status of the parent cannot be inferred on the basis of the obtainable information or by virtue of subsequent events within the family.

The method used to estimate the cumulative cancer risk over "t" decades of life is given by

$$\text{Risk} = 1 - \sum_{i+1}^{t} (1 - q_i)$$

where:

$$q_i = x_i/(n_i - \sum y_{ij}/10) \sum_{j=1}^{w_i}$$

x_i = the number of persons affected with cancer during the ith decade of life
n_i = the number of persons under observation and unaffected at the beginning of the ith decade
w_i = the number of withdrawals during the ith decade
y_{ij} = the number of years remaining in the ith decade for the jth withdrawal.

The risk is a function of the number of persons in a particular age group and the number of cancers occurring in that decade of life. Beyond the eighth decade of life, the number of persons in an interval becomes vanishingly small in relation to their chronic disease burden *vis-à-vis* other age groups. Consequently, any cancers in the interval will exaggerate the calculated lifetime risk of cancer for the entire sample. A more reasonable estimate of the lifetime risk is accomplished by either grouping everyone older than 79 into the seventieth to seventy-ninth decade of life or simply truncating the analysis at age 80. The latter was elected for this analysis.

Despite the inevitable lumping of subjects into somewhat arbitrary risk categories, some interesting findings did emerge (Fig. 4-5). In the case of endometrial cancer, risk was significantly ($p < 0.01$) greater for the high-risk group than the low-risk group, regardless of whether the subject showed colon cancer. One observes that the lifetime risk for the disease in high-risk patients is at least 15-fold greater than that in low-risk patients. This observation tends to support the position that has been taken in the past that endometrial carcinoma is a feature central to the tumor spectrum of CFS. However, some degree of caution must be exercised inasmuch as the risk figures make no specific attempt to deal with the question of ascertainment bias. The argument is as follows: to the extent that endometrial carcinoma has been regarded *a priori* as a feature of the syndrome, then the occurrence of such lesions could contribute to ascertainment of a given family. If calculation of risk for endometrial cancer imposes no limitations, then the nuclear family (typically classified as high risk according to the above criteria) would be differentially loaded with colon cancer, leading to artifactual results. Review of the pedigrees listed in the Appendix suggests that while this may indeed have been the case with respect to the initial classification of many families, the occurrence of endometrial cancer in subsequently affected patients from any particular family remained increased in the high-risk group relative to the subjects from cancer-free family branches.

One of the more curious findings suggested by Table 4-4 is the apparent excess of cancer of other anatomic sites in colon-cancer-affected and colon-cancer-free high-risk patients *vis-à-vis* the low-risk subjects. While every effort is made to fully document occurrence of cancer in *all* branches of a family, we must concede that probably more new diagnoses of cancer in high-risk branches are brought to our attention because these patients and relatives are more concerned than the low-risk group. In part, it is recognition of this tendency that necessitates periodic follow-up of all branches of the families comprising our registry.

The risk of breast cancer was greater among the high-risk subjects, but not significantly so. With respect to ovarian carcinoma, another tumor believed to be a part of the tumor spectrum of CFS, no valid comparison could be made inasmuch as no low-risk patients lacking colon cancer have manifested ovarian malignancy.

In general, the findings just discussed support the conclusion of endometrial carcinoma as a central feature of CFS. However, one is reluctant to attribute statistical significance to other specific adenocarcinomas since carcinoma of the breast and ovary, for example, tend to cluster in some families with colon cancer, but not others. Consequently, with the exception of colonic and endometrial cancer, one cannot generalize regarding risk of other tumors. Instead, one must regard each family in terms of those extracolonic malignancies that for presently unknown reasons occur in excess.

Table 4-4. Lifetime risk of Cancer of Selected Anatomic Sites among High- and Low-Risk Members of Nonpolyposis, Hereditary, Colon-Cancer Families

	HIGH RISK			LOW RISK			
	TOTAL # OF PEOPLE	TOTAL # OF CANCERS	LIFE RISK	TOTAL # OF PEOPLE	TOTAL # OF CANCERS	LIFE RISK	P-VALUE
LIFE RISK OF BREAST CANCER							
Lacking colon cancer	297	9	0.0911	996	6	0.0504	0.1423
± colon cancer	364	9	0.0712	1004	6	0.0493	0.2514
LIFE RISK OF ENDOMETRIAL CANCER							
Lacking colon cancer	297	24	0.1779	996	1	0.0116	<0.01
± colon cancer	364	43	0.2440	1004	1	0.0114	<0.01
LIFE RISK OF CANCER OF ANY EXTRACOLONIC SITE							
Lacking colon cancer	609	79	0.416	1961	56	0.2629	0.004
± colon cancer	750	101	0.3966	1976	58	0.267	0.0069

MISCELLANEOUS GENETIC DISORDERS IN WHICH NONPOLYPOTIC COLON CANCER HAS BEEN OBSERVED

Hereditary Brachydactyly

Certain clinically encountered developmental anomalies have been reported to cluster in affected members of colon-cancer-prone families. Macrae et al. reported an association between hereditary brachydactyly and colorectal cancer.[89] In the subject family, brachydactyly consisted of hypoplasia affecting the second, third, and fifth middle phalanges of both hands. Its severity varied within the kindred and it was present in five of seven siblings. Three of these brachydactyly-affected persons died of colorectal cancer, and the other two died from unrelated diseases at ages 29 and 68. Of the two siblings who did not manifest brachydactyly, one was living and well at age 69, and the other died at age 70 from coronary-artery disease. Unfortunately, no detail was given about the anatomic location of the colon cancers and whether or not polyps were present. Eleven of 16 members in the next generation (including 2 with brachydactyly) were screened for fecal occult blood and by flexible sigmoidoscopy at ages 45 to 54. One was found to have adenomatous polyps, while two had metaplastic polyps. Only one of the persons had brachydactyly. Macrae et al. concluded that while the concurrence of brachydactyly and colorectal cancer may have been due to chance, it may have represented a syndrome enabling identification of persons at risk for colorectal cancer.

Nail-Patella Syndrome

The nail-patella syndrome (NPS), or hereditary onycho-osteodysplasia, comprises nail and patella hypoplasia and iliac horn and elbow dysplasia.[90] The disease has been linked to the ABO blood groups and adenylate kinase.[91, 92]

Gilula and Kantor described a family with NPS and colon carcinoma.[93] The proband was a 46-year-old woman who had NPS. Her mother, maternal aunt, and maternal grandfather showed concordance for the NPS and colonic cancer, and one son also had NPS. Variable manifestations of NPS were observed in other relatives. The proband and her son had multiple epidermal cysts, prominent about the head and neck, but they lacked other features of Gardner's syndrome. In particular, no evidence of multiple polyposis coli was seen. The authors found no increased incidence of colon cancer in their review of other reported kindreds with NPS.

REFERENCES

1. Warthin, A.S.: Heredity with reference to carcinoma. *Ann. Int. Med.* **12:**546-555, 1913.
2. Warthin, A.S.: The further study of a cancer family. *J. Cancer Res.* **9:**279-286, 1925.
3. Hauser, I.J., and Weller, C.V.: A further report on the cancer family of Warthin. *Am. J. Cancer* **27:**434-444, 1936.
4. Lynch, H.T., and Krush, A.J.: Cancer Family "G" Revisited 1895-1970. *Cancer* **27:**1505-1511, 1971.
5. *Cancer Registration and Survival in California.* California State Tumor Registry, State of California, Dept of Public Health, 1963, p. 405.
6. Levin, I.: The influence of heredity on cancer: a study in eugenics. *Z. Krebsforschung* **11:**547-558, 1912.
7. Williams, W.R.: *The Natural History of Cancer,* London, 1908, p. 364.
8. Bashford, G.F., Heredity in cancer. *Lancet* **2:**1508-1512, 1908.
9. Cholewa, J.: Krebskrankheit und vererbung. *Z. Krebsforschung* **37:**5-23, 1932.
10. Paulsen, J.: Konstitution und krebs. *Z. Krebsforschung* **21:**119-130, 1924.
11. Bargen, J.A.; Mayo, C.U.; and Giffin, L.A.: Familial trends in hereditary cancer. *J. Hered.* **32:**7-10, 1941.
12. Lockhart-Mummery, J.P.: Cancer and heredity. *Lancet* **4:**427-429, 1925.
13. Dukes, C.E.: The hereditary factor in polyposis intestine or multiple adenocarcinoma. *Cancer Rev.* **5:**241-256, 1930.
14. Law, I.P.; Herberman, R.B.; Oldham, R.K.; Bouzoukis, J.; Hansom, S.M.; and Rhode, M.C.: Familial occurrence of colon and uterine carcinoma and of lymphoproliferative malignancies: clinical description. *Cancer* **39:**1224-1228, 1977.
15. Williams C.: Management of malignancy in "cancer families." *Lancet* **1:**198-199, 1978.
16. Cannon, M.M., and Leavell, B.S.: Multiple cancer types in one family. *Cancer* **19:**538-540, 1966.
17. Lynch, H.T.; Lynch, P.M.; and Harris, R.E.: Minimal genetic findings and their cancer control implications: a family with the cancer family syndrome. *JAMA* **240:**535-538, 1978.
18. Metzmaker, C.O., and Sheehan, P.: Report of a family with cancer family syndrome. *Dis. Colon Rect.* **24:**523-525, 1981.
19. Bulow, S.; Svendsen, L.B.; and Danes, B.S.: To familier med cancerfamilies-syndromet. *Vgeskrift for Laeger* **143:**2716-2718, 1981.
20. Mathis, M.: Familiares colonkarzinome. *Schweiz Med. Wochenschr.* **92:**1673-1678, 1962.
21. Dunstone, G.H., and Knaggs, T.W.: Familial cancer of the colon and rectum. *J. Med. Genet.* **9:**451-456, 1972.
22. Butt, H., and Schumacher, M.: Mehrfachkarzinome bei familiarer Haufung von genital-und intestinalkarzinomen. *Dtsch. Med. Wochenschr.* **96:**468-471, 1971.

23. Dubosson, J.D.; Klein, D.; Pettavel, J.; and Rey, C.D.: Syndrome du cancer familial a travers 4 generations. *Schweiz Med. Wochenschr.* **107:**875-881, 1977.
24. Mathis, M.: Familiares colonkarzinome. *Schweiz Med. Wochenschr.* **92:**1673-1678, 1962.
25. Kluge, T.: Familial cancer of the colon. *Acta. Chir. Scand.* **127:**392-398, 1964.
26. Peltokallio, P., and Peltokallio, V.: Relationship of familial factors to carcinoma of the colon. *Dis. Colon. Rect.* **9:**367-370, 1966.
27. Glidzic, V., and Petrovic, G.: Observations sur le caractere hereditaire des cancers du colon. *Bull. Cancer (Paris)* **55:**11-16, 1968.
28. Sarroca, C.; Quadrelli, R.; and Praderi, R.: Cancer colique familial. *Nouv. Presse. Med.* **7:**1412, 1978.
29. Innes, C.B.: A family with a high incidence of cancer. *NZ Med. J.* **87:**280-282, 1978.
30. Samter, B.: Beitrage zur kenntnis des erbfamiliaren krebses. *Arch. fur Gynakologie* **22:**679-691, 1924.
31. Macklin, M.T.: Inheritance of cancer of the stomach and large intestine in man. *JNCI* **24:**551-571, 1960.
32. Lynch, H.T.; Albano, W.A.; Recabaren, J.A.; Lynch, P.M.; Lynch, J.F.; and Elston, R.C.: Prolonged survival as a component of hereditary breast and nonpolyposis colon cancer. *Med. Hypotheses* **7:**1201-1209, 1981.
33. Woolf, C.M.: A genetic study of carcinoma of the large intestine. *Am. J. Hum. Genet.* **10:**42-47, 1958.
34. Lovett, E.: Family studies in cancer of the colon and rectum. *Brit. J. Surg.* **63:**13-18, 1976.
35. Lovett, E.: Familial cancer of the gastrointestinal tract. *Brit. J. Surg.* **63:**19-22, 1976.
36. Lynch, H.T.; Brodkey, F.D.; Lynch, P.; and Lynch, J.; Maloney, K.; Rankin, L.; Kraft C.; Swartz, M.; Westercamp, T.; and Guirgis, H.A.: Familial risk and cancer control. *JAMA* **236:**582-584, 1976.
37. Smith, W.G.: The cancer family syndrome and heritable solitary colonic polyps. *Dis. Colon. Rect.* **13:**362-367, 1970.
38. Lynch, H.T.; Lynch, P.M.; Albano, W.A.; and Lynch, J.F.: The cancer family syndrome: a status report. *Dis. Colon Rect.* **24:**311-322, 1981.
39. Lynch, H.T., and Lynch, P.M.: Tumor variation in the cancer family syndrome: ovarian cancer. *Am. J. Surg.* **138:**439-442, 1979.
40. Escobar, V., and Buxler, D.: Familial reticulum cell sarcoma and birth defects. *Original Article Series* **12:**151-158, 1976.
41. Lynch, P.M.; Lynch, H.T., and Harris, R.E.: Hereditary proximal colonic colon. *Dis. Colon. Rect.* **20:**661-668, 1977.
42. Lipkin, M.; Winawer, S.J.; and Sherlock, P.: Early identification of individuals at increased risk for cancer of the large intestine. Part I: Definition of high risk populations. *Clin. Bull.* **11:**13-21, 1981.
43. Lynch, H.T.; Harris, R.E.; Lynch, P.M.; Guirgis, H.A.; and Lynch, J.F.: The role of heredity in multiple primary cancers. *Cancer* **40:**1849-1854, 1977.
44. Lynch, H.T.; Guirgis, H.A.; Harris, R.E.; Lynch, P.M.; Lynch, J.F.; Elston, R.C.; Go, R.C.P.; and Kaplan, E.: Clinical, genetic and biostatistical progress in the cancer family syndrome. *Gastrointest. Res.* **4:**142-150, 1979.

45. Lynch, H.T.; Lynch, P.M.; Fusaro, R.; and Pester, J.: The cancer family syndrome: Rare cutaneous phenotypic linkage of Torre's syndrome. *Arch. Int. Med.* **141**:607-611, 1981.

46. Fahmy, A.; Burgdorf, W.H.C.; Schosser, R.H.; and Pitha, J.: Muir-Torre syndrome: Report of a case and reevaluation of the dermatopathologic features. *Cancer* **49**:1898-1903, 1982.

47. Lynch, H.T.; Bardawil, W.A.; Harris, R.G.; Lynch, P.M.; Guirgis, H.A.; and Lynch, J.F.: Multiple primary cancers and prolonged survival: Familial colonic and endometrial cancers. *Dis. Colon Rect.* **21**:165-168, 1978.

48. Lynch, P.; Lynch, H.T.; Harris, R.G.; Lynch, J.F.; and Guirgis, H.A.: Heritable colon cancer and solitary adenomatous polyps. In: *Prevention and Detection of Cancer I(2)* (Nieburgs, H.G., ed.). New York, NY: Marcel-Dekker Inc., 1978, pp. 1573-1589.

49. Third National Cancer Survey: Incidence Data. NCI Monograph 41. Biometry Branch Div. Cancer Causes and Prevention, NCI. (Cutler, S.J., and Young, J.H., eds.). *DHEW Pub. (NIH) 75-787,* Bethesda, MD, March 1975, pp. 454.

50. Correa, P., and Haenszel, W.: Comparative international incidence and mortality. In: *Cancer Epidemiology and Prevention: Current Concepts* (Schottenfeld, D., ed.). Springfield, ILL: Charles C. Thomas, 1975, p. 386.

51. Langlands, A.O., Kerr, G.R., and Bloomer, S.M.: Familial breast cancer. *Clin. Oncol.* **2**:41-45, 1976.

52. Albano, W.A.; Recabaren, J.A.; Lynch, H.T.; Campbell, A.S.; Mailliard, J.A.; Organ, C.H.; and Kimberling, W.J.: Natural history of hereditary cancer of the breast and colon. *Cancer* **50**:360-363, 1982.

53. Crifel, M.: Survival of cutaneous malignant melanoma patients at University of Iowa Hospitals 1950-1974. *Cancer* **47**:176-183, 1981.

54. Evans, J.T.; Vana, J.; Aronoff, B.L.; Baker, H.W.; and Murphy, G.P.: Management and survival of cancer of the colon: Results of a national survey by the American College of Surgeons. *Ann. Surg.* **188**:716-720, 1978.

55. Mayo, C.W.; Redentor, J.G.; and Pagtalunan, J.G.: Malignancy of colon and rectum in patients under 30 years of age. *Surgery* **53**:711-718, 1962.

56. Simstein, N.L.; Kovalcik, P.J.; and Gross, G.H.: Colorectal carcinoma in patients less than 40 years old. *Dis. Colon. Rect.***21**:169-171, 1978.

57. Howard, E.W.; Cavallo, C.; Hovey, L.M.; and Nelson, T.G.: Colon and rectal cancer in the young adult. *Am. Surgeon* **April**:260-265, 1975.

58. Torre, D.: Multiple sebaceous tumors. *Arch. Dermatol.* **98**:549-551, 1968.

59. Muir, E.G.; Yates-Bell, A.J.; and Barlow, K.A.: Multiple primary carcinomas of the colon, duodenum, and larynx associated with keratoacanthoma of the face. *Br. J. Surg.* **54**:191-195, 1967.

60. Rulon, D.G., and Helwig, D.G.: Multiple sebaceous neoplasms of the skin: an association with multiple visceral carcinomas, especially of the colon. *Am. J. Clin. Pathol.* **60**:745-752, 1973.

61. Reiffers, J.; Lougier, P.; and Hunziker, N.: Hyperplasies sebacees, keratoacanthomes, epitheliomas due visage et cancer due colon. *Dermatologica* **153**:23-33, 1976.

62. Bitran, J., and Pellettiere, E.V.: Multiple sebaceous gland tumors and internal carcinoma: Torre's syndrome. *Cancer* **33**:835-836, 1974.

63. Bakker, P.M., and Tjon-A-Joe, S.S.: Multiple sebaceous gland tumors with multiple tumors of internal organs, a new syndrome? *Dermatologica* **142:**50-57, 1971.

64. Jakobiec, F.A.: Sebaceous adenoma of the eyelid and visceral malignancy. *Am. J. Ophthalmol.* **78:**952-960, 1974.

65. Sciallis, G.F., and Winkelmann, R.K.: Multiple sebaceous adenomas and gastrointestinal carcinoma. *Arch. Dermatol.* **110:**913-916, 1974.

66. Leonard, D.D., and Deaton, W.R.: Multiple sebaceous gland tumors and visceral carcinomas. *Arch. Dermatol.* **110:**917-920, 1974.

67. Tschang, T.P.; Poulos, E.; Ho, C.K., et al.: Multiple sebaceous adenomas and internal malignant disease: A case report with chromosomal analysis. *Hum. Pathol.* **7:**589-594, 1976.

68. Poleksic, S.: Keratoacanthoma and multiple carcinomas. *Br. J. Dermatol.* **91:**461-462, 1974.

69. Stewart, W.M.; Lauret, P.H.; Hemet, J., et al.: Multiple keratoacanthomas and visceral carcinomas: Torre's syndrome. *Ann. Dermatol. Venereol.* **104:**622-626, 1977.

70. Housholder, M.S., and Zeligman, I.: Sebaceous neoplasms associated with visceral carcinomas. *Arch. Dermatol.* **116:**61-64, 1980.

71. Namio, H.; Koyama, Y.; Kodama, T.; Itabashi, M.; and Hirota, T.: A case of metachronous multiple carcinomas of the gastrointestinal tract and sebaceous gland. *Jpn. J. Clin. Oncol.* **10:**321-332, 1980.

72. Lynch, H.T., and Krush, A.J.: The cancer family syndrome and cancer control. *Surg. Gynecol. Obstet.* **132:**247-250, 1971.

73. Lynch, H.T.; Swartz, M.; and Lynch, J.: A family study of adenocarcinoma of the colon and multiple primary cancer. *Surg. Gyn. Obstet.* **134:**781-786, 1972.

74. Lynne-Davies, G., and Brown, J.: Multiple sebaceous gland tumors associated with polyposis of the colon and bony abnormalities. *Canadian Med. Assn. J.* **110:**1377-1379, 1974.

75. Schwartz, R.A.; Flieger, D.N.; and Saied, N.K.: The Torre syndrome with gastrointestinal polyposis. *Arch. Dermatol.* **116:**312-314, 1980.

76. Descalzi, M.E., and Rosenthal, S.R.: Sebaceous adenomas and keratoacanthomas in a patient with malignant lymphoma: A new form of Torre's syndrome. *Cutis* **28:**169-170, 1981.

77. Safai, B.; Grant, J.M.; and Good, R.: Cutaneous manifestation of internal malignancies (II): the sign of Leser-Trelat. *Int. J. Dermatol.* **17:**494-495, 1978.

78. Liddell, K.; White, J.E.; and Caldwell, I.W.: Seborrheic keratoses and carcinoma of the large bowel (three cases exhibiting the sign of Leser-Trelat). *Br. J. Dermatol.* **92:**449-452, 1975.

79. Gardner, E.J., and Richard, R.C.: Multiple cutaneous and subcutaneous lesions occurring simultaneously with hereditary polyposis and osteomatosis. *Am. J. Hum. Genet.* **5:**139-147, 1953.

80. Hornstein, O.P.; Knickenberg, M.; and Morl, M.: Multiple dermal perifollicular fibromas with polyps of the colon: report of a peculiar clinical syndrome. *Acta. Hepato-Gastroenterol.* **23:**55-58, 1976.

81. Hornstein, O.P.: Generalized dermal perifollicular fibromas with polyps of the colon. *Hum. Genet.* **33:**193-197, 1976.

82. Reed, W.B.; Nickel, W.R.; and Campion, G.: Internal manifestations of tuberous sclerosis. *Arch. Dermatol.* **87:**715-728, 1963.

83. Anderson, D.E.; Taylor, W.B.; Falls, H.F.; and Davidson, R.T.: The nevoid basal cell carcinoma syndrome. *Am. J. Hum. Genet.* **19:**12-22, 1967.

84. Winkelmann, R.E., and Brown, J.: Generalized eruptive keratoacanthoma. *Arch. Dermatol.* **97:**615-617, 1968.

85. Anderson, D.E.: An inherited form of large bowel cancer: Muir's syndrome. *Cancer* **45:**1103-1107, 1980.

86. Rulon, O.B., and Helwig, E.B.: Cutaneous sebaceous neoplasms. *Cancer* **33:**82-102, 1974.

87. Urban, F.H., and Winkelmann, R.K.: Sebaceous malignancy. *Arch. Dermatol.* **84:**63-72, 1961.

88. Elston, R.C., and Stewart, I.: A general model for the genetic analysis of pedigree data. *Hum. Hered.* **21:**523-542, 1971.

89. Macrae, F.A.; Roberts-Thomson, I.C.; Russell, D.; and St. John, D.J.B.: Familial colorectal cancer and hereditary brachydactyly. *Br. Med. J.* **282:**1431-1432, 1981.

90. Beals, R.K., and Eckhart, A.L.: Hereditary onycho-osteodysplasia. *J. Bone Joint Surg.* **51-A:**505-516, 1969.

91. Schleutermann, D.A.; Bias, W.B.; Murdock, J.L.; and McKusick, V.A.: Linkage of loci for nail-patella syndrome and adenylate kinase. *Am. J. Hum. Genet.* **21:**606-630, 1969.

92. Van Cong, H.; Rebourcet, R.; Weil, D.; Covillin, P.; Hors, M.C.; Jami, J., and Frezai, J.: Assignment of second locus of adenylate kinase to chromosome 1p: preliminary data. *Cytogenetics* **13:**173-178, 1974.

93. Gilula, Louis A., and Kantor, Owen S.: Familial colon carcinoma in nail-patella syndrome. *AJR* **123:**783-790, 1975.

ADDENDUM

Since this chapter was submitted for publication some of the data assembled by our consortium* has been analyzed by Drs. Kimberling, Elston, and Bailey-Wilson and is provided here.[1, 2]

---

*We respectfully acknowledge our consortium that was responsible for providing much of the biomarker data for this chapter. The members include Henry T. Lynch, M.D., Guy S. Schuelke, Ph.D., Jane F. Lynch, B.S.N., Karen A. Biscone, B.S.N., the late William A. Albano, M.D., and William J. Kimberling, Ph.D. (Departments of Preventive Medicine, Surgery, and Otolaryngology, Creighton University School of Medicine, Omaha); Martin Lipkin, M.D. and Eleanor E. Deschner, Ph.D. (Department of Gastroenterology and Laboratory of Digestive Tract Carcinogenesis, Memorial Sloan-Kettering Cancer Center, New York, NY); Yves B. Mikol, Ph.D. (Hunter College, New York, NY); Avery A. Sandberg, M.D. (Roswell Park Memorial Institute, Buffalo, NY); Robert C. Elston, Ph.D. and Joan E. Bailey-Wilson, Ph.D. (Department of Biometry, LSU Medical Center, New Orleans, LA); Thomas L. Drouhard, M.D. (Tuba City PHS Indian Hospital, Tuba City, AZ); and B. Shannon Danes, M.D., Ph.D. (Laboratory for Cell Biology, Cornell University Medical College, New York, NY).

BIOSTATISTICAL ANALYSIS OF CANCER PHENOTYPE IN HNPCC

We have investigated nine families with the Cancer Family Syndrome (CFS) and two families with the hereditary site-specific colorectal cancer (HSSCC) syndrome. Table 1 shows that there is a marked excess of cancer in the first degree relatives of cancer-affected individuals (colon and/or endometrial cancer in CFS or only colon cancer in HSSCC) in the eleven families studied. The paucity of cancer in nonbloodline relatives minimizes environmental significance and shows the importance of genotype contribution to the cancers within these families. Moreover, one of the HSSCC families was of pure Navajo Indian stock. The family is of particular interest in that this American Indian tribe has been characterized as having a low incidence of colorectal cancer.[3, 4] Thus, these observations lend further support to the primary role of genetic susceptibility in cancer expression in HNPCC families.

Known or suspected clinical aspects of HNPCC were confirmed by the most recent data presented in Table 1. These aspects include: an increased incidence of cancer among bloodline cancer-affected individuals and their siblings; a proclivity for proximal versus distal colonic cancer; early mean age of onset in all families; an earlier mean age of onset for proximal cancer versus distal cancer; and 95% gene penetrance of the cancer-prone genotype by 67.3 years of age.

BIOMARKER AND GENETIC DETERMINATIONS DONE IN HNPCC

The potentially informative parameters analyzed in these families included: in vitro tetraploidy of dermal fibroblast monolayer cultures; tritiated thymidine uptake (^{3}HdThd) labeling of colonic mucosa; cytogenetics of peripheral blood mononuclear leukocytes; and 25 landmark polymorphic serum and blood group markers. Segregation analysis of a subset of the putative biomarkers just discussed, and linkage analyses between each of the polymorphic markers and the cancer were performed.

IN VITRO TETRAPLOIDY AND TRITIATED THYMIDINE LABELLING OF COLONIC EPITHELIAL CELLS

Segregation Analysis

All eleven families were used in the segregation analysis of in vitro tetraploidy. The families were ascertained because of the presence of multiple cases of nonpolyposis colorectal cancer, each family having a single index case

Table 1. Characteristics of the HNPCC Families Studied

CHARACTERISTIC		FINDINGS	
Cancer status of living and deceased family members	9 CFS families	nonblood[a]	2.7% affected[b]
		Group 1[c]	20.4% affected
		Group 2	0.0% affected
	2 HSSCC families	nonblood	0.0% affected
		Group 1	18.8% affected
		Group 2	0.0% affected
Anatomic site of colon cancer	proximal	68.8% (N=66)	
	distal	31.2% (N=30)	
Mean age of cancer onset	45.9 years		
Mean ages of onset for proximal vs. distal colon cancer in HNPCC	proximal	43.7 yrs[d]	(N = 64)
	distal	48.9 yrs[d]	(N = 30)
Mean ages of onset for colon and endometrial cancer in the HNPCC families studied	colon	46 yrs[e]	(N = 130)
	endometrial	45 yrs[e]	(N = 33)

[a]Nonblood means an individual who married into the family or a relative of someone who married into the family.
[b]The percentage of individuals affected with either colon or endometrial cancer.
[c]Group 1 consists of living cancer-affected individuals and their siblings. Group 2 relatives are defined as children and grandchildren of a proven gene carrier.
[d]Means are significantly different at $p = 0.04$.
[e]Means not significantly different at $p. = 0.703$; however, there was a narrower range of age at onset for endometrial cancer. For example, 95% of the female gene carriers will have endometrial cancer by age 60.2 years, but one must go to 67.3 years to get 95% affected with colon cancer.

identified. For each of the three traits, the segregation analyses, which are preliminary in nature, were performed on the trait converted into a dichotomy, using the general transmission probability model,[5] and allowing for partial penetrance of each genotype. Three maximum likelihoods were calculated for each trait: with the transmission probabilities constrained to be Mendelian; with the transmission probabilities constrained to be equal; and under the unrestricted model of arbitrary (but between 0 and 1) transmission probabilities. Each of the first two likelihoods was compared to the third likelihood.

Shift of the Major Zone for ³HdThd Uptake in Colonic Crypts. For this trait, it was found that there is no significant departure from Mendelian autosomal dominant transmission, but there is significant departure from the hypothesis of no intergenerational transmission (i.e., equal transmission probabilities). The penetrance of the dominant genotype was estimated to be unity; that of the recessive genotype, representing sporadic cases, was estimated to be 0.03 at birth and increasing by a factor of 1.028 for each year of age.

³HdThd Uptake in 11 Colonic Crypt Divisions. For this trait, a significant departure from Mendelian autosomal dominant transmission was found, though the estimates of the genotypic frequencies and the penetrance of the dominant genotype under the Mendelian hypothesis were quite similar to those obtained for the shift of the major zone of ³HdThd uptake.

In Vitro Tetraploidy. For in vitro tetraploidy there was no significant departure from Mendelian autosomal dominant transmission, but there was significant departure from the hypothesis of no intergenerational transmission. The penetrance of the dominant genotype was estimated to be 0.44 at birth and increasing by a factor of 1.006 for each year of age. There were no sporadic cases.

Gene Linkage

Gene marker determinations were done on informative members in the kindreds. The markers typed were ABO, Rh, MNS, Kell, Fy, Jk, Le, Se, Di (in only the one American Indian kindred), Gm, Km, Hapt, C3, Bf, Gc, Pi, Tnf, PGM1, ACP, EsD, AK, PGD, ADA, GLO, and GPT. Linkage analysis was done using the linkage program LIPED.[6, 7]

Linkage analysis and the variable cancer test were done between each of these markers. For cancer, an individual was considered affected if he/she was affected with colon and/or endometrial cancer. Genotypic probabilities of CFS for each unaffected individual in the pedigree were calculated assuming CFS to be a rare autosomal-dominant gene with no sporadic cases and using a mean age of onset of 45 years with a standard deviation of 11 years. A normal distribution for age of onset was assumed.

In the linkage analysis results for HNPCC versus the standard set of markers, only one result was noteworthy. A maximum lod score of +1.88 was observed for all HNPCC kindreds taken together with the Kidd (Jk) blood group. Only one family gave a decidedly negative score. This family and one other family did not have any family members affected with endometrial cancer and may represent hereditary site-specific colonic cancer (HSSCC). Therefore, there was a legitimate basis for excluding these families from the analysis. When the HSSCC kindreds were removed, the lod score was 3.01 at recombination fraction $\theta = 0.0$. While significant, these results must be viewed cautiously because of the fact that two families were excluded from the summation of lod scores.

Cytogenetics.

Four families with HNPCC and one family characterized by a very low rate of cancer ("cancer resistant family") were evaluated. Leukocytes were cultured with PHA (phytohemaglutinin) for 72 hours, harvested, and prepared for chromosome analysis by established methods.[8] G- and C-banding was performed on each specimen; 25 metaphases were analyzed by C-banding and 15 metaphases were analyzed by G-banding.

In each case, the karyotype of the individual, the number of chromosome abnormalities (gaps, breaks, fragments, and deletions), and the nature of the pericentromeric heterochromatin were established. Polymorphisms of the latter were presumed to exist when inversion (partial or complete) or abnormally large amounts of heterochromatin were present on chromosomes #1, #9, and/or #16, in which such heterochromatin is readily identified because of their large size.

Interestingly, the mean incidence of chromosome abnormalities was found to be 10.5% in the control family versus 34.% in the HNPCC kindreds. Additionally, the mean incidence of heterochromatin polymorphisms was 21.1% in the control family versus 48.7% in the HNPCC kindreds. While these results are provocative, they must be viewed with caution as more control families need to be studied before their significance can be assessed. Chromosomal abnormalities have an association with neoplasia, as clearly evidenced in such disorders as the chromosome breakage syndromes. While we do not claim that the findings described in these families have comparable significance, it is nevertheless difficult to ignore the possibility that they may be contributing to susceptibility to neoplasia. In particular, we wonder about the effects of translocations (10.5% control vs. 34% in affected kindreds).

The cancer-affected families have a higher incidence of heterochromatin polymorphisms, but their interpretation remains elusive and will depend on proper control data. Nevertheless, the possibility remains that these changes, regardless of whether they occur in the affected or nonaffected individuals from these families, may interact with other genetic and/or cytogenetic events and thereby may have more etiologic significance than is presently appreciated.

COMMENT

It was not possible to allow completely for the mode of ascertainment of the pedigrees. However, both in vitro tetraploidy and a shift of the major zone for ^{3}HdThd uptake in colonic crypts appeared to fit a model of dominant Mendelian transmission, the former with reduced penetrance increasing with age. The lack of fit of ^{3}HdThd uptake in 11 colonic crypt divisions to a genetic model may or may not be significant; further data need to be collected before any definite conclusions regarding its mode of inheritance can be reached.

The biomarkers mentioned previously require extensive evaluation in both CFS and HSSCC kindreds before their utility can be assessed for purposes of both gene carrier identification and for classifying these disorders into distinct genetic entities as was suggested in the clinical data by differing mean ages of cancer onset, multiple primary cancer excess, and other facets of natural history (see Chapter 4). Continued investigations of cellular, biochemical and behavioral anomalies in such kindreds could help to elucidate the mechanisms responsible for cellular conversion from normal to malignant phenotypes.

The biomarker findings provide a major advance in the comprehension of HNPCC. Previously assignment of "affected" vs. "nonaffected" was dependent on the expression or lack of expression of the syndrome cancer phenotype, which was complicated by the age dependent penetrance. If these biomarker findings continue to display high sensitivity and specificity in the testing of additional HNPCC kindreds, we would then have a capability of our early genotype prediction, thereby indicating who will versus who will not manifest the phenotype (syndrome cancer).

In conclusion, this work provides a format for further investigations into the significant problem of genetically determined colon cancer. Specifically, these investigations should include as many potentially informative biological parameters as possible per sampling to: (1) assess concordance of putative biomarkers within kindreds; (2) assess differences in genotype and/or environmental influences between the various colon cancer-prone kindreds; and (3) obtain maximal information before patient participation may begin to decrease with additional samplings. As reliable genotype markers are elucidated, it should theoretically become possible to accurately determine both the contribution of genetically determined cancer to the total colon cancer burden and the incidence of colon cancer predisposing genotypes in the human population.

REFERENCES

1. Lynch, H.T., Kimberling, W.T.; Albano, W.A.; Lynch, J.F.; Biscone, K.A.; Schuelke, G.S.; Sandberg, A.A.; Lipkin, M.; Deschner, E.E.; Mikol, Y.B.; Elston, R.C.; Bailey-Wilson, J.E.; and Danes B.S.: Hereditary nonpolyposis colorectal cancer: Part I. Clinical description of resource. In preparation.
2. Lynch, H.T.; Schuelke, G.S.; Kimberling, W.J.; Albano, W.A.; Lynch, J.F.; Biscone, K.A.; Lipkin, M.L.; Deschner, E.E.; Mikol, Y.B.; Sandberg, A.A.; Elston, R.C.; Bailey-Wilson, J.F.; and Danes, B.S.: Hereditary nonpolyposis colorectal cancer: Part II. Biomarker studies. In preparation.
3. Sievers, M.L.: Cancer of the digestive system among American Indians. *AZ Med.* **33:**15-20, 1976.
4. Creagan, E.T., and Fraumeni, J.F.: Cancer mortality among American Indians. *JNCI* **49:**959-967, 1972.
5. Elston, R.C., and Stewart J.: A general model for the genetic analysis of pedigree data. *Hum. Hered.* **21:**523-542, 1971.
6. Ott, J.: Estimation of the recombination fraction in human pedigrees: efficient computation of the likelihood for human linkage studies. *Am. J. Hum. Genet.* **26:**588-597, 1974.
7. Morton, N.E.: Sequential tests for the detection of linkage. *Am. J. Hum. Genet.* **7:**277-318, 1955.
8. Sandberg, A.A.: *The Chromosomes in Human Cancer and Leukemia.* New York and Amsterdam: Elsevier, 748p.

5
Clinical Management of Hereditary Colon Cancer

William A. Albano, M.D. and Henry T. Lynch, M.D.

Hereditary colon cancer (HCC) is heterogeneous, encompassing a variety of distinct genetic entities. These entities are conveniently divided into two broad categories: syndromes where cancer is preceded by multiple polyps (polyposis syndromes) and syndromes without a polyp manifestation (nonpolyposis syndromes.)

The physician's responsibility begins with the recognition that HCC syndromes are not uncommon in clinical practice.[1] The suspicion of a potential hereditary syndrome is made on the basis of the modified nuclear family history (see *Modified Nuclear Pedigrees*), which can be easily performed on a patient's initial contact.[2] The elucidation of specific historical findings, that is, the cardinal features of HCC (early onset, multiple primary-cancer excess, vertical transmission, proximal colon cancer predominence, or a history of polyposis) within the modified nuclear family history, provide the nidus for such association. In these situations, consultation with knowledgeable specialists may allow the clinician to institute specific management protocols for already-affected persons and their high-risk, unaffected family members.

MODIFIED NUCLEAR PEDIGREES

A nuclear pedigree encompasses information regarding the proband's parents, siblings, and children. However, because of the young age of most cancer-affected probands, children are rarely old enough for cancer to be manifested, decreasing the efficacy of the nuclear pedigree as a screening test. To circumvent these problems, the modified nuclear pedigree, as we define it, is expanded to include grandparents, aunts and uncles (Fig. 5-1). Such a pedigree is easily compiled by either the attending physician or office personnel on the initial contact. It must be stressed that the key is to ask specific questions and record both pertinent positive and negative medical

99

ONCOLOGY PATIENT FAMILY HISTORY

Patient_____Attending Physician_____ Date_____

CRITERION A

1. Yes   No   2 or more 1st degree related
               persons with cancer among family
               members up to 2nd degree relatives
               other than the patient (If yes
               continue to Criterion B)

2. Yes   No   Clinical suspicion of hereditary
               cancer (If yes, follow up is
               needed)

CRITERION B

1. Yes   No   Vertical transmission

2. Yes   No   Bilaterality or multiple
               primaries

3. Yes   No   Site specific

4. Yes   No   Young age of onset,
               age 45 or younger

If yes to any of the above, extended
follow up is indicated.

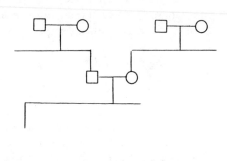

Interviewer_____ Physician Reviewer_____

INSTITUTE FOR FAMILIAL CANCER MANAGEMENT AND CONTROL, INC.
CREIGHTON UNIVERSITY SCHOOL OF MEDICINE
ONCOLOGY PATIENT FAMILY HISTORY

Figure 5-1.   Form used for obtaining the family history from a patient with suspected HCC. Arrow points to the index case *(Reprinted with permission from H.T. Lynch, P.M. Lynch, W.A. Albano, and J.F. Lynch. Hereditary colon cancer: Identifying the high risk person. Consultant 22:334, 1982.)*

data on relatives within the modified nuclear pedigree. Expansion of the nuclear pedigree provides the clinician with sufficient data to make any emergent clinical decisions and determines whether a full genetic consultation is indicated. Negative data including age and cause of noncancer death are essential for such decision making. We have found patient compliance to be excellent, but since recall is frequently poor, a second session is often necessary for completion of the modified nuclear pedigree.

The modified nuclear pedigree should be reviewed by an informed attending physician. Knowledge of the cardinal features of HCC and syndrome identification provide the tools necessary for evaluation. If one or more of the cardinal features are present, suspicion for the existence of a hereditary cancer syndrome is heightened. Families under suspicion should be referred for a detailed genetic consultation.[3] An extended pedigree (a detailed analysis of *all* family members with verification of each cancer) remains the best diagnostic tool available for definitive, HCC syndrome identification and confirmation. As previously stated, this objective is not feasible in most clinical practice settings. Often, such an evaluation is a long-term process of investigation and verification extending over several months. However, the clinician is frequently in a setting where management requires immediate attention. For purposes of medical expediency, a proband demonstrating any of the cardinal features of HCC who has one or more affected relatives in a modified nuclear pedigree should be considered as meeting presumptive criteria for the disease. The patient should be treated as if the syndrome has been confirmed, even though complete genetic evaluation and syndrome identification may still be pending. This might alter surgical management, and such probands, a total abdominal colectomy might be recommended rather than hemicolectomy.

NONPOLYPOSIS COLON CANCER SYNDROMES

The majority of families with HCC syndromes do not exhibit adenomatous polyposis of the colon—a fact not usually appreciated.[4] The major subclassifications of nonpolyposis hereditary cancer include the cancer family syndrome (CFS) and hereditary, site-specific colon cancer (HSSCC). Both CFS and HSSCC families exhibit the criteria listed under cardinal features. The CFS is characterized by carcinoma of the colon and endometrium, though adenocarcinoma of the ovary, stomach, breast, and other sites are seen within specific families. The CFS provides an excellent example of multiple organ susceptibility within a kindred, underscoring the need for indepth inquiry about family incidence of malignancies of *all* anatomic sites.[5] As the name implies, HSSCC *seems* to lack extracolonic manifestations, but in all other respects resembles CFS.

Management issues arise in four relatively distinct clinical settings: management of newly diagnosed cancer patients whose preoperative family history is compatible with a known hereditary cancer syndrome; management of previously, but perhaps incompletely, treated family members (i.e., cases in which the hereditary cancer syndrome diagnosis is not made until after the patient's initial treatment) management of high risk (50%) but unaffected family members; and management of patients in whom classification as hereditary or sporadic cancer cannot be made on the basis of existing information.

Management of Affected-Untreated Patients

When a diagnosis of a colon cancer is made in a member of a known or suspected hereditary colon-cancer-syndrome family, a complete evaluation of the entire colon is mandatory to exclude synchronous lesions (Fig. 5-2). A column barium enema is not adequate for detecting small lesions;[6] to fully evaluate the colon in such patients, an air-contrast barium study or colonoscopy should be performed. The choice of procedure will be determined by local experience, though we prefer colonoscopy when expertise is available. In certain cases, both procedures may be necessary to fully evaluate the entire colon.

The high incidence of subsequent colon cancer in these patients[7] underscores the need for a total abdominal colectomy with ileorectal anastomosis as the standard, initial treatment, rather than the traditional hemicolectomy. A curative, total-abdominal colectomy can be performed with no additional mortality and only a minimal increase in morbidity.[8] Most patients will ultimately have two to three bowel movements daily but will retain excellent continence and stool consistency.[9] An adequate lymphadenectomy should be performed in all areas draining invasive lesions. The amount of colon and rectum preserved should allow for subsequent follow-up with office proctosigmoidoscopy performed biannually for life. Data are insufficient at this time to estimate the frequency of subsequent malignant transformation in the rectum, though it appears to be uncommon enough as to not represent an indication for prophylactic proctectomy. However, this matter remains an area of ongoing investigation. Without question, the scope of surgery should *not* be extended in patients with metastatic or unresectable disease.[8]

The use of adjuvant treatment for advanced, resectable lesions must be approached cautiously, considering the poor efficacy of such treatment in general.[10] On the other hand, the relatively more benign clinical course in

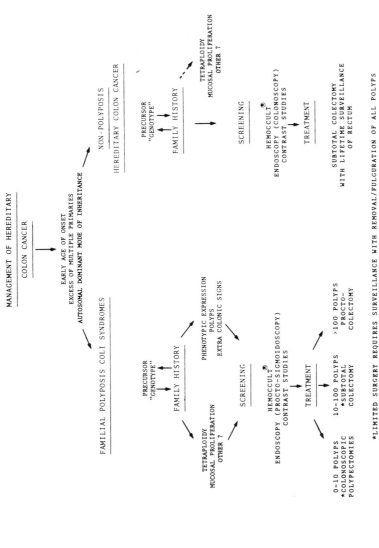

Figure 5-2. Diagram showing management protocol for FPC syndromes and for hereditary nonpolyposis colon cancer.

MANAGEMENT OF HEREDITARY

COLON CANCER

EARLY AGE OF ONSET
EXCESS OF MULTIPLE PRIMARIES
AUTOSOMAL DOMINANT MODE OF INHERITANCE

FAMILIAL POLYPOSIS COLI SYNDROMES

NON-POLYPOSIS

HEREDITARY COLON CANCER

PRECURSOR "GENOTYPE"

FAMILY HISTORY

PHENOTYPIC EXPRESSION
POLYPS
EXTRA COLONIC SIGNS

TETRAPLOIDY
MUCOSAL PROLIFERATION
OTHER ?

SCREENING

HEMOCCULT®
ENDOSCOPY (PROCTO-SIGMOIDOSCOPY)
CONTRAST STUDIES

TREATMENT

0-10 POLYPS
*COLONOSCOPIC
POLYPECTOMIES

10-100 POLYPS
*SUBTOTAL
COLECTOMY

>100 POLYPS
PROCTO-
COLECTOMY

PRECURSOR "GENOTYPE"

FAMILY HISTORY

TETRAPLOIDY
MUCOSAL PROLIFERATION
OTHER ?

SCREENING

HEMOCCULT®
ENDOSCOPY (COLONOSCOPY)
CONTRAST STUDIES

TREATMENT

SUBTOTAL COLECTOMY
WITH LIFETIME SURVEILLANCE
OF RECTUM

*LIMITED SURGERY REQUIRES SURVEILLANCE WITH REMOVAL/FULGURATION OF ALL POLYPS

103

heredofamilial cases may argue for aggressive treatment.[11-13] At present, we do not know whether the observed, improved survival in hereditary cases implies a better response to treatment or a less aggressive tumor.[12-13] Insight into this problem could be attained by redesigning adjuvant-therapy protocols for colorectal cancer. Specifically, patients could be stratified as to presence or absence of a family history of colon cancer, since those with such positive family histories may respond differently than sporadic cases.

In women from CFS families presenting with primary colon cancer, the endometrium assumes major importance.[14] Ideally, patients should be screened preoperatively with a pelvic exam and endometrial sampling to assess the possibility of an asymptomatic endometrial cancer. A variety of techniques for endometrial sampling have been devised, ranging from irrigation and aspiration for cytology, suctioning with devices enabling relatively thin-layer biopsy, and the more traditional dilatation and curettage.[15, 16] In certain families, there may be an additional risk for breast, ovary, gastric, and other neoplasms.[17, 18] If these sites are prominent within a family, specific radiographic studies should be performed even in the absence of historical or physical findings. In female patients with CFS, hysterectomy and bilateral oophorectomy should be performed at the time of initial colon surgery, as long as the patient has completed her family and no medical or psychological contraindications exist. Such a recommendation is based on the frequency of subsequent endometrial cancer.

Oophorectomy is recommended in specific CFS families because of increased risk of primary malignancy, lack of early diagnostic measures, aggressive behavior of the tumors, and the possible occurrence of ovarian metastases from primary colon cancer.[19] The role of hormonal replacement following oophorectomy in these patients presents a difficult problem. Currently, no increase in malignant disease has been reported with replacement hormones following hysterectomy, and the positive effects, including amelioration of surgical menopause symptoms and a decrease in osteoporosis, are well documented.[20] Although no well-documented evidence exists of an increased incidence of breast cancer among castrated patients given estrogens, the issue nevertheless remains controversial. Consequently, we avoid the use of replacement hormones, especially if breast cancer is a known problem within the family. If such agents are to be used, patients should be placed in a breast surveillance program, including monthly breast self-examination, biannual physical examination, and mammography every two years.

Management of Affected–Previously Treated Patients

A frequently encountered clinical situation is the patient who has undergone standard hemicolectomy for colon cancer in the past, with recognition of the hereditary cancer risk occurring later. If the initial tumor has been success-fully treated, a complete evaluation of the remaining colon is the major concern, with subsequent assessment of additional organs at risk. In HSSCC, the remaining colon should be evaluated with colonoscopy or air-contrast barium enema as a baseline. In CFS, colonic evaluation should be supplemented with endometrial sampling. A modest number of patients from registry families who have had colonic cancer in the past have elected to undergo prophylactic removal of the remaining colon with ileorectal anastomosis. However, *surveillance* rather than prophylactic surgery is our primary rec-ommendation in this clinical setting. Contemporary advances in screening and diagnostic technology (i.e., colonic endoscopy and radiographic procedures, as well as the relative ease of endometrial sampling) enable us to support such an option more strongly. This position is bolstered by the observation of improved survival in both categories of nonpolyposis HCC.[11-13] The presence of recurring colonic adenomas or atypical endometrial changes should increase clinical suspicion, thereby making the option of prophylactic sur-gery a viable one. The probability of compliance with aggressive screen-ing as well as the patient's express wishes must also be taken into considera-tion when a specific treatment or surveillance plan is formulated.

In patients with an initial negative screening, reevaluation should include biannual fecal-occult-blood testing, annual colonoscopy, and, in women with CFS, endometrial sampling. Additional organs at risk, based on the family-specific tumor spectrum, should also be evaluated. If subsequent cancer is found, therapy is instituted according to the previously described guidelines.

It is essential that the surgeon and pathologist communicate well in order to provide meticulous sectioning and careful histologic examination of all specimens removed. Even when a complete preoperative evaluation has been performed, occult synchronous lesions have been identified on careful pathological examination.[21]

Management of Unaffected High-Risk Relatives

The clinician, though skilled in caring for the patient with a specific lesion, may lack experience when confronted with a cohort of high-risk family members.[22] When an autosomal-dominant HCC syndrome is identified in a given kindred, the cancer risk approaches 50% in those people in the direct genetic line.

Ideally, family physicians should be provided with a complete pedigree of the subject kindred. This pedigree should indicate the genetic risk for cancer of specific target organs in their individual patients. Physicians should also be provided with a detailed management protocol. Periodic updates are desirable so that all physicians involved in the management of a specific family understand the scope of the problem. Centralized hereditary-cancer registries would facilitate such functions, but unfortunately, such ideal circumstances rarely exist. Thus, our pragmatic emphasis is on the utility of the modified nuclear pedigree.

Counseling should begin in the second decade to cement the patient-physician relationship. All aspects of cancer risk should be fully discussed. Surveillance in the nonpolyposis hereditary syndromes should begin in earnest during the third decade. Of course, without question, any family member who is symptomatic should be competely evaluated, regardless of age. Since most of these colon cancers are proximal in location,[23] standard screening with sigmoidoscopy and rectal exam is inadequate and may give a false sense of security. An initial baseline colonoscopy or air-contrast barium enema should be performed by age 30 and repeated every two to three years thereafter. Fecal-occult-blood determination (guaiac slide test) is an important component of our recommended surveillance program. These studies are performed every six months using the standard technique of a red-meat-free diet and sampling of stools on three consecutive days.[22] Patients with a positive study should be reevaluated by the same technique. The presence of confirmed fecal occult blood mandates a complete colon evaluation, preferably with endoscopy. All polyps or mucosal abnormalities must be sampled, with specific treatment instituted if cancer is detected. In patients with recurrent adenomas, especially if atypia or carcinoma *in situ* is found, the surveillance program should be modified to provide an even more intensive approach. Strong consideration for prophylactic surgery (total abdominal colectomy) should be given in this clinical setting, though the correlation with subsequent cancer is not well delineated. We currently advise any patient from such families with biopsy evidence of dysplasia or carcinoma *in situ* to undergo prophylactic surgery.

Women at high risk (50%) for CFS should undergo biannual pelvic exams with annual endometrial sampling. Care must be taken to correlate such sampling with the menstrual cycle to avoid potential fetal harm in early gravid patients. Patients with possible ovarian masses or those with body conformations precluding accurate bimanual pelvic exam, should undergo pelvic ultrasonography. Computerized tomography has also been increasingly helpful, especially with obese patients. Laparotomy is indicated for the evaluation of any suspected, solid, or persistent ovarian lesion.

Management of Unaffected Family Members when 50% Risk Cannot be Confirmed

The clinician is often confronted with a situation in which hereditary syndrome is suspected but not amenable to verification by pedigree analysis alone. Typical situations are adoption, dubious paternity, early death in a family *not* due to cancer, or technical inability to verify an extended pedigree. An indeterminate risk also applies to members of confirmed nonpolyposis HCC families that are the offspring of direct-line parents who are or were at 50% risk but are either young themselves or died at a young age. Though classically the computed risk of such people would have to be reckoned at 25%, the factors entering into such estimates must be kept in mind, and the clinician must be able to explain their basis to interested patients. Our approach has been to enter all such persons into high-risk protocols for surveillance. Because of the high penetrance of the cancer gene, if parents are unaffected by age 60, risk to offspring is considered to decrease with each subsequent, cancer-free year in the parent.

We are convinced of the urgent need to reassess traditional surveillance-management protocols for nonpolyposis HCC. The approach presented here uses some of the most sophisticated screening and diagnostic modalities in concert with cancer-family-history status. Surveillance of available high-risk kindreds may substantially decrease cancer mortality when specific measures are promptly instituted and followed faithfully. In specific clinical situations where prophylactic surgery is performed, the incidence of cancer may also be decreased. These protocols will undoubtedly be modified if and when the discovery of cancer genotype-specific biomarkers is accomplished.

HEREDITARY POLYPOSIS SYNDROMES

Variability in polyp expression has been demonstrated in FPC kindreds (see Fig. 5-2), somewhat complicating clinical management (see also Chap. 12).[24, 25] Although the colon is the predominant site of malignant transformation, an increased tumor spectrum, including periampullary carcinoma, gastric cancer, sarcoma, thyroid cancer, and brain tumors has been appreciated. In the typical patient, there will be polyp formation by the second decade of life, with cancer development in the third and fourth decades. Consequently, surveillance programs should begin before the age of 20. However, since the polyps are most commonly present in the rectosigmoid, these patients are more amenable to screening than their counterparts with nonpolyposis syndromes.

Screening Nonpolyp-Affected, High-Risk Family Members

Because of the early onset of polyps, screening must be instituted at a young age. Proctosigmoidoscopy is difficult in young children and should be reserved for symptomatic persons but by age 15, it should be performed biannually in all high-risk patients, with or without symptoms. However, screening with stool guaiac studies can easily be introduced by age 10 and performed routinely three times a year. A full evaluation is indicated if fecal occult blood is documented. A baseline colonoscopy or air-contrast barium enema is performed at age 20 and repeated at three-year intervals and when indicated by clinical findings. The presence of multiple adenomatous polyps should place the person in the "syndrome-affected" category. All family members should be well informed as to their potential for harboring the polyposis gene.

Polyposis-Affected Family Members

Due to the observed variability of polyp presentation within kindreds, a patient should be presumed to have the syndrome even if only one to ten polyps are found. However, because of age dependency, it may be clinically impossible to differentiate sporadic polyp formation from limited phenotypic expression of the polyposis syndrome. In such situations, individual acceptance of prophylactic surgery may be less acceptable than in patients with a florid polyposis presentation, though cancer risk may be similar. Surgical options include polypectomies, subtotal colectomy with repeated rectal-polyp fulguration, proctocolectomy, or the use of sophisticated sphincter-saving procedures that involve removal of the rectal mucosa with an ileal pull-through and anastomosis to the anus.[26] All treatment regimens have in common the prevention of subsequent cancer. Patient compliance with potentially lifelong surveillance programs, if any rectal or colonic mucosa is positive, may be paramount to decision-making as is physician expertise within the community. At this time, with the exception of ulcerative colitis, no colon cancer has been identified as arising in flat mucosae. Based on the guidelines discussed, we follow the strategy outline next.

Patients with 1 to 10 Polyps.   If fewer than 10 adenomas are encountered, endoscopic removal of *all* polyps may be the treatment of choice. This approach mandates biannual colonoscopic evaluations. If atypia is noted or technical difficulties preclude total excision of all polyps, resection should be considered. This alteration of approach is also indicated if the rate of polyp formation increases or patient compliance wanes. Surgical approaches in such clinical settings would involve total abdominal colectomy with preservation of the rectum and repeated office proctosigmoidoscopy wuth fulguration of rectal polyps.

Patients with 10 to 100 Polyps.   Patients with 10 to 100 polyps *must* be considered for resection. If the rectum is not extensively involved (less than ten polyps), total abdominal colectomy with ileorectal anastomosis (IRA) is advocated with subsequent office proctosigmoidoscopy. More intensive involvement of the rectum necessitates a more aggressive approach. In younger patients who are more compliant, this approach might include deferring the second, third, and fourth decades. Alternatively, standard combined resection has been the usual treatment. We have been impressed with the recent results of sphincter-preserving procedures in that they remove all at-risk colon–rectal mucosae but preserve fecal continency and avoid colostomy.[24, 25] Such procedures are not in widespread use but should no longer be considered experimental surgery.

Patients with More than 100 Polyps.   In patients with more than 100 polyps preservation of an intact rectum is impossible if the cancer risk is to be eliminated. Again, standard combined resection is the traditional treatment, but sphincter-preserving procedures should be given increased attention.

The increasing tumor spectrum observed within the polyposis syndromes mandates follow-up even when all colorectal mucosae have been removed. However, with the exception of continued fecal-occult-blood testing, no specific screening program can be recommended for asymptomatic patients. The physicians expertise and knowledge of the tumor spectrum provides the best assurance for good patient follow-up.

REFERENCES

1. Lynch, H.T.; Lynch, P.M.; and Harris, R.E.: Minimal genetic findings and their cancer control implications. *JAMA* **240:**535-538, 1978.
2. Lynch, H.T.; Follett, K.L.; Lynch, P.M.; Albano, W.A.; Mailliard, J.A.; and Pierson, R.L.: Family history in an oncology clinic: Implications concerning cancer genetics. *JAMA* **242:**1268-1272, 1979.
3. Lynch, H.T.; Lynch, P.M.; and Lynch, J.F.: Genetic counselling and cancer. In: *Genetic Counselling: Psychological Dimensions* Kessler, S., (ed). New York, NY: Academic Press, 1979, pp. 221-241.
4. Lovett, E.: Family studies in cancer of the colon and rectum. *Br. J. Surg.* **63:**13-18, 1976.
5. Lynch, H.T.; Lynch, P.M.; Albano, W.A.; Edney, J.; Organ, C.H.; and Lynch, J.: Hereditary cancer: ascertainment and management. *Cancer* **29:**216-232, 1979.
6. Wehin, S.: Results of Malmo technique of colon exam. *JAMA* **199:**119, 1967.
7. Lynch, H.T.; Harris, R.E.; Organ, Claude, Jr.; Guirgis, H.A.; Lynch, P.M.; Lynch, J.F.; and Nelson, E.J.: The surgeon, genetics and cancer control: The cancer family syndrome. *Ann. Surg.* **185:**435-440, 1977.
8. James, A.G.: *Cancer Prognosis Manual.* New York, NY: American Cancer Society, 1970, 82p.
9. Falterman, K.W.; Hill, C.B.; Markey, J.C.; Fox, J.W.; and Cohn, I.: Cancer of the colon, rectum, and anus: A review of 2313 cases. *Cancer* **34:**951, 1974.

10. Bedikiaun, A.Y.; Bodey, G.P.; Valdivieso, M.; Stroehlein, J.R.; and Karlin, D.A.: Chemotherapeutic management of colorectal cancer and prospects for new agents. In: *Gastrointestinal Cancer* (Stroehlein, J.R., and Romsdahl, M.M., eds.). New York, NY: Raven Press, 1981, pp. 365-380.

11. Lynch, H.T.; Bardawil, W.A.; Harris, R.E.; Lynch, P.M.; Guirgis, H.A.; and Lynch, J.F.: Multiple primary cancers and prolonged survival: familial colonic and endometrial cancers. *Dis. Colon Rect.* **21:**165-168, 1978.

12. Lynch, H.T.; Albano, W.A.; Recabaren, J.A.; Lynch, P.M.; Lynch, J.F.; and Elston, R.C.: Prolonged survival as a component of hereditary breast and nonpolyposis colon cancer. *Med. Hypotheses* **7:**1201-1209, 1981.

13. Albano, W.A.; Recabaren, J.A.; Lynch, H.T.; Campbell, A.S.; Mailliard, J.A.; Organ, C.H.; Lynch, J.F.; and Kimberling, W.J.: Natural history of hereditary cancer of the breast and colon. *Cancer* **50:**360-363, 1982.

14. Lynch, H.T.; Krush, A.J.; Larsen, A.L.; and Magnuson, C.W.: Endometrial carcinoma: Multiple primary malignancies, constitutional factors, and heredity. *Am. J. Med. Sci.* **252:**281-290, 1966.

15. Reagan, J.W., and Ng, A.B.P.: *The Cells of Uterine Adenocarcinoma,* 2nd ed. New York, NY: Karger, 1973.

16. Ng, A.B.P.: Diagnostic cytopatholoqy. In: *Gynecologic Oncology* Coppleson, M., ed. New York, NY: Churchill-Livingstone, 1981, pp. 187-204.

17. Lynch, H.T., and Lynch, P.M.: Tumor variation in the cancer family syndrome: Ovarian cancer. *Am. J. Surg.* **138:**439-442, 1979.

18. Lynch, H.T.; Harris, R.E.; Lynch, P.M.; Guirgis, H.A.; and Lynch, J.F.: The role of heredity in multiple primary cancer. *Cancer* **40:**1849-1854, 1977.

19. Stearns, M.W.J., and Deddish, M.R.: Five year results of abdomino pelvic lymph node dissection for carcinoma of the rectum. *Dis. Colon Rect.* **2:**169-172, 1959.

20. Byrd, B.F., and Vaugn, W.K.: What happens after 15 years of estrogen replacement therapy — a report of 402 patients (Paper delivered at the Society for Surgical Oncology, San Diego, CA, 1978).

21. Ruma, T.A.; Lynch, H.T.; Albano, W.A.; and Sterioff, S.: Total colectomy and the cancer family syndrome: A case report. *Dis. Colon Rect.* **25:**582-585, 1982.

22. Lynch, H.T.; Lynch, P.M.; Albano, W.A.; and Lynch, J.F. Hereditary colon cancer: Identifying the high risk person. *Consultant* **22:**331-343, 1982.

23. Lynch, P.M.; Lynch, H.T.; and Harris, R.E.: Hereditary proximal colon cancer. *Dis. Colon Rect.* **20:**661-668, 1977.

24. Lynch, H.T.; Lynch, P.M.; Follett, K.L.; and Harris, R.E.: Familial polyposis coli: Heterogeneous polyp expression in 2 kindreds. *J. Med. Genet.* **6:**17, 1979.

25. Heimann, T.; Beck, R.; and Greenstein, A.J.: Familial polyposis coli: Management by total colectomy with preservation of continence. *Arch. Surg.* **113:**1104-1106, 1978.

26. Wolfstein, I.H.; Dreznik, Z.J.; and Avigad, I.S.: Total colectomy and anal ileostomy in multiple polyposis coli. *Arch. Surg.* **113:**1101-1103, 1978.

6
Epithelial-Cell Kinetics in Colorectal Mucosa of Patients at High Risk for Colon Cancer

Eleanor E. Deschner, Ph.D.

The proliferation of epithelial cells in the colorectal mucosa of patients believed to be at increased risk of heritable colon cancer (HCC) is thought to contain some clues that would characterize the future development of a tumor.[1, 2] Recognition of a common alteration in the pattern of cell renewal in cancer-prone patients could provide a useful device in the selection of high-risk colon cancer candidates.

The data based on that assumption and derived from cell kinetic studies of human colorectal mucosa form the backbone of this chapter. However, this information has also been augmented and confirmed with studies of animal models for colon cancer. These studies have been influenced by the recognition of the action of cycasin and its byproducts, 1,2-dimethylhydrazine (DMH) and methylazoxymethanol (MAM), which appear to be organotropic for the induction of intestinal neoplasia.[3] However, other known carcinogens have also been adapted for this purpose by direct installation intrarectally, as in the case of N-methyl-N-nitrosourea (MNU) and N-methyl-N-nitro-N-nitrosoguanidine (MNNG). Synthesis of data from all these sources reinforces the concept that colon cancer induction and development follows a similar or parallel course in both humans and animals.

METHODOLOGY

Initially, cell proliferation studies in humans were carried out on sequential biopsies obtained from patients with limited life expectancies who were injected with labeled deoxyribonucleic acid (DNA) precursors, such as tritiated thymidine (^{3}HTdR). Because of the difficult nature of this type of protocol and the severe limitations of the technique, data derived from such studies have not accumulated rapidly. However, a technique of *in vitro* propagation has emerged that allows ^{3}HTdR and other radioactive compounds to be incorporated into epithelial cells so that alterations in the pattern of DNA, ribonucleic acid (RNA), and protein synthesis can be followed over time.

This *in vitro* technique requires the fragmentation of a biopsy into units of approximately 1 mm. The tissue fragments are incubated at 37°C in nutrient medium, namely Eagle's basic salt solution, to which 10% fetal calf serum and ³HTdR have been added. Each tissue fragment encompasses five to seven crypts, which allows proper diffusion of ³HTdR into all portions of the tissue when 95% O_2 and 5% CO_2 is bubbled into the media. This last procedure provides the necessary oxygen required for ³HTdR to become incorporated into the new DNA being formed in every S-phase cell.

After an hour, specimens are fixed in neutral, buffered formalin, dehydrated, embedded in paraffin, and then sectioned at 3 microns. Following removal of the paraffin and rehydration, slides are dipped in NTB_2 emulsion (manufactured by Kodak) and placed in light tight boxes at 4°C for a suitable exposure time. The slides are developed in D19 (by Kodak) and stained with hematoxylin and eosin.

Lavage samples from the large bowel can also be studied if the cellular material is collected in normal saline; then cells are spun down before being introduced into the nutrient isotope mixture. After an hour of incubation they are respun, decanted, fixed in Mucolexx, and paraffin blocks are prepared. From this point on, the slides are handled in the same way as the biopsy specimens.

To accumulate data, slides of biopsy material are examined microscopically and all longitudinally sectioned crypts are counted for several parameters. These parameters include the number and position of ³HTdR-labeled cells, the total number of epithelial cells per crypt column (one-half a crypt), and the number and position of mitotic figures. When a nucleus has four or more grains over it, the cell is included among the labeled cell population. To avoid the inclusion of the same cells in the compiled data, at least five sections are skipped between scored material.

Lavage material is analyzed to determine the presence of ³HTdR incorporation among the well-differentiated, columnar, epithelial cell population sloughed from the luminal surface of the colonic mucosa. When the lavage technique is effectively carried out, the sample will contain cells derived from both the right and left sides of the colon, thus providing a very representative sample of the entire organ.

NORMAL COLONIC EPITHELIAL CELL KINETICS

The crypts of Lieberkühn, which are lined with epithelial cells, are the basic glandular structure of the colon and rectum. Cells at the base of the crypt

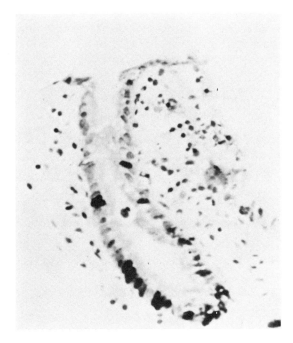

Figure 6-1.   Microautoradiograph of a single, normal, colorectal crypt with ³HTdR-labeled cells in lower two-thirds of the gland. (× 250)

are histologically more immature than those lining the upper luminal portion of the gland. Cells synthesizing DNA have been found to occupy the lower 65% of the crypt, a position similar to that seen in other animal species (Fig. 6-1). The lower two-thirds of these glands is also the region where mitotic figures appear; therefore, the presence of ³HTdR-labeled cells in this area merely confirmed this as the site of cell proliferation from which cells migrated to the surface.

When a labeled precursor was injected into patients with limited life expectancy, the percentage of epithelial cells involved in DNA synthesis in colorectal crypts, that is, the labeling index (LI) was determined to be approximately 15 to 25% of the total population of cells. Studies using the *in vitro* technique have shown LI values ranging from 3.4% to 15.4%.[4] The duration of S phase was also found to be shorter when estimated from *in vitro* data (7.2-8.9hr)[5] rather than by direct measurement of *in vivo* data (9-20hr).[6,7] The average turnover time for this tissue ranged from 3 to 4 days[6] to 6 to 8 days.[8]

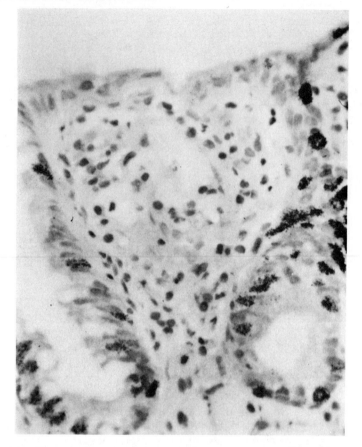

Figure 6-2.   Two colonic crypts demonstrating extension of the ^{3}**HTdR-labeled cells to the upper third and along the surface of the gland.** ($\times$ 540)

EARLY PROLIFERATIVE CHANGES

Expansion of the Proliferative Compartment (Stage I Abnormality)

The earliest microscopic hint that the flat, normal-appearing mucosa expresses an altered pattern of cell proliferation in certain colorectal crypts was reported in 1963, when two separate groups described the presence of ^{3}HTdR-labeled, epithelial, DNA-synthesizing cells in the upper third and along the luminal surface of glands (Fig. 6-2). One group reported data obtained from *in vivo*-labeled specimens of a patient with familial polyposis,[9] while the other group had carried out *in vitro* pulse labeling of tissue from a patient with multiple polyposis.[10] While the observation of DNA-synthesizing

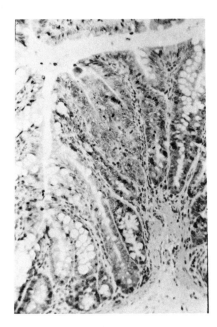

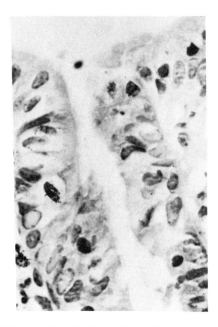

Figure 6-3. Portion of colorectal crypt of DMH-treated mouse showing labeled epithelial cells along the upper third and luminal surface. ($\times$ 665)

Figure 6-4. Section of the distal colon of mouse 6 weeks after initiation of weekly subcutaneous injections of DMH (20 mg/kg body weight). An area of focal atypism is seen involving two crypts. ($\times$ 70)

cells at the surface and upper third of crypts was first made in patients with multiple or familial polyposis, the finding was later reported in patients with single, isolated adenomatous polyps,[11] in relatives of familial polyposis patients,[12, 13] and occasionally in patients in the general population with no history of gastrointestinal disease.[12] The latter finding may be compatible with the percentage of people over age 45 in whom polyps are found.[14] This expanded proliferation compartment was thought to be the earliest sign of the possible future development of a neoplasm.

This observation was later found to have a direct counterpart in the DMH animal model and added credence to its possible significance.[15-17] When the colon carcinogen DMH was injected subcutaneously into CF_1 mice on a weekly schedule at a dose level of 20 mg/kg body weight, one of the first changes noted in colonic, epithelial cell renewal was an extension of the proliferative compartment to the surface (Fig. 6-3). This change was accompanied by the appearance of areas of focal atypism, which were seen as early as 3 weeks after the initiation of DMH treatment (Fig. 6-4).

Normal, well-differentiated surface epithelial cells engaged in DNA synthesis could also be demonstrated at this time by a simple lavage procedure. Using a fine catheter, normal saline was introduced into the rectum of the DMH-treated mice, and exfoliated cells were retrieved under negative pressure.[18] After incubation with [3]HTdR, in addition to unlabeled, normal-appearing epithelial cells, the presence of well-differentiated labeled cells indicated an alteration in some cells' ability to terminate or repress DNA synthesis in the upper region of colonic crypts. Unlike aging humans, (i.e., over 45) aging rodents have never evidenced labeled cells at the surface or upper third of colonic crypts.

The merits of saline lavage have been known for many years.[19] The technique has recently been improved and is now employed on a regular basis in high-risk patients when early diagnosis of colonic neoplasia is important.[20] The role normally filled by exfoliative cytology has been expanded decidedly by combining it with the isotopic labeling technique. The existence of DNA synthesis in mature, well-differentiated exfoliated cells was first successfully demonstrated in asymptomatic members of two familial polyposis families[21] as well as one asymptomatic sibling of a patient with multiple polyps.[22] Labeled cells at the surface and upper third of crypts were shown in biopsies from each of these cases, indicating a strong correlation between procedures. Thereafter, labeled colonic lavage samples as well as biopsies were employed in evaluation of persons at high risk. The lavage technique may well prove to be extremely important, since the sampling of exfoliated cells is from a wider area than that provided by a single or multiple biopsy.

These preliminary findings have been expanded extensively within the high-risk categories previously mentioned, with the addition of several groups of Hemoccult-positive patients.[23] These are patients over age 45 who showed blood in the feces on one or more of the six slides tested over a 3-day period while on a meat-free diet. Radiological and colonoscopic examination revealed the Hemoccult-positive groups to include patients with one or more adenomatous polyps, adenocarcinoma, diverticulosis, and diverticular disease and polyps, as well as those with no overt disease or lesion. A significant number of the patients in these groups demonstrated this abnormal zone of DNA synthesis or expansion of the proliferative zone. Patients with adenomatous polyps or cancer showed a higher frequency of the pheomenon than other groups, although some symptom-free relatives of familial polyposis patients exhibited equally high frequencies.[12]

This aberrant zone of DNA synthesis does not occur in all crypts of a biopsy of the large intestine. Indeed, multiple samples from the same patient have revealed this phenomenon to be an extremely patchy one. Such a finding is most reasonable in light of the sporadic development of neoplasia along the length of the large intestine[23] and also confirms findings reported previously among the familial polyposis population studied.[12]

Altered Distribution of DNA-Synthesizing Cells (Stage II Abnormality)

Labeled cells in the upper third and along the luminal surfaces of colorectal crypts were found to occur in 60 to 90% of biopsies from high-risk groups. In other words, biopsies from patients in these groups demonstrated normal incorporation in the lower two-thirds of crypts at a frequency of approximately 10 to 40%.

A more discriminating kinetic parameter was needed to pinpoint later events in the neoplastic sequence, and such an observation was reported by Maskens and Deschner.[4] The proliferation patterns of epithelial cells of normal-appearing colorectal mucosa from cancer patients was compared with patients with no large bowel disease. A higher mean-labeling index was demonstrated in the cancer group than in the control group (11.9 vs. 7.7%), but because of wide individual variations, this difference was not significant. However, an alteration in the distribution of labeled epithelial cells was seen. A highly significant upward shift of the proliferative compartment was observed in the cancer group, resulting in a specific modification of the ^{3}HTdR-labeling pattern. One such cancer patient is depicted in Figure 6-5. DNA synthesis predominated in the middle or middle and upper thirds of the crypts rather than in the lower third, as observed in controls. A shift in the major zone of DNA synthesis to the middle third may also have occurred in the crypt on the right in Figure 6-2.

This patchy alteration of epithelial-cell renewal within colonic crypts has also been seen in DMH-treated mice after approximately 4 to 6 weekly subcutaneous injections of carcinogen.[17] In this animal model, when the acute effects of the DMH are followed, replacement of lethally damaged cells 2 to 4 days after initial injection of DMH involved DNA synthesis in an increased number of epithelial cells in the mid portion of colonic crypts with some activity of cells in the upper crypt. By the 7th day a normal distribution of cells was again present. However, following a fourth, fifth, and sixth injection of DMH, this shift of the major portions of the proliferative compartments to the mid and upper portions of the crypts was still in evidence a week later (Fig. 6-6). This would indicate the existence of a more permanent defect in the regulatory control of cell proliferation at a time when focal areas of atypism were increasing in number (Fig. 6-4).[16]

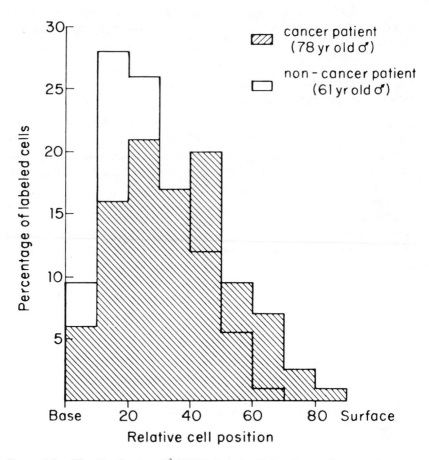

Figure 6-5. The distribution of ³HTdR-labeled cells in colorectal crypts of a cancer patient and a control patient. A shift in the major zone of DNA synthesis upward toward the surface is found in the cancer patient. *(From E. E. Deschner. Cell proliferation as a biological marker in human colorectal neoplasia. In: Colorectal Cancer: Prevention, Epidemiology, and Screening. (S. Winawer, D. Schottenfeld, and P. Sherlock, eds.). Raven Press, New York, 1980. Copyright © 1980 by Raven Press.)*

Elevated Crypt Labeling Indices (Stage III Abnormality)

A later stage in the evolution of the mucosa toward neoplasia was recognized when the behavior of individual crypts was examined in patients with no gastrointestinal disease, patients with a history of colon cancer, and patients with a previous isolated adenoma.

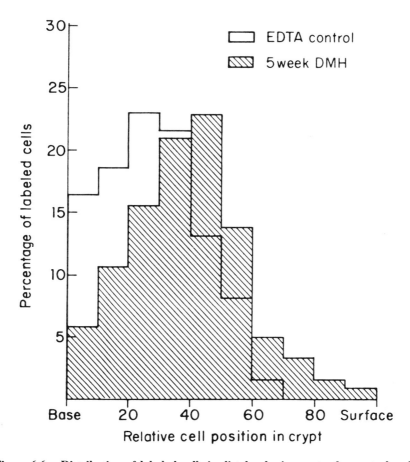

Figure 6-6. Distribution of labeled cells in distal colonic crypts of a control and a mouse treated with five weekly subcutaneous injections of DMH. An upward shift of the major zone of proliferation is seen compared with the distribution in the control mouse. *(From E. E. Deschner. Cell proliferation as a biological marker in human colorectal neoplasia. In: Colorectal Cancer: Prevention, Epidemiology, and Screening. (S. Winawer, D. Schottenfeld, and P. Sherlock, eds.). Raven Press, New York, 1980. Copyright © 1980 by Raven Press.)*

One control patient out of 13 had glands with an LI over 15% whereas 17 out of 26 patients with colorectal tumors were characterized by this high level of epithelial cell proliferation ($p < 0.05$).[24] When the distribution of labeled cells in these crypts with an LI of 15% was compared with those having an LI of 6-8%, it was seen that both catagories of glands showed extension of the proliferative compartment (Stage I abnormality) and a shift of the major zone of DNA synthesis (Stage II abnormality). However, both defects were expressed to a greater degree in crypts with extremely elevated LIs. Among the cancer patients, for example, crypts with a 6-8% LI had 6.3% of the labeled cells in the upper third while crypts with an LI greater than 15% had 12.4% of them in this region. Similarly, 49.1% of labeled cells occupied the lower third of crypts with a 6-8% LI but only 42.8% of them were present in crypts with an LI greater than 15%, indicating a greater shift of S phase cells to the middle and upper third of hyperactive glands (Stage II abnormality).

Mice treated with DMH demonstrated distal colonic crypts with LIs of 21-38%, values above that of control mice. Examination of the distribution of labeled cells revealed a greater number of labeled cells in the upper third of crypts with a high LI as well as a reduced number of S phase cells in the lower third of hyperactive glands. Thus increased replication within crypts appears to emphasize their existing proliferative defects.

The presence of the Stage I and Stage II abnormalities in crypts with both a low and high LI suggests that increased proliferative activity is a later stage in the neoplastic potential of the mucosa. Moreover, these observations would highlight the importance of individual glands and would signify the earlier involvement of hyperactive crypts in neoplastic transformation.

Microscopic Adenoma Formation

Perhaps one further piece of information derived from the simultaneous analysis of a biopsy and lavage specimen should be mentioned. An exfoliated-cell sample from a proctoscopically normal-appearing colon may, on examination, contain fragments of an adenoma or adenocarcinoma (Fig. 6-7). Such was the case in the lavage sample from a symptom-free relative of a patient with familial polyposis. A fragment of an adenoma was retrieved from an area beyond the field of the proctoscope helping to clarify the patient's involvement with the disease.

The occasional recognition of clumps of abnormal-appearing epithelial cells in the cytology specimen, foci of atypism in the biopsy, or both, occurred with a frequency of 10 to 15% among the high-risk groups surveyed.[23] This figure may not be surprising in the light of reports on the incidence of synchronous and metachronous lesions of the colon. Kirsner et al.[25] as well as Brahme et al.[26] have shown that patients with a history of an isolated polyp have a 21 to 41% greater likelihood of a future excrescence than the general population. However, this value may be reduced in the future with the increasing use of the flexible colonoscope. The incidence of synchronous polyps has been found to be markedly elevated in Hemoccult-positive patients given a complete colonoscopic examination (Winawer, personal communi-

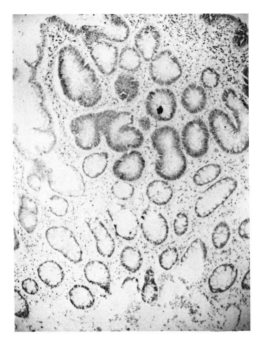

Figure 6-7.   A fragment from a lavage specimen obtained from an asymptomatic member of a familial polyposis family. A focus of adenomatous epithelium occupies the upper portion of the mucosa. ($\times$ 73)

cation). As a corollary, one might predict the frequency of metachronous polyps in these patients on follow-up examinations to be far lower than the values previously reported.

COMMON DEVELOPMENTAL PATTERNS

Further reinforcement of these observations to prove a common evolution in the breakdown or disruption of regulatory control of cell proliferation have been obtained by the study of specimens of ulcerativer-colitic colons. This inflammatory bowel disease, marked by continued ulceration and regeneration of the mucosa, has serious consequences including a higher risk for colon cancer. Foci adenomatous epithelium and adenomatous polyps have been reported.[27, 28] The presence of adenomatous epithelium in this disease state is viewed as an early stage in the progression to cancer and acts as the connecting or unifying link among diseases of the large bowel that demonstrate a high risk for cancer.

Rectal biopsies from patients with ulcerative colitis have shown faster migrations of labeled epithelial cells to the luminal surface as well as a two-fold increase in the number of cells involved in DNA synthesis.[29, 30] A proliferative compartment extended toward the surface was another abnormality reported by these investigators.

Information on the distribution of labeled cells in colonic crypts in a patient with longstanding ulcerative colitis has recently been developed.[31] Of ten progressively spaced biopsies taken in a proximal-to-distal fashion along the length of a colectomy specimen, two biopsies demonstrated marked shifting in the proliferative compartment with predominant DNA synthesis in the middle and upper third of crypts as well as marked elevation of the LI. An invasive adenocarcinoma was found in the region of one of these biopsies and an area of severe dysplasia was located near the other.

Theoretical Progression Leading to Colon Cancer

In the light of the more recent studies of flat, normal-appearing mucosa, an increased frequency of DNA synthesis in colonic crypts may be looked on as a further step in the evolution of the mucosa toward the formation of a neoplasm. How, then, do we view the overall progression of a colorectal mucosa towards colon cancer as it is presumed to occur in human and mouse models?

Table 6-1 presents a schematic outline of the possible sequence of kinetic events leading to colon cancer as deduced from our knowledge at the present time. What brings about the progression from one stage to the next is unknown, although genetic inheritance undoubtedly plays a significant role

Table 6-1. Theory of Progressive Histologic and Kinetic Events Leading to Colon Cancer

NORMAL-APPEARING COLONIC CRYPTS

Cell proliferation in lower $^2/_3$ with lower $^1/_3$ major zone of DNA synthesis

Stage 1: Expanded proliferative compartment to surface with lower $^1/_3$ major zone of DNA synthesis

Stage 2: Shift in major distribution of S-phase cells to middle and upper zones

Stage 3: Increased L.I. in individual crypts

NEOPLASIA

Stage 4: Adenomatous epithelium arising in crypts (neoplastic transformation)

Stage 5: Adenomatous polyp (exophytic growth)

Stage 6: *In situ* cancer within polyp

Stage 7: Invasive cancer

as do environmental factors. A number of environmental factors have been suggested as important in the etiology of colon cancer. These would include gut bacterial flora, diet, and bile acids.[32] All of these factors are interrelated — the number and type of bacterial organisms depends on the diet, and the concentration of bile acids depends on the amount of dietary fat. Bacteria have been postulated to produce carcinogens or cocarcinogens from fats, bile acids, and neutral steroids within the gut. Feces of normal persons have been found to contain mutagens active in the Ames salmonella test system, although these mutagens were more frequently observed in patients with colonic cancer.[33] Demonstration of the endogenous synthesis of nitrites and nitrates in human intestine suggests that formation of reputedly carcinogenic N-nitroso compounds may be an additional contributing factor in the induction of cancer.[34]

Bile acids or their bacterial metabolites have themselves the capacity to act as colon-tumor promotors when intrarectally instilled in animals treated with carcinogens[35] or when administered as a dietary supplement.[36] Cholic-acid fed rats showed enhanced colonic-epithelial-cell proliferation over control values.[37] In carcinogen-treated animals, this heightened cell proliferation allowed the progression of malignancy to occur earlier and with greater frequency.

The progression of neoplasia from benign to malignant colon cancer has not only been shown to occur by means of a polyp-to-cancer sequence as seen in the DMH model mentioned previously in mice,[18] but it has also been induced in BDIX rats without the previous formation of an excrescence.[38] The carcinogen effectively elicited the formation of small foci of dysplasia that eventually invaded the muscularis mucosa. Adhering to the thesis that colon cancer in humans closely parallels its development in animals, the concept of the cancer's dual site of origin must be considered.

The absence of DNA synthesis in the upper third and along the surface of crypts (Stage 1), even in people of advanced years, is well documented. This is the natural and normal state of colorectal mucosa. A mild deviation from this pattern appears to be visible within a large spectrum of the population, that is, a cell or cells capable of DNA synthesis escape and migrate to the upper third and along the luminal surface of normal-appearing crypts (Stage 1). The frequency of DNA-synthesizing cells in this aberrant zone of DNA synthesis can rise and coexist with a redistributed population of proliferative cells (Stage 2). This shifting of the major zone of S-phase cells from the lower third to the middle and upper third can be followed by a markedly elevated level of DNA synthesis within individual crypts (Stage III abnormality). This proliferative hyperactivity may lead to eventual transformation of cells into foci of adenomatous epithelium as well as the budding of new crypts from the middle and upper region (Stage 4) (Figs. 6-7 and 6-8).

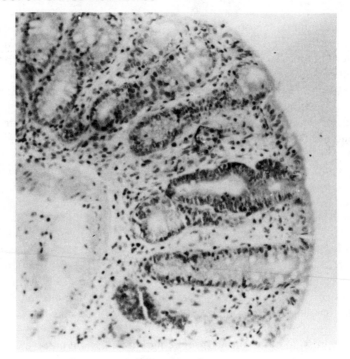

Figure 6-8. Segment of mouse colon treated with DMH. After three injections, a crypt with cellular atypia and formation of new glands from middle and upper third. (× 100)

The continued formation of adenomatous glands in the middle and upper portions of the colonic mucosa results in an upward expansion and creation of a polyp or an adenomatous excrescence (Stage 5, exophytic growth).[39] Continued proliferation and transformation of cells within the polyp may cause a severely dysplastic tissue to arise, and an *in situ* carcinoma may be formed within the excrescence (Stage 6). Eventually this tumor may become invasive (Stage 7).

Alternatively, it is also possible that a malignancy may arise *de novo* intramucosally. Obviously, this sequence carries the more serious consequences since current endoscopic and radiologic techniques may be insufficient to pick up changes within this mucosa. Unless parameters other than endoscopic and radiological can be devised, only the emergence of an excrescence can offer a good opportunity for early detection of potential cancer. Hopefully, the field of cell kinetics can provide the type of marker that will be sufficiently sensitive to select not only persons already affected but also those at high risk for future tumorigenesis.

Acknowledgements.   The author is grateful to Florence C. Long for her many helpful contributions.

REFERENCES

1. Lynch, P.M.; Lynch, H.T.; and Harris, R.E.: Hereditary proximal colonic cancer, *Dis. Colon Rect.* **20:**661-668, 1977.
2. Winawer, S.J.; Sherlock, P.; Schottenfeld, D.; and Miller, D.G.: Screening for colon cancer. *Gastroenterology* **70:**783-789, 1976.
3. Druckrey, H.: Production of colonic carcinomas by 1,2-dialkylhydrazines and azoxyalkanes. In: *Carcinoma of the Colon and Antecedent Epithelium* (Burdette, W.J., ed. Springfield, ILL: C.C. Thomas, 1970, pp. 267-279.
4. Maskens, A.P., and Deschner, E.E.: Tritiated thymidine incorporation into epithelial cells of normal-appearing colorectal mucosa of cancer patients. *JNCI* **58:**1221-1224, 1977.
5. Galand, P.; Mainguet, P.; Arguello, M.; Chretien, J.; and Douxfils, N.: *In vitro* autoradiographic studies of cell proliferation in the gastrointestinal tract of man. *J. Nuclear Med.* **9:**37-39, 1968.
6. Lipkin, M.; Bell, B.; and Sherlock, P.: Cell proliferation kinetics in the gastrointestinal tract of man. I. Cell renewal in colon and rectum. *J. Clin. Invest.* **42:**767-776, 1963.
7. Lipkin, M.; Sherlock, P.; and Bell, B.: Cell proliferation kinetics in the gastrointestinal tract of man. II. Cell renewal in colon and rectum. *Gastroenterology* **45:**721-729, 1963.
8. Cole, J.W., and McKalen, A.: Observations of cell renewal in human rectal mucosa *in vivo* with thymidine-H^3. *Gastroenterology* **41:**122-125, 1961.
9. Cole, J.W., and McKalen, A.: Studies on the morphogenesis of adenomatous polyps in the human colon. *Cancer* **16:**998-1002, 1963.
10. Deschner, E.E.; Lewis, C.M.; and Lipkin, M.: *In vitro* study of human epithelial cells. I. Atypical zone of H^3-thymidine incorporation in mucosa of multiple polyposis. *J. Clin. Invest.* **42:**1922-1928, 1963.
11. Deschner, E.E.; Lipkin, M.; and Solomon, C.: *In vitro* study of human epithelial cells. II. H^3-thymidine incorporation into polyps and adjacent mucosa. *JNCI* **36:**849-857, 1966.
12. Deschner, E.E., and Lipkin, M.: Proliferative patterns in colonic mucosa in familial polyposis. *Cancer* **35:**413-418, 1975.
13. Bleiberg, H.; Mainguet, P.; and Galand, P.: Cell renewal in familial polyposis. Comparison between polyps and adjacent healthy mucosa. *Gastroenterology* **58:**851-855, 1970.
14. Enquist, I.F.: The incidence and significance of polyps of the colon and rectum. *Surgery* **42:**681-688, 1957.
15. Thurnherr, N.; Deschner, E.E.; Stonehill, E.H.; and Lipkin, M.: Induction of adenocarcinomas of the colon in mice by weekly injection of 1, 2-dimethylhydrazine. *Cancer Res.* **33:**940-945, 1973.

16. Deschner, E.E.: Experimentally induced cancer of the colon. *Cancer* **34:**824-828, 1974.

17. Deschner, E.E.: Early proliferative defects induced by six weekly injections of 1,2-dimethylhydrazine in epithelial cells of mouse distal colon. *Z. Krebsforschung* **91:**205-216, 1978.

18. Deschner, E.E.; Winawer, S.J.; Long, F.C.; and Boyle, C.C.: ³H-thymidine labeled colonic epithelial cells and mucosa in mice and men. *Am. J. Dig. Dis.* **23:**305-311, 1978.

19. Wisseman, C.L.; Lemon, H.M.; Laurence, L.B.: Cytologic diagnosis of cancer of the descending colon and rectum. *Surg. Gynecol. Obstet.* **89:**24-30, 1949.

20. Katz, S.; Sherlock, P.; and Winawer, S.J.: Rectocolonic exfoliative cytology. *Am. J. Dig. Dis.* **17:**1109-1116, 1972.

21. Deschner, E.E.; Long, F.C.; and Katz, S.: Autoradiographic method for an expanded assessment of colonic cytology. *Acta Cytologica* **17:**435-438, 1973.

22. Deschner, E.E.; Long, F.C.; and Katz, S.: The detection of aberrant DNA synthesis in a member of a high risk cancer family. *Am. J. Dig. Dis.* **20:**418-424, 1975.

23. Deschner, E.E.; Winawer, S.J.; Long, F.C.; and Boyle, C.C.: Early detection of colonic neoplasia in patients at high risk. *Cancer* **40:**2625-2631, 1977.

24. Deschner, E.E., and Maskens, A.P.: Significance of the labeling index and labeling distribution as kinetic parameters in colorectal mucosa of cancer patients and DMH treated animals, *Cancer* **50:**1136-1141, 1982.

25. Kirsner, J.B.; Rider, I.A.; Moeller, H.C.; Palmer, W.L.; and Gold, S.S.: Polyps of the colon and rectum—statistical analysis of a long term follow up study. *Gastroenterology* **39:**178-182, 1960.

26. Brahme, F.; Ekelund, G.R.; Norden, J.G.; and Wenckert, A.: Metachronous colorectal polyps—comparison of development of colorectal polyps and carcinomas in persons with and without histories of polyps. *Dis. Colon Rect.* **17:**166-171, 1974.

27. Teague, R.H.; and Read, A.E.: Polyposis in ulcerative colitis. *Gut* **16:**792-795, 1975.

28. Fenoglio, C.M., and Pascal, R.R.: Adenomatous epithelium, intraepithelial anaplasia, and invasive carcinoma in ulcerative colitis. *Dig. Dis.* **18:**556-562, 1973.

29. Eastwood, G.L., and Trier, J.S.: Epithelial cell renewal in cultured rectal biopsies in ulcerative colitis. *Gastroenterology* **64:**383-390, 1973.

30. Bleiberg, H.; Mainguet, P.; Galand, P.; Chretien, J.; and Dupont-Mairesse, N.: Cell renewal in the human rectum: *In vitro* autoradiographic study on active ulcerative colitis. *Gastroenterology* **58:**851-855, 1970.

31. Deschner, E.E., unpublished findings.

32. Hill, M.J.: Bacteria and the etiology of colonic cancer. *Cancer* **34:**815-823, 1974.

33. Sand, P.C., and Bruce, W.R.: Fecal mutagens: A possible relationship with colorectal cancer. Abstract #668. *Am. Assn. Cancer Res.* **19:**167, 1978.

34. Tannenbaum, S.R.; Fett, D.; Young, V.R.; Land, P.D.; and Bruce, W.R.: Nitrite and nitrate are formed by endogenous synthesis in the human intestine. *Science* **200:**1487-1489, 1978.

35. Reddy, B.S.; Narisawa, T.; Weisburger, J.H.; and Wynder, E.L.: Promoting effect of deoxycholate on colon adenocarcinomas in germfree rats. *JNCI* **56:**440-442, 1976.

36. Cohen, B.I.; Raicht, R.F.; Deschner, E.E.; Takahashi, M.; Sarwal, A.N.; and Fazzini, E.: Effect of cholic acid feeding on N-methyl-N-nitrosourea induced colon tumors and cell kinetics in rats. *JNCI* **64:**573-578, 1980.

37. Deschner, E.E.; Cohen, B.I.; and Raicht, R.F.: Acute and chronic effect of dietary cholic acid on colonic epithelial cell proliferation. *Digestion* **21:**290-296, 1981.

38. Maskens, A.P.: Histogenesis and growth pattern of 1,2-dimethylhydrazine induced rat colon adenocarcinoma. *Cancer Res.* **36:**1585-1592, 1976.

39. Maskens, A.P.: Histogenesis of adenomatous polyps in the human large intestine. *Gastroenterology* **77:**1245-1251, 1979.

7
Identification of Populations with Increased Susceptibility to Cancer of the Large Intestine

Martin Lipkin, M.D.

FAMILIAL POLYPOSIS

At present, the *Memorial Sloan-Kettering Registry of Population Groups at High Risk for Cancer of the Large Intestine* (Table 7-1) is comprised of 39 families with familial polyposis. These include 79 symptomatic persons, 319 asymptomatic persons at risk, and 71 spouses.

Familial polyposis is a disease with an autosomal-dominant mode of inheritance that is characterized by the development of large numbers of adenomatous polyps throughout the entire colon and rectum. Carcinomas eventually develop in virtually all affected persons. The cancers occur with highest frequency in the distal colon, a distribution that is similar to that of colorectal cancer in the general population.

While the existence of intestinal polyposis has been recorded for 250 years, only during the last century have researchers further delineated the condition into subgroups.[1] In 1721, Menzel may have described the first case, one that was probably inflammatory in type. By 1881, Woodward had

Table 7-1. Registry of Population Groups at High and Low Risk for Cancer of the Large Intestine

Familial polyposis	Single and multiple sporadic
Inherited adenomatosis	colorectal adenomas
Gardner's syndrome	Primary colorectal cancer
Turcot's syndrome	in the general population
Peutz-Jeghers syndrome	Ulcerative colitis
Juvenile polyposis	Crohn's disease
Familial colon cancer	Familial aggregates cancer free
without polyposis	for two or more generations
Multiple cancers including	
colorectal	

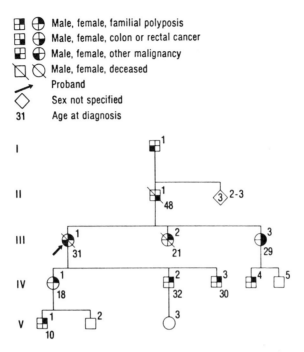

Figure 7-1.   Typical pattern of inheritance in familial polyposis together with ages of onset of polyposis in family members. *(From M. Lipkin, S. Scherf, L. Schechter, and D. Braun, Jr. Memorial hospital registry of populations at high risk for cancer of the large intestine: Age of onset of neoplasms. Prev. Med. 9:3, 1980.)*

divided polyposis into two categories: primary or adenomatous (i.e., hyperplastic or neoplastic) and inflammatory. At about the same time, researchers observed that primary polyposis had hereditary tendencies—hence, "familial polyposis coli." Within 30 years, it became clear that this was a precancerous, hereditary condition in the large intestine. In 1882, Cripps observed two siblings with polyposis coli, and by 1900 the division was apparent: familial (adenomatosis) versus nonfamilial (inflammatory) polyposis.

Familial polyposis, an autosomal-dominant genetic defect affecting each generation, is expressed phenotypically about 80% of the time. A typical pattern of inheritance in familial polyposis is shown in Figure 7-1. The probable genetic background of familial polyposis and its various associated syndromes has been debated by many investigators. There appears to be general agreement that classic familial polyposis is caused by a single dominant gene. However, there is less agreement as to the genetics of sporadic cases and the various associated syndromes. Some investigators believe that

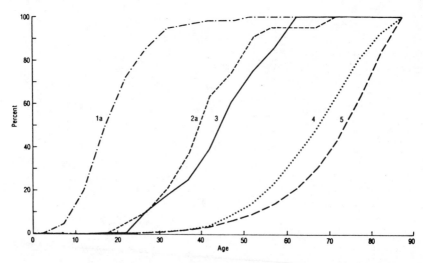

Figure 7-2. Cumulative percent of incident cases at various ages having familial polyposis, compared to cumulative age incidence of colon cancer in other population groups. Curve 1a shows the onset of nonmalignant polyposis and Curve 2a, the onset of cancer in familial polyposis, derived from data of 38 cases seen at Memorial Hospital. Curve 3 shows early age of onset of cancer in 28 affected persons from Memorial Hospital series who have familial colon-cancer-prone disease without polyposis. Curve 4 illustrates the age of onset of colon and rectal cancer in the general population of the United States from the Third National Cancer Survey, National Cancer Institute and includes both white and black males and females. Curve 5 illustrates the onset of colon and rectal cancer in males and females in Japan from data supplied by Dr. T. Hirayama. *(After M. Lipkin, S. Scherf, L. Schechter, and D. Braun, Jr. Memorial hospital registry of populations at high risk for cancer of the large intestine: Age of onset of neoplasms. Prev. Med. 9:3, 1980.)*

sporadic cases can be explained by new mutations. Others disagree, maintaining that a minor fraction of all sporadic cases would result from a fresh mutation. It has also been suggested that environmental modification would render the expression of disease and inheritance virtually polygenic.

Records of the incidence of polyposis coli exist in Great Britain, the United States, and northern Europe; that is, among Caucasians who have access to advanced medical services. The disease has also occurred, however, in Arabs, West Indians, American and African blacks, Orientals, and American Indians. Analysis of age at onset of disease is an important determinant in the identification of familial polyposis and other diseases where familial predisposition increases the risk of colorectal cancer.[2] Figure 7-2 gives the cumulative age distributions of onset of familial polyposis and subsequent colon cancer, and comparisons are made with other population groups. From these data, the magnitude of increased risk at every age level can be estimated.

Environmental factors in polyposis coli have not been identified; however, it is possible that the known genetic predisposition could be modified by the environment. In our conceptual understanding of the development of cancer, the concept of a multistage evolution of neoplasms, with promotor or cocarcinogenic agents having a role, has become widely accepted.[3-5] Environmental or physiological stimuli may contribute to the steps leading to neoplastic change, adenomas, and malignancy. In familial polyposis, although adenomas are scattered throughout the colon, carcinomas develop mainly in the distal colon. This is a pattern similar to that seen in the general population.

Gardner's Syndrome

Gardner's syndrome (GS), a variant of familial polyposis, is an autosomal-dominant disorder showing a high degree of penetrance. Adenomatous polyps of the colon and, occasionally, of the small intestine are formed, and there is a propensity for development of adenocarcinoma. Recognized today on the basis of characteristic clinical findings, the incidence of the syndrome is lower than familial polyposis and is estimated at 1 in 14,000 births.

Adenomatosis of the large intestine, multiple osteomata of the skull and mandible, and multiple epidermoid cysts and soft-tissue tumors of the skin were the symptoms reported by Gardner in 1951.[6] Previously studied cases were in 1912,[7] 1938,[8] and 1943.[9] Gardner did follow-up work in 1952,[10] 1953, 1962, and 1969, when the original case was reviewed. New observations showed impacted teeth, early dental caries, cysts and abnormal bone structure of the mandible and tibia, desmoid tumors of the abdominal wall, and small-intestinal mesentery. It should be noted that an epidermoid cyst, uncommon before the age of puberty, may indicate polyposis.

Other possible associated lesions include carcinoma of the thyroid, ampulla of Vater, duodenum, and adrenal glands, adenomas of the small intestine, carcinoma *in situ* of the gallbladder, carcinomatous tumors of the small intestine, tumors of the brain and central nervous system, and lymphoid polyps of the ileum. Adenomas are distributed in the colon and rectum; they can, however, also occur in the small intestine, especially in the region of the ampulla of Vater, and in the stomach.

Gene expression in GS is variable, with some persons with hereditary polyposis having the various manifestations of the major triad of the syndrome and others having only intestinal neoplasms. Periampullary carcinomas have been reported in the recent literature.

The desmoid tumors that arise following surgery present a particular problem. These can erupt between one and three years after an operation for polyposis, appearing in the abdominal wall or the mesentery of the small intestine. They may be large and multiple, and on occasion, they may precede the phenotypic expression of polyposis. At the Mayo Clinic, desmoid tumors developed in 3.5% of patients after surgery.[11] Similar observations have been made elsewhere. Clinically, desmoid tumors appear as carcinomatous recurrences, but they are considered benign or low-grade malignancies. Histologically, these intra-abdominal tumors often reach a stable size and afterward remain unchanged. They can obstruct the intestine or urinary tract.

The incidence of GS among families in which more than one member has polyposis has been estimated at 14 to 18%. Only one or several family members may have obvious clinical manifestations of the disease. The expression of the disease is incomplete, so diagnoses made on the basis of clinical findings are limited. As will be noted, abnormalities of epidermal cells and fibroblasts can be observed in family members lacking clinical manifestations of disease.

It is not yet clear whether features of the syndrome result from one dominant gene or from two or more genes. There are also questions about the number, nature, and location of polyps in polyposis patients showing manifestations of GS compared to those with the typical non-Gardner familial polyposis. In terms of pathogenesis, the syndrome described by Gardner could represent the full manifestation of a spectrum of pathologic changes affecting all patients with multiple polyposis. It is possible that a single mutation may be responsible for most of the various associated syndromes. On that basis, GS would include all adenomatous polyposis, with subsidiary lesions expressed in different degrees.

Turcot's Syndrome

Turcot's syndrome (TS) has been described by Turcot as polyposis coli associated with malignant tumors of the central nervous system.[12] In this study, two family members, a boy and a girl with polyposis, died from medulloblastoma of the spinal cord and a cerebral tumor, respectively. Several other similar instances have been reported and may be examples of the tumor association found in GS.

Peutz-Jeghers Syndrome

Peutz-Jeghers syndrome (PJS), an additional autosomal-dominant, inherited disease with variable expression, was first described by Peutz in 1921 and later elaborated on by Jeghers et al.[13] In this disease, pigmented spots often appear on the lips and buccal mucosa and also on the dorsal aspect of the hands and feet. Dozens of intestinal tumors (although not as many as in familial polyposis) are found throughout the gastrointestinal tract and can intussuscept and obstruct the small intestine. Because of their composition (normal intestinal epithelium and abnormal amounts and arrangement of smooth muscle), these tumors are considered hamartomas. Juvenile polyps are similar, except for the smooth muscle arrangement. The disease can occur with polyps and without pigmentation or vice versa.

The tumors were originally considered benign and without high potential for malignancy. However, more than 15 cases of cancer (stomach, duodenum, and colon) have been reported, and adenomas have been found to coexist with the other lesions. Most patients have been under the age of 40, a further indication of the tumor's malignant potential. In this disease, when carcinoma of the colon has developed, it is believed to arise from the adenomas.

Juvenile Polyposis

Distribution of the polyps in juvenile polyposis is not as extensive as that seen in adenomatous polyposis. Although the polyps occur indiscriminately throughout the gastrointestinal tract, they are seen more often in the large intestine. They are not precancerous, and a major operation is not necessarily required. Average age of onset of the disease is 6 years, but it has been diagnosed earlier, often in infants. The main symptom is bleeding, which can be accompanied by severe anemia, hypoproteinemia, malnutrition, and retarded development.

Found singly or in small numbers, the polyps consist of normal mucosal epithelium in irregular glandular patterns, surrounded by an increased amount of lamina propria. The mucous glands may be cystic and distended. Hemorrhage and secondary inflammation are additional symptoms. Some tumors have exhibited the combined characteristics of juvenile polyps and adenomas. Adenomatous tumors have been discovered in patients with juvenile polyposis (one patient also had rectal cancer), and a higher incidence of colon carcinomas may occur in family members. Thirty-seven cases of multiple juvenile polyposis were recorded in 29 families. In six of these cases more than one member was affected, and in one family, the disease spanned three generations.[14] Most cases have been solitary rather than familial, and such patients have also shown a high incidence of other congenital abnormalities.

FAMILIAL COLON CANCER WITHOUT POLYPOSIS

Despite the identification of familial polyposis, it is difficult to identify or analyze other forms of gastrointestinal cancer that may result from hereditary predisposition. This is because members of familial groups with high frequencies of colorectal and other cancers often do not make information readily available. Also, the widespread recognition of environmental and dietary factors that may contribute to the occurrence of colorectal cancer has prevented a simple classification of susceptibility based on genetic patterns. The long length of human life, the small number of progeny, in many families, and the fear of cancer that often develops make long-term analyses difficult. But despite these problems, important advances have been made in recent years toward recognition of the existence of this condition in colon-cancer etiology.

Recent studies show that numerous Mendelian-inherited diseases have previously undiscovered cancer associations. Mulvihill estimated that 9% of the 2,000 diseases in McKusick's catalog of Mendelian inheritance in humans have neoplastic associations.[15] Of related importance is the term "ecogenetics" to emphasize host-environmental interactions.[16]

In terms of cancer of the large intestine, findings developed in recent years indicate that familial associations in colon cancer are higher than in control groups, suggesting that inherited factors may play a greater role in the genesis of colorectal cancer than was previously believed.[17, 18]

Our population registry of familial groups having high frequencies of colon cancer without familial polyposis includes 32 families with mainly site-specific colon cancer, 54 affected family members, and 681 asymptomatic persons at risk. The pedigree of a typical familial aggregate is shown in Figure 7-3. These persons do not have the extensive colonic polyposis that characterizes familial polyposis, but they are believed to have a hereditary form of cancer with an autosomal-dominant mode of inheritance.[19, 20] The early age of onset for cancer of the large intestine is also shown in Figure 7-2.

Systematic surveillance has recently been started at Memorial Hospital to detect additional pedigrees of familial cancer. We are now able to identify new familial groups and to continue to enlarge our registry. Verification is made of individual and family history of previous colorectal cancer and other pathological findings by obtaining pathology records and death certificates and by consulting physicians' records of affected family members.

Criteria for a familial syndrome of this type associated with cancer of the large intestine include: increased numbers of all types of adenocarcinomas in affected patients, especially colonic and endometrial carcinomas; early age of cancer development as compared with that noted for the same organ sites in the general population; a tendency to multiple, primary, malignant neoplasms in affected persons; and segregation ratios consistent with an autosomal-dominant mode of inheritance.

In early work, Warthin reported on the first "family G" that corresponded to the above criteria,[21] a study that was subsequently updated.[22] Other investigations in the United States and Europe were undertaken in the 1950s,

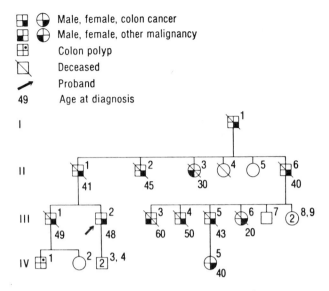

Figure 7-3.   **Typical pattern of inheritance of cancer in a Memorial-Hospital familial aggregate highly predisposed to colon cancer without polyposis together with ages of onset of cancer in some family members.** *(From M. Lipkin, S. Scherf, L. Schechter, and D. Braun, Jr. Memorial hospital registry of populations at high risk for cancer of the large intestine: Age of onset of neoplasms. Prev. Med. 9:3, 1980.)*

1960s, and 1970s, and increasing numbers of familial aggregations of this type are now being recognized.

Figure 7-4 shows the early age at onset of colon cancer in a familial aggregate with site-specific colon cancer, and Table 7-2 shows the nearly 50% cancer risk to children of affected parents in a recent series.[23] In both instances, the average age is in the 40- to 50-year range for onset of cancer, a characteristic finding illustrated earlier (see Fig. 7-2). An autosomal-dominant mode of inheritance has been suggested, and the findings are consistent with a hereditary, precancerous disorder such as familial polyposis.

A classic study that exemplified hereditary, site-specific colon cancer in the absence of classic familial polyposis coli (FPC) was carried out by Woolf et al.[24] Individual polyps were present in the colon along with colonic cancer. Many other kindreds with site-specific colon lesions have also been reported. Lynch's reports on "family R"[19, 23] seemed consistent with findings on this disease observed in Europe and the United States over the past 20 years. Colon cancer risk in the R family segregated with ratios consistent with that of a single, autosomal-dominant gene with complete penetrance. All but 1 of 33 family members with cancer of the gastrointestinal tract had a parent

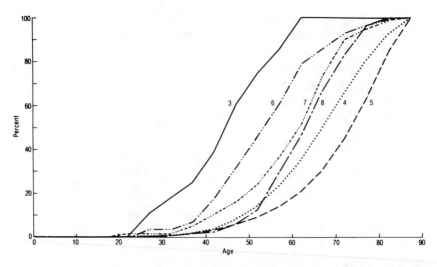

Figure 7-4.   Cumulative percent of incident cases at various ages having multiple cancers, including colorectal, from Memorial-Hospital series. Curves 3, 4, and 5 show the same population groups seen in Figure 2. Curve 6 shows the onset of colorectal cancer in persons with multiple primary cancers and family history of colorectal cancer. Curve 7 shows the onset of colorectal cancer in persons with multiple primary cancers and family history of cancer other than colorectal. Curve 8 shows onset of colorectal cancer in persons with multiple primary cancers and no family history of cancer. *(After M. Lipkin, S. Scherf, L. Schechter, and D. Braun, Jr. Memorial hospital registry of populations at high risk for cancer of the large intestine: Age of onset of neoplasms. Prev. Med. 9:3, 1980.)*

Table 7-2. Risk for Colon Cancer in Offspring of Affected Parents

FAMILY	TOTAL NO. OF RELATIVES ASCERTAINED	RISK % OF SYNDROME TO PROGENY OF AFFECTED PARENT IN AGE INTERVAL $(x \pm 2\ sd)$
1	931	48 ± 5
2	177	54 ± 13
3	184	47 ± 9
4	1139	59 ± 6
5	79	59 ± 13
6	127	53 ± 9
7-11	124	60 ± 8
12[a]	232	54 ± 9
Total	2993	54 ± 5

Source: After H.T. Lynch. *Cancer Genetics.* Springfield, IL: Charles C. Thomas, 1976.
[a]Site-specific colon cancer. All others consistent with cancer family syndrome (CFS).

with the same disease. In another family with 2 affected members, surgery was recommended for an asymptomatic member, and an occult adenocarcinoma of the cecum was subsequently discovered. The family as a whole showed a high risk (50%) for development of primary, malignant neoplasms of the colon subsequent to carcinoma.

Along with many cancer family patients, Lynch's R family revealed a strong tendency towards developing cancer of the proximal colon. The mean frequency of proximal colon cancer is higher in that group than in either patients with familial polyposis or the general population. Also, the frequency of colon cancer is three to four times that of FPC patients'. Examination of high-risk patients of this type should include hemoccult and radiologic and endoscopic evaluations that assess the status of the right side of the colon and cecum. Endoscopic examination may have to start at age 30 or 35, depending on the previous pattern of inheritance or current findings.

MULTIPLE CANCERS INCLUDING COLORECTAL

Our registry includes 324 patients who have colorectal cancer in addition to other primary tumors. The associated neoplasms include breast (21%), genital (women) (16%), genitourinary (11%), and other regions of the gastrointestinal tract (9%). These patients experienced an early age of onset of colorectal cancer (Figure 7-4).

SINGLE AND MULTIPLE, SPORADIC, COLORECTAL ADENOMAS

The presence of one or more adenomas occurs in 5 to 10% of all persons in the general population and is associated with the development of adenocarcinomas. Kindreds have been reported that show an association of single and multiple adenomas with adenocarcinomas, thus suggesting a genetic susceptibility.[24]

According to estimates, 5% of adenomas become malignant, and the development of villous characteristics in the adenomas is associated with increased frequency of malignancy. Colonic adenomas have a peak incidence 5 to 10 years earlier than in colon cancer in the general population. This would be consistent with their being precursors to the malignant neoplasms. These adenomatous polyps have an epidemiologic distribution similar to that seen in colon cancer.[25, 26] Our registry of single and multiple adenomas now includes 634 persons, and we are developing age–incidence data for the appearance of multiple adenomas in these persons.

Further correlations between adenomatous polyps and cancer have been observed in Hawaiian citizens of Japanese extraction who show an increased susceptibility both to polyps and to colonic cancer. The larger the polyps and the more there are, the more malignant the change. A study of two prefectures in Japan—Akita and Miyagi—showed a 13.7% incidence of multiple polyps to 7.5% respectively, with colon cancer being more frequent in Akita. Twenty-three percent of patients from Akita had moderate to severe epithelial cell atypia; the figure in Miyagi was 12.7%. In other investigations, Japanese and Swedish researchers found more advanced atypical and dysplastic changes in the sigmoid colon than in the cecum, implying more exposure to endogenous or environmental carcinogenic or promoter elements.[27-29] The largest adenomas and carcinomas in familial polyposis also occur in the distal colon. Hyperplastic polyps are not generally considered precancerous, although a possible role for these polyps in large bowel carcinogenesis has been considered.[30]

PRIMARY COLORECTAL CANCER IN THE GENERAL POPULATION

Persons in this category who have had colorectal cancer without other malignant disease are not included in the familial or genetic groups just discussed. Within our registry, this group is also divided into three subcategories: persons with primary colorectal cancer plus a family history of colorectal cancer; persons with a family history of cancer other than colorectal; and persons with no family history of cancer (Fig. 7-5). The age-incidence distributions in these groups are closer to the age incidence for colon cancer in the general population of the United States and Japan. Within our population registry, the group is now comprised of 374 patients having primary colorectal cancer. In this group, 59 have a family history of colorectal cancer, 123 have a family history of cancer other than colorectal, and 192 have no family history of cancer. Further subdivisions are being made for persons with colon cancer and rectal cancer. Several studies show that familial associations of colorectal cancer among index cases of colorectal cancer in the general population are higher than in control groups. Environmental as well as inherited factors could also be associated with the development of neoplasms in these groups.

ULCERATIVE COLITIS

The lifetime cancer risk with this disease is about 57%,[31] beginning after the first 10 years and then increasing in total frequency. The number of colorectal carcinomas arising from ulcerative colitis is believed to be comparable to or

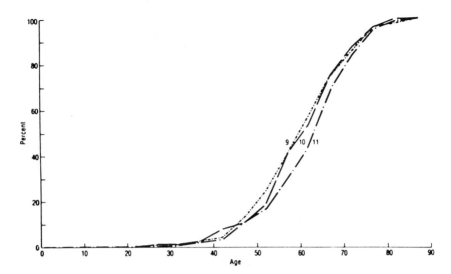

Figure 7-5.   Cumulative percent of incident cases in Memorial Hospital series having primary colorectal cancer without a second tumor. Curve 9 shows primary colorectal cancer and family history of cancer other than colorectal. Curve 10 shows primary colorectal cancer and family history of colon cancer. Curve 11 shows primary colorectal cancer and no family history of cancer. *(After M. Lipkin, S. Scherf, L. Schechter, and D. Braun, Jr. Memorial hospital registry of populations at high risk for cancer of the large intestine: Age of onset of neoplasms. Prev. Med. 9:3, 1980.)*

even greater than the number arising from familial polyposis. Many of the cancers arising before the age of 45 are believed to be preceded by ulcerative colitis.[32] Inflammatory changes are also present in the colonic mucosa of familial polyposis. Although ulcerative colitis is a chronic and relapsing disease, the possibility of risk increases in patients with continuous disease, total colonic involvement, and an early age at onset. Carcinomas appearing in ulcerative colitis are often flat, infiltrating, and poorly differentiated, and a high multicentricity rate has been reported. A registry of subjects with ulcerative colitis is also being developed at Memorial Hospital.

CROHN'S DISEASE

Like ulcerative colitis, Crohn's disease is chronic and inflammatory. Unlike ulcerative colitis, it affects the entire bowel wall and is granulomatous, primarily affecting the small bowel and, at times, the large intestine. Until recently, Crohn's disease had generally not been regarded as a premalignant condition, however, during the past decade, there has been increasing recognition of the development of adenocarcinoma in association with the disease.[33, 34] The adenocarcinomas have been noted to occur in young patients and in areas similar to the distribution of Crohn's disease rather than the usual distribution of large bowel cancer. This registry is also currently being developed.

FAMILIAL AGGREGATES CANCER-FREE FOR TWO OR MORE GENERATIONS

Familial aggregates with 41 persons cancer-free for two or more generations have also been identified and are available for study of risk factors. In addition, spouses of persons in the population groups mentioned and medical student volunteers are available as control subjects. Measurements have also been begun on populations at low risk for colorectal cancer in geographic areas that include Medellin, Colombia and various regions in Japan,

Table 7-3. Phenotypic Characteristics Recently Reported in Population Groups at Increased Risk for Colorectal Cancer

PHENOTYPIC CHARACTERISTIC

1. Colonic epithelial cells
   a) Etopic development of adenoma leading to adenoma cancer sequence[43, 73-75]
   b) Abnormal proliferation of cells in persons with familial polyposis and GS[35-40]
2. Extraintestinal neoplasms[71]
3. Immunoparameter—Inappropriate suppression of lymphocyte response to allogeneic stimuli in nonpolyposis familial aggregates and GS[57]
4. Cutaneous cells
   a) Heteroploidy of cutaneous epithelial cells in persons with GS[55]
   b) Growth changes in cutaneous fibroblasts in familial polyposis and GS[56]
5. Fecal contents
   a) Decreased fecal cholesterol degradation in familial polyposis and in some persons in the general population[58-61]
   b) Fecal microflora conversion of bile acids and cholesterol and modifications of fecal bacterial-enzyme activities[69, 70]
   c) Mutagenic activity in feces of human subjects in the general population[63-67]
   d) Conversion of nitrites to nitrosamines with carcinogenic activity[72]

for further comparison with the high-risk population groups in the Center's registry.

Thus, the major population groups at increased risk for colorectal cancer have been identified together with persons at lower risk. Furthermore, the development of these population registries has enabled us to call up individual patients and familial aggregates in the categories just mentioned for measurements of phenotypic abnormalities associated with high-frequency and early-age development of colorectal cancer. With these studies, a series of biological characteristics associated with a genetic predisposition to large bowel cancer, not only during the growth of benign and malignant neoplasms, but also before the appearance of clinically detectable lesions, has now been found by our group and others. These are summarized in Table 7-3 and are further discussed in the following sections.

PROLIFERATIVE ABNORMALITIES IN COLONIC EPITHELIAL CELLS

An early abnormal characteristic of colonic epithelial cells that we have identified in persons with a genetic predisposition to colorectal cancer, is modified, epithelial-cell, proliferative activity. During progressive stages of abnormal development, cell phenotypes are seen in which epithelial cells gain an increased ability to proliferate and to accumulate in the mucosa.[35-40] The identification of these changes has aided our understanding of events that occur during neoplastic transformation of cells in colorectal cancer.

In the normal human colon, these cells proliferate in the lower regions and midregions of the colonic crypts as shown in Figure 7-6. About 15 to 20% of the proliferating cells are in synthesizing deoxyribonucleic acid (DNA) simultaneously, and they migrate to the surface of the mucosa to be extruded. Our earlier studies in humans showed that the colonic mucosa is replaced by new cells in 4 to 8 days.[41, 42] During migration of these cells, the number that continue to proliferate decreases as they progress to the luminal region of the crypts; they undergo terminal differentiation within hours, and proliferation ceases as they migrate to the crypt surfaces.[42]

However, in subjects with familial polyposis, patches of flat mucosa are found having colonic epithelial cells that fail to repress DNA synthesis during migration to the surface of the mucosa.[35-40] This is illustrated in Figures 7-6 and 7-7 and occurs in normal-appearing colonic epithelial cells before as well as after the cells develop adenomatous changes and begin to accumulate as polyps. Observed in over 80% of random biopsy specimens,[41, 42] a failure of cells to repress DNA synthesis has now been shown to occur with higher frequency in patients with familial polyposis than in population groups at

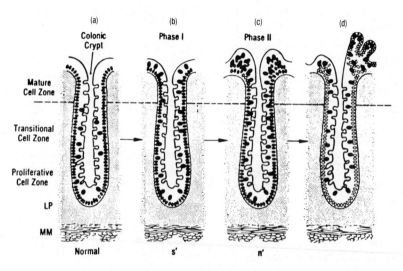

Figure 7-6. Sequence of events to account for the location of abnormally proliferating colonic-epithelial cells before and during the formation of polypoid neoplasms in humans. (a) Shows location of proliferating and differentiating epithelial cells in normal colonic crypt. Dark cells illustrate thymidine labeling in cells that are synthesizing DNA and preparing to undergo cell division. As cells pass from the proliferative zone through the transitional zone, DNA synthesis and mitosis are repressed, and migrating epithelial cells leave the proliferative-cell cycle to undergo normal maturation before they reach the surface of the mucosa. (b) Shows the development of a Phase I proliferative lesion in the colonic epithelial cells as they fail to repress the incorporation of thymidine ³H into DNA and begin to develop an enhanced ability to proliferate. The mucosa is flat, and the number of new cells born equals the number extruded without excess cell accumulation in the mucosa. (c) Shows the development of a Phase II proliferative lesions in colonic epithelial cells. The cells incorporate thymidine ³H into DNA and also have developed additional properties that enable them to accumulate in the mucosa as neoplasms begin to form. (d) Shows further differentiation of abnormally retained, proliferating epithelial cells into pathologically defined neoplastic lesions, including adenomatous polyps and villous papillomas. *(From M. Lipkin. Phase 1 and phase 2 proliferative lesions of colonic epithelial cells in diseases leading to colon cancer. Cancer 34:878, 1974.)*

low risk for colorectal cancer. More recently, a significant increase in abnormal proliferative activity has also been noted in the colonic mucosa of strongly colon-cancer-prone families without polyposis (Table 7-4). This finding, in a highly cancer-prone population group that does not develop the early warning signals provided by the appearance of adenomas, has led to

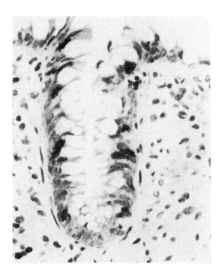

Figure 7-7.   Thymidine ^{3}**H incorporation into epithelial cells near the crypt surface of flat colonic mucosa in a biopsy specimen from a high-risk subject.** *(From M. Lipkin, S.J. Winawer, and P. Sherlock. Early identification of individuals at increased risk for cancer of the large intestine, Part II: Developments of risk factor profiles. Clin. Bull. 11:66, 1981.)*

newer measurements. Thus, our current work is now focusing on these findings in other high-, average- and low-risk populations and on the development of discriminatory indices in subjects at risk in colon-cancer-prone families. For this purpose, these and related measurements, as will be described, are being automated and extended into a larger epidemiologic study in which both genetic and environmental contributions to abnormal cell development are identified. To facilitate this work, the data from specific population groups are analyzed using computer-assisted methods to evaluate differences between population groups of interest. An example of the type of computer-generated output that is now possible is shown in Figure 7-8.

In familial polyposis, the further modifications of proliferative activity believed to occur before the development of malignancy also are shown in Figure 7-6. Following the failure of cells that have inherited the germinal mutation to repress DNA synthesis during migration in the colonic crypts, additional events take place, giving rise to new clones from the original cell population.   An early event leads to the development of the well-known

Table 7-4. Labeling Distribution % of TdR³H-Labeled Cells in Upper 1/3 of Colonic Crypts (LD μl/3) in Flat, Normal-Appearing Mucosa of High- and Low-Risk Populations

POPULATION GROUP	NO. OF PERSONS	RATIO OF MEAN VALUE OF (LD μ1/3) IN-TEST GROUP TO MEAN VALUE IN CONTROL GROUP (C)
Familial polyposis		
Symptomatic (FP$_s$)[a]	10	2.49[c]
Asymptomatic (FP$_a$)[b]	11	2.68[c]
Polyp-free branch	10	1.22[d]
Familial colon cancer		
Symptomatic (FCC$_s$)[a]	8	3.21[c]
Asymptomatic (FCC$_a$)[b]	23	3.16[c]
Cancer-free branches	16	1.72[d]
Nonfamilial colon cancer	13	1.41[d]
Normal subjects	15	1.00[d]

Source: After M. Lipkin, E. Deschner, W. Blattner, J.F. Fraumeni, Jr., and H. Lynch. Triatiated thymidine incorporation into colonic epithelial cells of subjects in cancer-prone families. *Proceedings Am. Assn. Cancer Res.* **21**:188, 1980.
[a] Affected persons
[b] Possible carriers (about 50% risk of developing disease)
[c] Percentage of labeled cells significantly greater than normal subjects, nonfamilial colon-cancer cases, or polyp-free and cancer-free branches of families ($p < 0.05$)
[d] Percentage of labeled cells not significantly greater than normal subjects

adenomatous cells that proliferate and accumulate near the surface of the mucosa (Figure 7-6). In familial polyposis, according to this concept, additional changes then occur in the cells, giving rise to modifications in cell surface and related properties that lead to invasive malignancy. This concept allows for a contribution of endogenous or exogenous carcinogenic or promoter elements interacting with the cells having a hereditary predisposition to neoplasia. This concept also allows for the introduction of preventive measures to inhibit the steps leading to malignant transformation of the cells.

In the familial-polyposis model of human cancer development, as epithelial cells develop an increased capacity to proliferate and to accumulate in the mucosa, areas of microscopic hyperplasia and adenomatous foci develop. As these adenomatous foci become recognizable lesions, they are seen to consist of an overgrowth of hyperplastic, mucus-secreting intestinal epithelium together with a stroma of loose connective tissue and blood vessels. As

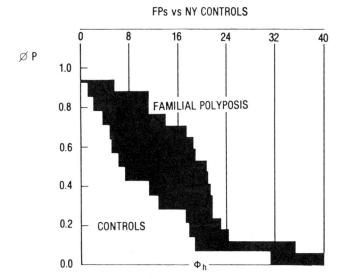

Figure 7-8. Diagram of computer-generated curves comparing crypt-column-occupancy fractions of tritiated, thymidine-labeled epithelial cells in a high-risk and a low-risk group. Abscissa records ϕ_h, the fraction-labeled cells found within the upper 40 percent of assayed crypt columns adjacent to and including the luminal surface. The ordinate ϕP records the fraction of all persons in a given group whose measured ϕ_h values equal or exceed the abscissa value. Significant differences are present between high and low risk groups ($P < 0.005$). *(Data from M. Lipkin, E. Deschner, W. Blattner, J.F. Fraumeni, Jr., and W. Lynch. Tritiated thymidine incorporation into colonic epithelial cells of subjects in colon cancer-prone families. Proc. Adm. Assoc. Cancer Res. 21, 1980.)*

a further indication of enhanced cell proliferation, the epithelial cells exhibit hyperchromatism, stratification, and decreased mucus production as well as increased mitotic activity. Studies have shown that only a single crypt of Lieberkühn, or part of its surface, can be affected. Occasionally, the epithelium buds as a small diverticulum from the main glandular spaces lined by one layer of normal mucus-secreting cells. The transition from normal to abnormal epithelium can be an abrupt process halfway up the crypts of Lieberkühn.[43] When the tubules have branched sufficiently and have expanded to about 3 mm in diameter with 3 mm above the mucosal surface, the lesion can be recognized as an adenoma that will differentiate further into one of the three characteristic types: tubular, villous, or villotubular.

The same process of adenoma tubule growth is believed to occur in intramucosal hyperplasia, which also occasionally develops as a concave depression. Following further malignant transformation of the cells, it may lead to the small, rare, cancerous ulcers described as *de novo* cancer. Another mode of adenoma development is extensive adenomatous formation on the mucosal surface, degenerating into "surface" cancer.[43] Both hyperchromatism and decreased mucus production are present during the period when these tumors become either sessile or villous adenomas.

COMPARISON OF CARCINOGEN-INDUCED PROLIFERATIVE ABNORMALITIES AND PATHOLOGIC CHANGES IN COLONIC MUCOSA

Proliferative and pathologic abnormalities in colonic-epithelial cells similar to those observed in humans have now been observed to be induced in rodent colonic-epithelial cells. Like humans, rodent strains have different susceptibilities to the induction of colon cancer. In rodents, the cell transformations can be induced by 1, 2-dimethylhydrazine (DMH), methylazoxymethanol (MAM), N-methyl-N^1-nitro-N-nitrosoguanidine (MNNG), and N-methyl-N-nitrosourea (MNU).[44-47] Tumor nodules develop in mice following exposure to DMH. The main site of activity is the distal colon, the same distribution noted to occur in humans. In mice, multifocal tumors ranging from adenomatous polyps to metaplasias and carcinomas grow from the mucosa and then protrude into the lumen of the rectosigmoid. Early focal atypias and hyperplasias located mainly on the folds, adenomatous polyps, and carcinomas appear to be part of the progressive pathologic changes in mice and rats that develop following administration of DMH. These changes are accompanied by an increased proliferative activity in the cells. DMH and MNNG both induce an extension of the proliferative zone of the flat mucosa toward the surfaces of the colonic crypts as seen in Figure 7-9.

Thus, some of the colonic epithelial cells of rodents exposed to repeated injections of DMH also develop the capacity to continue to synthesize DNA throughout most of their lifespan. Thymidine-labeled cells show an increase in both their position up from the crypt base and in their total number; these cells also show a shift into expanding adenomas and carcinomas. The tumors that develop show a proliferation of neoplastic epithelial cells near the surface of the lesion, with a continued expansion into the colonic lumen.

A failure of colonic epithelial cells to repress DNA synthesis also occurs in epithelial cell-renewing tissues in other human diseases, including ulcerative colitis of the colon.[48] In atrophic gastritis, a condition associated with the development of gastric malignancy of the stomach, epithelial cells also fail to repress DNA synthesis and undergo abnormal maturation as they migrate through the gastric mucosa (Fig. 7-10).[49, 50] Analogous changes are found in the stomachs of rodents after exposure to a chemical carcinogen.[51] A similar

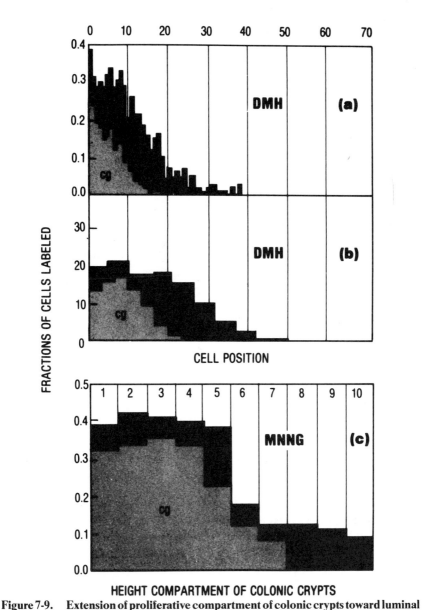

Figure 7-9. Extension of proliferative compartment of colonic crypts toward luminal surface of crypts, after repeated exposure to chemical carcinogens. Control groups = cg; carcinogenic groups = black areas. (a) Fraction of cells labeled at various cell positions within colonic crypts, 1 hour after injection of thymidine-^{3}H and 8 days after start of weekly DMH injections into mice (20 μg/g).[10] (b) Fractions of cells labeled at various cell positions within colonic crypts, 125 days after beginning of DMH treatment in mice.[12] (c) Fraction of cells labeled in segments of colonic crypt after rectal installation of MNNG in rats.[11] *(From M. Lipkin, S.J. Winawer, and P. Sherlock. Early identification of individuals at increased risk for cancer of the large intestine, Part II: Developments of risk factor profiles. Clin. Bull. 11:66, 1981.)*

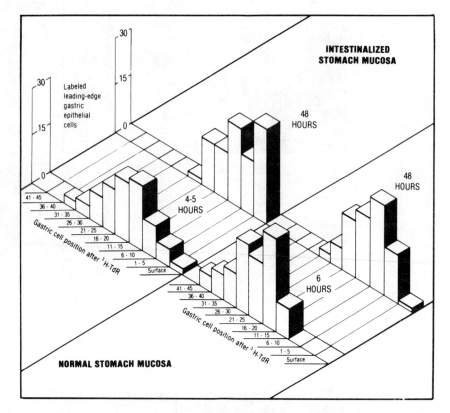

Figure 7-10.   Cell position below surface of gastric pits occupied by labeled leading-edge, gastric epithelial cells at early and late periods after *in vivo* pulse injection of tritiated thymidine into two human subjects. In contrast to normal stomach mucosa, in intestinalized stomach mucosa, the zone of labeled cells extends to the surface of the gastric pits after pulse injection. *(From M. Lipkin, S.J. Winawer, and P. Sherlock. Early identification of individuals at increased risk for cancer of the large intestine, Part II: Developments of risk factor profiles. Clin. Bull. 11:66, 1981.)*

event occurs in precancerous disease of the human cervical epithelium[52] and in the cervixes of rodents after introduction of a chemical carcinogen.[53] Thus, during the development of neoplasms in organs that contain renewing epithelium other than the colon, persistent DNA synthesis occurs in cells that normally would be terminal or end cells. As occurs in the colon in familial polyposis, similar pathological changes accompany this development and also lead to atypias, dysplasias, and malignancy.[54]

STUDIES OF CUTANEOUS CELLS OF PATIENTS WITH FAMILIAL POLYPOSIS

Phenotypic expressions of the genetic defect leading to familial polyposis have also been found in cutaneous cells. Increased heteroploidy in cutaneous epithelial cells derived from persons with GS has been reported.[55] Several recent studies have shown differences in the distribution of the cytoskeletal protein actin within cultured skin fibroblasts from persons with familial polyposis when compared to normal subjects.[56]

IMMUNOLOGIC STUDIES

An immunologic abnormality has recently been reported in persons from colon-cancer-prone families without polyposis.[57] When cancer-free persons from families predisposed to large bowel cancer, but without familial polyposis, were studied to determine the nature of their cell-mediated immune capacities, 44% showed failure of potentially normal lymphocytes to react to an allogeneic stimulus. This *in vitro* defect in recognitive immunity was similar to that seen in persons with established malignancies. Several patients with GS also showed the defect in recognitive immunity. These findings, as well as those just noted, are being applied in evaluations of asymptomatic persons in familial aggregates having the various disorders leading to large bowel cancer, in order to develop the risk factor profiles described next.

EXAMINATION OF FECAL CONTENTS

In familial polyposis and related disorders, still other studies are in progress to identify constituents of fecal contents that may be abnormal and to examine their potential carcinogenic activity on cells in the colon. A group of compounds currently under examination consists of the bile acids and their bacterial-conversion products. Accordingly, several recent reports have compared the fecal neutral sterols and bile acids in patients with familial polyposis to those of controls.[58-61] Persons with familial polyposis excreted significantly higher amounts of cholesterol and lower levels of the degradation products of cholesterol, which are mainly coprostanol and coprostanone. This is illustrated by our recent data on fecal cholesterol degradation in these high-risk subjects (Table 7-5). Nondegradation of cholesterol has also been found in a minor fraction of persons in the general population whose background and related characteristics have not been defined.[62]

Current results have also suggested differences in metabolic activity of

Table 7-5. Fecal Neutral Sterols in Subjects at High Risk for Cancer of the Large Intestine and in Controls [a]

POPULATION GROUPS	NO. OF PERSONS	AGE RANGE	SEX M	SEX F	CHOLESTEROL (mg/g DRY FECES)	% DEGRADATION
Familial polyposis						
Symptomatic (FP_s)	9	12-51	5	4	13.29 ($\pm$ 1.65)	20.4[a] ($\pm$ 8.1)
Asymptomatic (FP_a)						
Low converters	5	17-46	3	2	12.85 ($\pm$ 2.83)	11.2[a] ($\pm$ 5.8)
High converters	9	12-23	5	4	1.6 ($\pm$ 0.23)	90.2 ($\pm$ 2.8)
Familial colon cancer						
Symptomatic (FCC_s)	5	31-59	1	4	16.42 ($\pm$ 1.97)	32.6[a]1 ($\pm$ 7.7)
Asymptomatic (FCC_a)						
Low converters	9	7-43	2	7	15.34 ($\pm$ 1.87)	25.1[a] ($\pm$ 5.6)
High converters	4	23-59	1	3	3.92 ($\pm$ 1.88)	82.4 ($\pm$ 6.7)
Normal subjects	31	10-62	17	14	3.2 ($\pm$ 0.50)	84.9 ($\pm$ 2.2)

Source: After M. Lipkin, B.S. Reddy, J. Weisberger, and L. Schechter. Nondegradation of fecal cholesterol in subjects at high risk for cancer of the large intestine. *J. Clin. Invest.* 67:304-307, 1981.
[a] Average values ($\pm$ SE) of cholesterol and degradation products in each population group are shown. In the last column for each population group, the average percent degradation is shown where a given patient's percent degradation is defined as degradation products divided by total neutral sterols $\times$ 100. Superscript[a] indicates that the percent degradation of cholesterol in the group differs significantly from the controls ($p < .001$) with the student test. A tentative lower limit of 60% for degradation of cholesterol in the control group has been derived from the mean value minus two standard deviations. Low converters have been defined as having percent degradation below 60% and high converters as having values above.

fecal microflora in members of familial polyposis aggregates when compared to age- and sex-matched controls who have consumed similar western-style diets. Differences in metabolic activity of fecal microflora have previously been shown in population groups at increased risk for large bowel neoplasia.[58, 59] Thus, newer studies are also in progress to extend these findings to persons in the familial colon-cancer-prone groups, in order to further assess the usefulness of these variations in metabolic activity of fecal microflora and in cholesterol and its metabolites.

Recently, an additional and potentially important lead to the identification of factors involved in colon-cancer development was provided by detection of mutagenic activity in the feces of humans.[63] Studies of this type have analyzed mutagenic activity with the well-known Ames assay.[64] Wilkins et al. had shown that fecal specimens from the population of the United States were more mutagenic than those from South-African blacks.[65] Bruce and Dion have also described how much of the mutagenic activity in humans, as detected with the Ames test, is due to the presence of a single compound.[66]

Table 7-6. Fecal Mutagens in High-Risk Populations

POPULATIONS GROUPS	NO. OF PERSONS	AGE	NO. WITH HIGH ACTIVITY		ELEVATED MUTAGENIC RATIOS			
			M	F	TA 98	98 S	100	100 S
Familial polyposis								
Symptomatic (FP$_s$)	11	22	1			2		
Asymptomatic (FP$_a$)	8							
Familial colon cancer								
Symptomatic (FCC$_s$)	2	70	1					2
Asymptomatic (FCC$_a$)	27	39		1	2.4	1.5		
		60		1				2
		28	1				>9	
		63		1	1.9			
		41	1		2.1			
		36		1	2.3			
		41	1		3.2		2.6	2.2
		28	1		2.3			1.9
Normal subjects	9			1		2.4		

Source: Data from study in progress by T.D. Wilkins and M. Lipkin.

Recent findings on fecal-mutagenic activity in subjects with familial polyposis and familial colon cancer without polyposis are shown in Table 7-6.[67] Findings have not thus far revealed striking differences between high-risk groups and controls, and larger numbers of subjects are being studied. Thus, in addition to the evaluation of cellular and secretory parameters, a variety of approaches to the analysis of fecal contents of persons in high and low-risk groups for cancer of the large intestine are under way.

DEVELOPMENT OF RISK-FACTOR PROFILES

These current findings have led to the development of the risk-factor profiles previously described characterizing the first of the high-risk populations with increased susceptibility to colorectal cancer.[68] Further risk-factor profiles are being developed for the other population groups with increased susceptibility to cancer of the large intestine.

In current measurements, we are carrying out multivariate analyses of these various risk factors in subjects who have been affected by cancer and in those who are unaffected and at high risk in the population groups just described. Simultaneous measurements are underway in subjects whose families have been cancer-free for two or more generations as well as others in the general population. Dietary and related variables are being analyzed. We are attempting to determine whether these findings represent general trends within the high-risk population groups or whether any of them may be an absolute marker for identifying persons destined to develop cancer of the large intestine. In this context, subjects in these populations, in whom neoplastic lesions occur at early ages, are being identified for future prospective analyses. A concurrent program of long-term surveillance of these persons is also being developed.

REFERENCES

1. Bussey, H.J.R.: *Familial Polyposis Coli.* Baltimore, MD: The John Hopkins University Press, 1975.
2. Lipkin, M.; Scherf, S.; Schechter, L.; and Braun, D., Jr.: Memorial Hospital registry of populations at high risk for cancer of the large intestine: Age of onset of neoplasms. *Prev. Med.* **9:**3, 1980.
3. Lipkin, M.: Biology of large bowel cancer. *Cancer* **36:**2319, 1975.
4. Knudsen, A.G., Jr.: Genetic and environmental interactions in the origin of human cancer. In: *Genetics of Human Cancer* (Mulvihill, J.J.; Miller, R.W.; and Fraumeni, J.F. eds.). New York, NY: Raven Press, 1977, pp. 391-399.
5. Fraumeni, J.F.: Clinical patterns of familial cancer. In: *Genetics of Human Cancer* (Mulvihill, J.J.; Miller, R.W.; and Fraumeni, J.F. eds.). New York, NY: Raven Press, 1977, pp. 223-233.
6. Gardner, E.J.: A genetic and clinical study of intestinal polyposis, a predisposing factor for carcinoma of the colon and rectum. *Am. J. Hum. Genet.* **3:**167, 1951.
7. Devic, A., and Bussy, M.: Un cas de polypose adenomateuse generalisee a tout l'intestin. *Arch. Mal. App. Dig.* **6:**278-289, 1912.
8. Cabot, R.C.: Case records of the Massachusetts General Hospital, case no. 21061. *N. Engl. J. Med.* **212:**263, 1935.
9. Fitzgerald, G.M.: Multiple composite odontomas coincidental with other tumorous conditions: report of a case. *J. Am. Dent. Assn.* **30:**1408, 1943.
10. Gardner, E.J., and Plenk, H.P.: Hereditary pattern for multiple osteomas in a family group. *Am. J. Hum. Genet.* **4:**31, 1952.
11. Smith, W.G.: Desmoid tumors in familial multiple polyposis. *Mayo Clin. Proc.* **34:**31, 1959.
12. Turcot, J.; Despres, J.P.; and Pierre, F.: Malignant tumors of the central nervous system associated with familial polyposis of the colon. *Dis. Colon Rect.* **2:**465, 1959.
13. Jeghers, H.; McKusick, V.A.; and Katz, K.H.: Generalized intestinal polyposis and melanin spots of the oral mucosa, lips and digits. *N. Engl. J. Med.,* **241:**993, 1949.

14. Smilow, P.C.; Pryor, C.A., Jr.; and Swinton, N.W.: Juvenile polyposis coli: A report of three patients in three generations of one family. *Dis. Colon Rect.* **9:**248, 1966.

15. Mulvihill, J.J.: Congenital and genetic disease. In: *Persons at High Risk for Cancer: An Approach for Cancer Etiology and Control* (Fraumeni, J.F., Jr., ed.). New York: NY: Academic Press, 1975, pp. 3-35.

16. Mulvihill, J.J.: Host factors in human lung tumors: an example of ecogenetics in oncology. *J. Natl. Cancer Inst.* **57:**3, 1976.

17. Lovett, E.: Family studies in cancer of the colon and rectum. *Intern. J. Surg.* **63:**13, 1976.

18. Anderson, D.E., and Romsdahl, M.D.: Family history: A criterion for selective screening. In: *Genetics of Human Cancer* (Mulvihill, J.J.; Miller, R.W.; and Fraumeni, J.F., Jr., eds.). New York, NY: Raven Press, 1977, pp. 257-262.

19. Lynch, H.T.: *Cancer Genetics.* Springfield, ILL.: Charles C Thomas, Co., 1976.

20. Anderson, D.E.: *Proceedings of the 23rd Annual Symposium of Fundamental Cancer Research,* 1970, pp. 85-109.

21. Warthin, A.S.: Heredity with reference to carcinoma as shown by the study of the cases examined in the pathological laboratory of the University of Michigan, 1895-1913. *Arch. Int. Med.* **12:**546, 1925.

22. Warthin, A.S.: The further study of a cancer family. *J. Cancer Res.* **9:**279, 1925.

23. Lynch, H.T., and Lynch, P.M.: Heredity and gastrointestinal tract cancer. In: *Gastrointestinal Tract Cancer* (Lipkin, M., and Good, R.A., eds.). New York, NY: Plenum Publishing Corporation, 1978.

24. Woolf, C.M.; Richards, R.C.; and Gardner, E.J.: Occasional discrete polyps of colon and rectum showing inherited tendency in kindred. *Cancer* **8:**403, 1955.

25. Morson, B.C., and Bussey, J.R.: Predisposing causes of intestinal cancer. *Curr. Probl. Surg.* Feb, 1970.

26. Correa, P., and Haenszel, W.: Epidemiology of large bowel cancer. *Adv. Cancer Res.* **26:**1, 1978.

27. Haenszel, W., and Correa, P.: Cancer of the colon and rectum and adenomatous polyps. *Cancer* **28:**14, 1971.

28. Sato, E.; Ouchi, A.; Sasano, N.; and Ishidate, T.: Polyps and diverticulosis of large bowel in autopsy population of Akita Prefecture, compared with Miyagi. High risk for colorectal cancer in Japan. *Cancer* **37:**1316, 1976.

29. Ekelund, G., and Lindstrom, C.: Histopathological analysis of benign polyps in patients with carcinoma of the colon and rectum. *Gut* **15:**654, 1974.

30. Stemmermann, G.N., and Yatani, R.: Diverticulosis and polyps of the large intestine: a necropsy study of Hawaii Japanese. *Cancer* **31:**1260, 1973.

31. DeDombal, F.T.; Watts, J.; Watkinson, G.; and Goligher, J.C.: Local complications of ulcerative colitis; stricture, pseudopolyposis, and carcinoma of the colon and rectum. *Br. Med. J.* **1:**1442, 1966.

32. Edwards, F.C., and Truelove, S.C.: The course and prognosis of ulcerative colitis. III Complications. *Gut* **5:**1, 1964.

33. Lightdale, C.J.; Strenberg, S.S.; Posner, J.B.; and Sherlock, P.: Carcinoma complicating Crohn's disease. *Am. J. Med.* **59:**262, 1975.

34. Karlin, D.A., and Kirsner, J.B.: Premalignant diseases of the colon and rectum. In: *Carcinomas of the Colon and Rectum* (Enker, W.L., ed.). Chicago, IL: Year Book Medical Publishers, 1978.

35. Deschner, E.E.; Lewis, C.M.; and Lipkin, M.: *In vitro* study of human rectal epithelial cells. I. Atypical zone of H_3 thymidine incorporation in mucosa of multiple polyposis. *J. Clin. Invest.* **42:**1922, 1963.

36. Cole, J.W., and McKalen, A.: Studies on the morphogenesis of adenomatous polyps in the human colon. *Cancer* **16:**998, 1963.

37. Deschner, E.E., and Lipkin, M.: Study of human rectal epithelial cells *in vitro*. III. RNA, protein, and DNA synthesis in polyps and adjacent mucosa. *J. Natl. Cancer Inst.* **44:**175, 1970.

38. Iwana, T.; Utsunomiya, J.; and Sasaki, J.: Epithelial cell kinetics in the crypts of familial polyposis of the colon. *Jpn. J. Surg.* **7:**230, 1977.

39. Bleiberg, H.; Mainguet, P.; and Galand, P.: Cell renewal in familial polyposis: comparison between polyps and adjacent healthy mucosa. *Gastroenterology* **63:**240, 1972.

40. Lipkin, M.: Phase 1 and phase 2 proliferative lesions of colonic epithelial cells in diseases leading to colon cancer. *Cancer* **34:**878, 1974.

41. Lipkin, M.: Susceptibility of human population groups to colon cancer. *Adv. Cancer Res.* **27:**281, 1978.

42. Lipkin, M.: Growth kinetics of normal and premalignant gastrointestinal epithelium. In: *Growth Kinetics and Biochemical Regulation of Normal and Malignant Cells* (Drwinko, B., and Humphreys, R.M., eds.). Baltimore, MD: Williams & Wilkins Co., 1977, pp. 562-589.

43. Bussey, H.J.R.: *Familial Polyposis Coli.* Baltimore, MD: The Johns Hopkins University Press, 1975, p. 104.

44. Thurnherr, N.; Deschner, E.E.; Stonehill, E.; and Liplin, M.: Induction of adenocarcinomas of the colon in mice by weekly injections of 1, 2-dimethylhydrazine. *Cancer Res.* **33:**940, 1973.

45. Kikkawa, N.: Experimental studies on polypogenesis of the large intestine. *Med. J. Osaka Univ.* **24:**293, 1974.

46. Chang, W.W.L.: Histogenesis of sym. 1-2 DMH-induced neoplasms of the colon in the mouse. *J. Natl. Cancer Inst.* **60:**1405, 1978.

47. Deschner, E.E. and Long, F.C.: Colonic neoplasms in mice produced with six injections of 1, 2-dimethylhydrazine. *Oncology* **34:**255, 1977.

48. Eastwood, G.L., and Trier, J.S.: Epithelial cell renewal in cultured rectal biopsies in ulcerative colitis. *Gastroenterology* **64:**383, 1973.

49. Winawer, S., and Lipkin, M.: Cell proliferation kinetics in the gastrointestinal tract of man. IV. Cell renewal in intestinalized gastric mucosa. *J. Natl. Cancer Inst.* **42:**9, 1969.

50. Deschner, E.E.; Winawer, S.; and Lipkin, M.: Patterns of nucleic acid and protein synthesis in normal human gastric mucosa and atrophic gastritis. *J. Natl. Cancer Inst.* **48:**1567, 1972.

51. Deschner, E.E.; Tamura, K.; and Bralow, S.P.: Early proliferative changes in rat pyloric mucosa induced with N-methyl-N-nitro-N-nitrosoguanidine. *Frontiers Gastrointest. Res.* **4:**25-31, 1979.

52. Wilbanks, G.D.; Richart, R.M.; and Terner, J.Y.: DNA content of cervical intraepithelial neoplasm studied by two-wave length Feulgen cytophotometry. *Am. J. Obstet. Gynecol.* **98:**792, 1967.

53. Hasegawa, I.; Matsumira, Y.; and Tojo, S.: Cellular kinetics and histological changes in experimental cancer of the uterine cervix. *Cancer* **36:**359, 1976.

54. Maskins, A.P.: Histogenesis and growth patterns of 1, 2-dimethylhydrazine-induced rat colon adenocarcinoma. *Cancer Res.* **36:**1585, 1976.

55. Danes, B.: Brief communication: The Gardner syndrome: A family study in cell culture. *J. Natl. Cancer Inst.* **58:**771, 1977.

56. Kopelovich, L.; Lipkin, M.; Blattner, W.; Fraumeni, J.F., Jr.; Lynch, H.; and Pollack, R.: Organization of actin-containing cables in cultured skin fibroblasts from individuals at high risk of colon cancer. *Intern. J. Cancer* **26:**301. 1980.

57. Berlinger, N.T.; Lopez, C.; Vogel, J.; Lipkin, M.; and Good, R.A.: Defective recognitive immunity in family aggregates of colon carcinoma. *J. Clin. Invest.* **59:**761, 1977.

58. Drasar, B.S.; Bone, E.S.; Hill, M.F.; and Marks, C.G.: Colon cancer and bacterial metabolism in familial polyposis. *Gut* **16:**824, 1975.

59. Reddy, B.S.; Mastromarino, A.; Gustafson, C.; Lipkin, M.; and Wynder, E.L.: Fecal bile acids and neutral sterols in patients with familial polyposis. *Cancer* **34:**1694, 1976.

60. Watne, P.L.; Lai, H.L.; Mance, T.; and Core, S.: Fecal steroids and bacterial flora in polyposis coli patients. *Am. J. Surg.* **131:**42, 1976.

61. Lipkin, M.; Reddy, B.S.; Weisburger, J.; and Schechter, L.: Nondegradation of fecal cholesterol in subjects at high risk for cancer of the large intestine. *J. Clin. Invest.* **67:**304-307, 1981.

62. Wilkins, T.D., and Hackman, A.S.: Two patterns of neutral steroid conversion in the feces of normal North Americans. *Cancer Res.* **34:**2250, 1974.

63. Varghese, A.J.; Land, P.; Furrer, R.; and Bruce, W.R.: Proc. 68th annual meeting, *Am. Assn. Cancer Res.* **18:**317, 1977.

64. Ames, B.N.; McCann, J.; and Yamasaki, E.: Method of detecting carcinogens and mutagens with the Salmonella/Mammalian-microsome mutagenicity test. *Mutat. Res.* **31:**347, 1975.

65. Wilkins, T.D.; Lederman, M; and Van Tassel, R.L.: Isolation of a mutagen producer in the human colon by bacterial action. In: *Banbury Report 7, Gastrointestinal Cancer* (Bruce, W.R.; Correa, P.; Lipkin, M.; Tannenbaum, S.; and Wilkins, T.D., eds.). Cold Spring Harbor, NY: Cold Spring Harbor Laboratory Publications, 1981.

66. Bruce, W.R., and Dion, P.: Studies related to a fecal mutagen. *Am. J. Clin. Nutr.* **33:**2511, 1980.

67. Lipkin, M., and Wilkins, T.D.: Unpublished observations.

68. Lipkin, M.; Sherlock, P.; and DeCosse, J.: *Risk Factors and Preventive Measures in the Control of Cancer of the Large Intestine. Current Problems in Cancer 4.* No. 10. Chicago, IL: Medical Publishers Year Book, 1980, pp. 1-57.

69. Reddy, B.S.; Weisburger, J.; and Wynder, E.L.: Effects of high risk and low risk diets for colon carcinogenesis on fecal microflora and steroids in man. *J. Nutr.* **105:**878, 1975.

70. Hill, M.J.: The role of colon anaerobes in the metabolism of bile acids and steroids, and its relation to colon cancer. *Cancer* **36:**2387, 1975.

71. Gardner, E.J., and Richards, R.C.: Multiple cutaneous and subcutaneous lesions occurring simultaneously with hereditary polyposis and osteomatosis. *Am. J. Hum. Genet.* **5:**139, 1953.

72. Tannenbaum, S.R.; Fett, D.; Young, V.R.; Land, P.D.; and Bruce, W.R.: Nitrite and nitrate are formed by endogenous synthesis in human intestine. *Science* **200:**1487, 1978.

73. Morson, B.C., and Bussey, H.J.R.: Predisposing causes of intestinal cancer. *Curr. Probl. Surg.* 1970.

74. Lane, N., and Lev, R.: Observations on the origin of adenomatous epithelium of the colon: Serial reaction studies of minute polyps in familial polyposis. *Cancer* **16:**751, 1963.

75. Utsunomiya, J.; Iwana, T.; Ichikawa, T.; Maki, T.; Miyanga, T.; and Hirayama, T.: Present studies of familial polyposis of the colon in Japan. In: *Pathophysiology of Carcinogenesis in Digestive Organs* (Farber, E. et al., eds.) Tokyo, Japan: University of Tokyo Press, 1977, pp. 305-321.

76. Lipkin, M.; Deschner, E.; Blattner, W.; Fraumeni, J.F., Jr.; and Lynch, H.: Tritiated thymidine incorporation into colonic epithelial cells of subjects in colon cancer-prone families. *Proc. Am. Assn. Cancer Res.* **21:**188, 1980.

77. Lipkin, M.; Winawer, S.J.; and Sherlock, P.: Early identification of individuals at increased risk for cancer of the large intestine. Part II: Development of risk factor profiles. *Clin. Bull.* **11:**66, 1981.

8
In Vitro Family Studies of Heritable Colon Cancer

B. Shannon Danes, M.D., Ph.D.,
Thor Alm, M.D., Steffen Bulow, M.D.,
and Lars Bo Svendsen, M.D.

Hereditary cancer syndromes have provided indisputable evidence for the role of heredity in the etiology of some forms of cancer. In the majority of cancer cases, however, hereditary factors are not apparent in the etiology and are the subjects of controversy. Much of this stems from our inability to detect genetic predisposition (germinal or somatic mutations) to different cancers before their clinical expression.

Since a person's somatic cells all have the same genome (i.e., genetic information) then any cell, irrespective of its *in vivo* expression, could express such cancer-prone mutations *in vitro*. If such cellular changes occur solely or more frequently in cells cultured from affecteds and persons at risk than from matched controls, then identification of increased cancer risk before clinical expression would be possible.

The family unit contains members who share genes and members by marriage who do not, living under the same or different cultural-environmental conditions. Consequently, to employ the family approach involves finding enough members in consecutive generations who are willing to participate; thoroughly describing, and accurately, the clinical phenotype of each affected member within each family; and collecting, using interdisciplinary expertise, family data, clinical evaluation, and laboratory techniques to study the expression of the cancer genotype of such families.

Families with heritable cancer syndromes such as those involving the colon offer models for studying the nature of such genetic expression (i.e., cancer cell phenotypes) and the operation of trigger mechanisms for gene expression.

HERITABLE COLON CANCER SYNDROMES

Two common features of the heritable colon cancer (HCC) syndromes are autosomal-dominant mode of inheritance, and colonic adenocarcinomas with or without colonic polyposis (single, multiple, or adenomatosis).

On clinical evaluations (based on colonoscopy, histopathological examination, skeletal survey, dermatological evaluations, and physical examination) and family pedigree data derived from medical records and parish registers, the HCC syndromes have been divided into the following groups: (1) those with only colonic lesions (familial polyposis coli [FPC])[1] and discrete colonic adenomas;[2] (2) those also having extracolonic lesions (Gardner's syndrome [GS],[3] Oldfield syndrome [OS],[4] and Turcot's syndrome [TS];[5] and (3) those with heritable colon cancer without polyposis coli (HCC).[6, 7]

IN VITRO METHODOLOGY

Establishment of Cultures

Skin biopsies were obtained from each family member studied. A coded number was assigned to each biopsy—the only identification used until studies were completed. Skin cultures were established from these split-thickness biopsies by standard culture methods (Fig. 8-1).[8, 9] Cultures were grown in Falcon plastic petri dishes in Eagle's Minimal Essential Medium (MEM) with 20% (vol) fetal calf serum in an atmosphere of 5% CO_2 in air. To enhance the migration of epithelial cells from the dermis, a minimum amount of medium (approximately 1 ml—just enough to cover the biopsy and floor of the culture dish) was used in the first culture weeks. The pH of the medium was kept between 7 and 7.4 during the culture period. After two culture weeks, the initial explant culture was examined microscopically to verify that both sheets of epithelial cells, presumably from the epidermis, and fibroblasts from the dermis were present in the migration zone surrounding the explant. The cells were then dispersed by a 5- to 10 minute exposure to a solution of 0.05% trypsin and 0.02% versene in calcium-magnesium-free saline at 37°C to obtain subcultures. Cultures were routinely checked for bacterial and mycoplasma contamination.

In Vitro Tetraploidy

Only explant cultures containing epithelium before the first subculture were included as it had been determined that increased tetraploidy was observed only in cultures containing epithelium.[10] Cells were grown in culture for 4 to 29 weeks (two to ten subcultures after the primary explant culture) before mitotic activity was studied. *In vitro* tetraploidy had been demonstrated to be an *in vitro* phenomenon, and false, negative results might have been recorded if the occurrence of *in vitro* tetraploidy had been determined solely before the fifteenth culture week after the establishment of the primary explant culture (Table 8-1).[11]

Chromosome preparations were made and evaluated for the occurrence

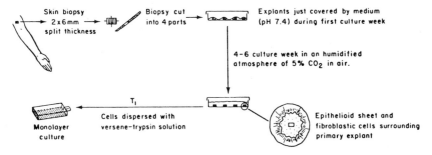

Figure 8-1. Methodology used in the establishment of monolayer (mixed fibroblastic and epithelioid) cultures from human skin biopsies. *(From H. T. Lynch, W.A. Albano, B.S. Danes, J. Lynch, and P.M. Lynch. Precursor conditions and monitoring of high colon cancer risk patients. In: Gastrointestinal Cancer. J.R. Stroehlein and M.M. Romsdahl, eds. New York: Raven Press, 1981, p. 303. Copyright © 1981 by Raven Press.)*

Table 8-1. Occurrence of Increased In Vitro Tetraploidy in Cultures Established from Skin Biopsies Taken From 20 Patients with FPC, 10 Patients with GS, and 8 Normals [a]

	PRESENCE OF INCREASED IN VITRO TETRAPLOIDY[a]			
		WEEKS IN CULTURE		
	PERSONS STUDIED	4-9	9-15	15-29
Normals	8	−	−	−
GS	2	−	+	+
	8	+	+	+
FPC	1	+	+	+
	1	−	+	+
	18	−	−	−

[a]Range of tetraploidy in cultures derived from normals not-at-risk: 0-7%. Increased tetraploidy: + = present; − = absent.

of tetraploidy for each culture during three culture periods (4-9, 9-15, and 15-29 wk in culture). For such preparations, cells were dispersed into suspension, approximately 10^4 cells in 5 ml of medium without antibiotics inoculated into small, Falcon petri dishes and incubated in an atmosphere of 5% CO_2 in air. After 48 hours, when a burst of mitosis was observed, chromosome preparations were made with and without the addition of colchicine and stained in aceto-orcein.

Two slides of each preparation were made on two different cultures of each subculture examined. Mitoses on the entire slide were examined, as it was found that bias could be introduced if only part of a slide was studied. Since it was considered that a slide had to contain 100 mitoses to reflect the mitotic activity of a culture, slides with less than 100 mitoses were not included.

The occurrence (%) of tetraploidy in a culture was expressed as the number of metaphases showing tetraploidy divided by the total number of metaphases counted.

Assays of Growth Properties

Cells were grown in culture 15 to 25 weeks (five to nine subcultures after the primary explant culture) before growth assays were performed.

Serum Requirement for Growth

Subcultures, grown to confluency in petri dishes, were dispersed to obtain single-cell suspensions. Each cell sample was plated at an initial cell concentration of 1×10^4 into duplicate 28 cm² Falcon petri dishes containing medium with either 15% or 1% (vol) fetal calf serum. The medium was changed every third day, and each culture examined microscopically for a 14-day culture period.

Density-Dependent Regulation of Growth in Subconfluent and Confluent Monolayers

Each cell sample was plated at an initial cell concentration of 1×10^3, 1×10^4, and 1×10^5 into duplicate 28 cm² Falcon petri dishes containing medium with 15% (vol) fetal calf serum. The medium was changed after the first culture day and then every third day for 21 days. Cell counts were done daily using a Coulter counter on duplicate cell samples from single petri dish cultures. In addition, cell samples were counted in hemocytometer chambers on days 1, 7, 14, and 21 for technical verification of cell counts. Generation time was determined from the slope of logarithmic growth curve in the density ranges 0.04 to 0.4, 0.4 to 4.0, and 4.0 to 40.0 $\times 10^3$ cells/cm² growth area before saturation density. Influence of cell density on cell growth was expressed as a ratio of generation time in two density ranges.

$$\left(\frac{\text{g.t. at } 4.0\text{-}40.0 \times 10^3 \text{ cells/cm}^2}{\text{g.t. at } 0.4\text{-}4.0 \times 10^3 \text{ cells/cm}^2} \right)$$

Saturation density was the equilibrium density that the cells maintained for the last 3 to 4 days of the growth experiment.[12] Each time a cell count was done or the medium changed, the morphological appearance of the monolayer was examined for random arrangement of cells (crisscrossing and multilayering). These evaluations were done independently by several investigators for objectivity.

Anchorage Requirement for Growth

Cells were plated in 1 ml of medium containing 1.2% methylcellulose at densities of 1×10^3, 1×10^4, and 1×10^5 cells per 28 cm^2 in a plastic culture dish over an underlay of 0.9% agarose in the same culture medium in duplicate cultures. Cultures were fed with an additional 1 ml of methocel medium at weekly intervals for 7 weeks. Growth was based on the increase in size of colonies measured microscopically by use of an eyepiece reticle.

Tumorigenicity

Washed cells at 2×10^6, suspended in 0.2 ml of phosphate-buffered saline, were injected at a single subcutaneous site into the dorsum of a male, congenitally athymic BABL/c nu/nu 4 to 8-week-old mouse. Treated mice were checked weekly for tumor development over a 6-month period.

IN VITRO OBSERVATIONS

Occurrence of *In Vitro* Tetraploidy

Increased tetraploidy has been observed in normal and tumor tissues.[13-16] Colonic adenomas without evidence of neoplastic changes from GS patients have been reported to show chromosome abnormalities including tetraploidy.[17] *In vitro,* the human cell maintains a stable diploid karyotype with from 1 to 7% tetraploid cells observed in skin cultures (see Fig. 8-2).[10, 18-20]

Increased tetraploidy appeared to be an *in vitro* rather than *in vivo* phenomenon since occurrence of tetraploidy was constant in cultures derived from some persons in the first subculture, but in cultures from other persons, the occurrence of tetraploidy increased during the first 15 culture weeks after initiation of the explant culture (Table 8-1).[11] The occurrence of tetraploidy in all subcultures derived from a single explant culture was similar (Table 8-2).[8, 20, 21] False, negative results could have been recorded if the occurrence of *in vitro* tetraploidy was determined only before the fifteenth culture week.[11] Therefore, chromosome preparations were made

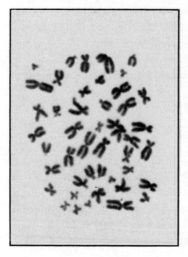 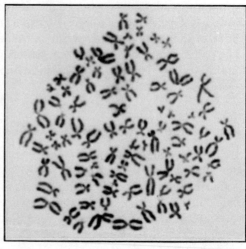

DIPLOID   TETRAPLOID

Figure 8-2. Metaphase preparations of cells having diploid and tetraploid chromosome complements from a monolayer skin culture derived from a GS affected.

during three culture periods (4-9, 9-15, and 15-29 wk in culture). Ingredients of the culture medium such as serum from different species has been known to influence stability of chromosomes.[22] For this reason, fetal calf serum has been used in both primary and monolayer cultures.

Culture conditions that did not influence the occurrence of tetraploidy were variations in the pH of the medium in the acid of alkaline ranges; presence of chronic mycoplasm (*M. hyorhinis*) infection; and presence in the medium of a mitotic inhibitor, colchicine, for 1 to 3 hours before chromosome preparations. The age or sex of the skin donor irrespective of genotype did not influence the presence of tetraploidy. (Fig. 8-3).[23]

Normals (Family Members by Marriage)

The occurrence of tetraploidy in dermal cultures established from 90 (aged 9-73) of the 97 normals was 0 to 7% (Fig. 8-4). The percentage of cells showing tetraploidy was approximately the same in all subcultures established from a single biopsy from all of these normals, and stayed within this range through 29 culture weeks. Age (Fig. 8-3) and sex of the normal skin

Table 8-2. Percentage of Dividing Cells Showing Tetraploidy in Subcultures Derived from Separate Skin Biopsies Taken from Each of Two GS Affecteds and Two FPC Affecteds over a 2-year Period

PATIENT	YEAR BIOPSY TAKEN AND SUB-CULTURES ESTABLISHED	SN^a	1	2	3	4	5
			PERCENTAGE OF DIVIDING CELLS SHOWING TETRAPLOIDY^b SUBCULTURES ESTABLISHED FROM PRIMARY EXPLANT CULTURE				
GS #1	1978	4	10	9	11	14	10
		10	12	10	11	15	14
	1979	6	11	14	9	15	12
		12	16	12	12	15	10
GS #2	1978	5	17	19	19	21	22
		18	15	22	24	20	18
	1979	6	22	27	29	22	20
		20	20	29	32	20	18
FPC #1	1978	4	1	0	1	1	0
		20	1	1	0	0	0
	1979	7	2	2	2	1	2
		18	1	1	2	1	0
FPC #2	1978	5	3	2	2	3	0
		20	2	2	2	0	3
	1979	8	0	0	1	1	0
		22	1	0	2	0	0

^{a}SN = subculture number after establishment of primary explant culture
^{b}Based on number of metaphases showing tetraploidy divided by total number of metaphases scored blind on slides having at least 100 divisions

donor did not influence the occurrence of tetraploidy. Cultures from the other 7 normals (aged 16-53) showed increased tetraploidy (8-19%). Cultures established from a second biopsy from each of these normals showed approximately the same percentage of tetraploidy. None of the 7 had a family history of colonic cancer, but 4 had a family history of other solid tumors (breast, skin, ovary, and urogenital tract).

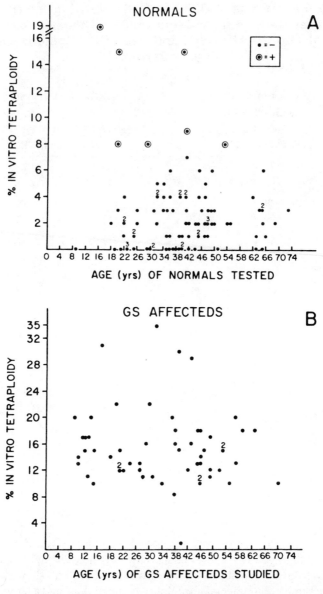

Figure 8-3.   Comparison of the occurrence of *in vitro* tetraploidy in skin cultures with the ages of the donors of skin biopsies from which the cultures were derived. (A) 97 normals from age 9-74; (B) 57 clinically affected GS patients from age 10-70. *(From B.S. Danes. Occurrence of in vitro tetraploidy in the heritable colon cancer syndromes. Cancer 48:1597, 1599, 1981.)*

NORMALS STUDIED

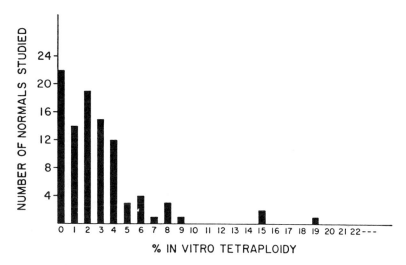

Figure 8-4.   **Percentage of dividing cells showing tetraploidy in cultures from skin biopsies from 97 normals (family members by marriage without a family history of colon cancer).** *(From B. S. Danes. Occurrence of in vitro tetraploidy in the heritable colon cancer syndrome. Cancer 48:1597, 1981.)*

Familial Polyposis Coli

Cultures established from 28 FPC affecteds from 16 of the 19 FPC families studied (Fig. 8-5A) showed no increased tetraploidy (0-7%). Of the 14 family members at increased risk from 8 of these FPC families, none showed increased tetraploidy (0-7%) (Fig. 8-5B). Cultures established from 5 affecteds from 3 families with FPC, who were clinically indistinguishable from the other FPC affecteds studied, showed increased tetraploidy (8-14%) (Fig. 8-5A). Of the 6 family members at increased risk from 2 of these FPC families, 3 had increased *in vitro* tetraploidy (10%, 11%, and 18%) and 3 did not (1%, 3%, and 7%) (Fig. 8-5B).

Familial Colon Cancer in Association with Discrete Polyps

In the 3 families studied (Figs. 8-6), the cultures from the 3 affecteds showed increased tetraploidy (9-13%). Of the 4 at-risk family members studied, 1 affected showed increased *in vitro* tetraploidy (11%) and 3 did not (0-4%).

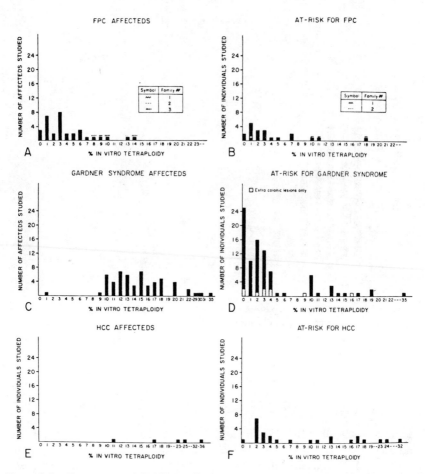

Figure 8-5. Percentage of dividing cells showing tetraploidy in cultures derived from skin biopsies from (A) 33 clinically affected FPC patients; (B) 20 at-risk members from 19 FPC families; (C) 57 clinically affected GS patients; (D) 91 at-risk members from 16 GS families; (E) 5 clinically affected HCC patients and (F) 26 at-risk members from 4 HCC families. *(From B. S. Danes. Occurrence of in vitro tetraploidy in the heritable colon cancer syndromes. Cancer 48:1598, 1981.)*

Gardner's Syndrome

In the 16 GS families studied (Figs. 8-5C and D), increased *in vitro* tetraploidy (9-35%) was observed in cultures from 56 of the 57 GS affecteds. One affected male, aged 40, who had all the clinical stigmata of GS but whose family history was unknown, did not have increased *in vitro* tetraploidy (1%). Cultures derived from a second biopsy obtained two years later showed a

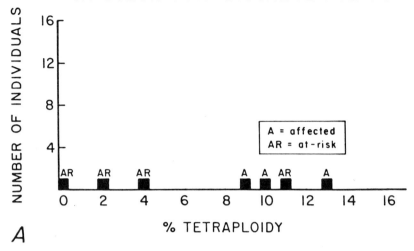

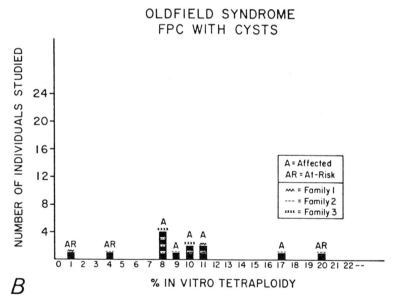

Figure 8-6.   Percentage of dividing cells showing tetraploidy in cultures derived from skin biopsies from (A) 3 clinically affected patients and 4 members at risk for HCC in association with discrete polyps in 3 families and (B) 10 clinically affected patients and 3 members at risk for OS in 3 OS families studied. *(From B. S. Danes. Occurrence of in vitro tetraploidy in the heritable colon cancer syndromes. Cancer 48:1600, 1981.)*

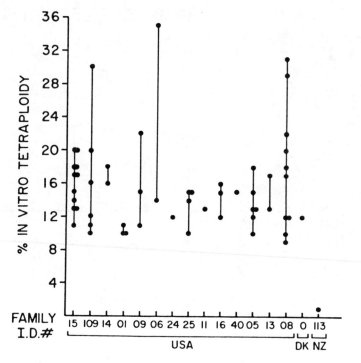

Figure 8-7. The ranges of *in vitro* tetraploidy in skin cultures derived from 57 affected members within 16 GS families studied. *(From B. S. Danes. Occurrence of in vitro tetraploidy in the heritable colon cancer syndromes. Cancer 48:1600, 1981.)*

similar percentage of tetraploid mitoses. Of the 91 family members at risk from 15 unrelated GS families (Fig. 8-5D), 18 showed increased *in vitro* tetraploidy (9-35%) and 73 did not (0-6%). The ranges of *in vitro* tetraploidy within each of the 15 GS families with increased *in vitro* tetraploidy were similar (Fig. 8-7).

Oldfield Syndrome

In the 3 families with OS (Fig. 8-6B), all 10 affecteds showed increased *in vitro* tetraploidy (8-17%). Of the 3 at-risk members from 2 OS families studied, 1 showed increased tetraploidy (20%) and 2 did not (1%, 4%).

Turcot's Syndrome

Two TS affecteds studied did not show increased *in vitro* tetraploidy (0%, 1%).

HCC Syndrome without Polyposis

In the 4 HCC families studied (Figs. 8-5E and F), 5 affecteds showed increased *in vitro* tetraploidy. Of the 26 members at risk from 4 HCC families studied, the cultures from 11 showed increased tetraploidy (10-32%) and 15 did not (0-7%).[24]

Assays of Growth Properties

Growth of human fibroblasts in culture has been found to be dependent on the presence of serum and nutrients and influenced by cell density and anchorage to a solid substrate. Assays of *in vitro* growth requirements have been used to identify any change in these properties. Each assay has been considered to reflect a different biological change that disrupts the regulation of *in vitro* growth.[25]

Four growth properties—lower serum requirement for growth; density-independent regulation of growth in subconfluent and confluent monolayers; anchorage dependency; and nontumorigenicity in athymic nude mice—have been observed in two laboratories for cultured FPC skin cells.[26-29] Two other properties—increased saturation density of growth and random cellular arrangement in monolayers have been reported for these cells from one of these laboratories.[26, 27]

The six syndromes studied had differences in the growth properties studied (Table 8-3). These *in vitro* assays supported the concept, long assumed on the basis of clinical differences, that they are not all due to the same mutation but, rather, represent distinct genetic entities, and that this genetic difference is detected *in vitro*.[8]

COMMENTS

Since there are no symptoms specific to HCC syndromes before clinical expression, and, from a practical standpoint, proctosigmoidoscopy is not feasible for the general population, a specific cell marker is needed to identify subjects who have a genotype for heritable colon cancer syndrome and who should receive periodic colonic examinations, and eventually, when required, preventive colonic surgery.

Identifying through cell-culture studies family members who have inherited a cancer-prone gene depends on the age at which the clinical signs are recognized within such families. In GS[3] and OS, the extracolonic expression (connective tissue growths) usually appears early in life. For example, of the 57 GS affecteds studied (Fig. 8-3B), 12 were between 8 and 18 years. As a consequence, only 18 of the 91 members at risk had increased *in vitro*

Table 8-3. Panel of Biological Properties Associated with Transformation Studied in Skin Cultures Derived from Affecteds with FPC, GS, and TS and without HCC

BIOLOGICAL PROPERTIES	PERSONS STUDIED							ASSAY PROCEDURES
	NL (−) 19 pts.	FPC (−) 9 pts.	FPC (+) 8 pts.	GS (−) 1 pts.	GS (+) 7 pts.	TS (−) 2 pts.	HCC (+) 4 pts.	
Increased *in vitro* tetraploidy	−	−	+	−	+	−	+	Danes 1976,[10] 1978[21]
Lower serum requirement for growth	+	+	−	+	−	−	+	Smith et al. 1971[30] and Holley and Kiernan 1968[31]
Density-dependent regulation of growth in subconfluent and confluent monolayers	+	−	−	+	−	+	−	Kruse and Miedema 1965[32] and Levin et al. 1965[33]
Increased saturation-density of growth	−	−	−	−	−	+	−	Todaro et al. 1964[34] and Risser and Pollack 1974[12]
Random arrangement in monolayers	+	+	+	+	+	+	+	Kruse and Miedema 1965[32] and Pfeffer et al. 1976[26]
Anchorage-independent growth	−	−	−	−	−	−	−	Macpherson and Montagnier 1965[35] and Stoker and O'Neill 1968[36]
Tumorigenic in athymic nude mice	−	−	−	−	−	−	−	Freedman and Shin 1974[37]

Abbreviations: NL = normal (family member by marriage)
FPC = familial polyposis coli
GS = Gardner's syndrome
TS = Turcot's syndrome
HCC = heritable colon cancer without polyposis coli
+ = present
− = absent

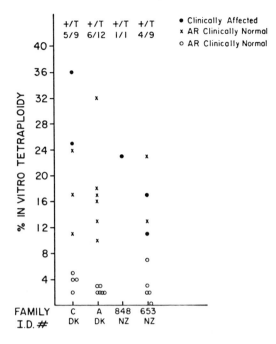

Figure 8-8.   The occurrence of *in vitro* tetraploidy in skin cultures derived from 4 HCC families clinically affected, at risk for HCC, and without increased tetraploidy. Family identification numbers were used in the clinics where the family members were seen. *(From B. S. Danes. Occurrence of in vitro tetraploidy in the heritable colon cancer syndromes. Cancer 48:1601, 1981.)*

tetraploidy (Fig. 8-5D), since the majority of those family members having the GS gene had been identified through their extracolonic lesions in the first decade of life. When the total GS affecteds with increased tetraploidy (56) were added to those detected *in vitro* (18), 74 of the total of 147 GS family members (affecteds and at risk) studied had increased *in vitro* tetraploidy— the 50% expected to have inherited the GS gene in this autosomal-dominant disorder.

However, in HCC there are no clinical signs to identify those family members who have inherited an increased risk for colonic cancer. Therefore, identification of members in such families through cell-culture studies before the disease's clinical expression as a colonic adenocarcinoma producing colonic symptoms would have clinical value. Although only 4 families have been studied (Fig. 8-8), all 5 affected and 42% (11 out of 26) of at-risk family members studied have shown increased *in vitro* tetraploidy.

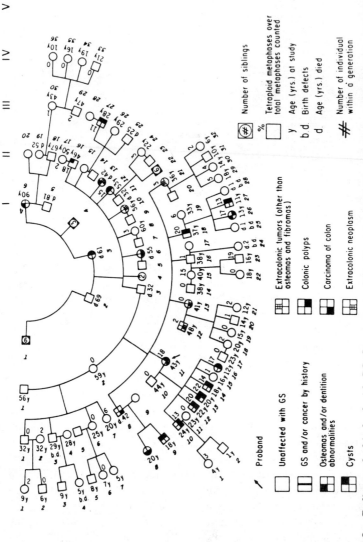

Figure 8-9. Pedigree of a kindred with GS. Occurrence of *in vitro* tetraploidy in cultures established from skin biopsies taken from 52 members of the GS kindred. Fourteen clinically affected members (11-53 yr), 8 family members at risk (4-90 yr), and 30 family members not at risk (6-59 yr). (*From B.S. Danes, T. Alm, and A.M.O. Veale. In: Colorectal Cancer: Prevention, Epidemiology, and Screening. S.J. Winawer, D. Schottenfeld, and P. Sherlock, eds. New York: Raven Press, 1980, p. 77. Copyright © 1980 by Raven Press.*)

Increased *in vitro* tetraploidy was found not to be useful in detecting the polyposis gene in the majority of FPC families. In 16 of 19 FPC families studied, none of the affecteds (28) or at-risk persons (14) showed increased *in vitro* tetraploidy. However, in those 3 FPC families in which increased *in vitro* tetraploidy *was* found in all affecteds studied (Fig. 8-5A, Table 8-3), this cellular abnormality was informative. All 19 families studied were considered to have FPC on the basis of adenomatosis of the colon without any extracolonic pathology. The finding that 3 showed increased *in vitro* tetraploidy and 16 did not, suggested that the clinical phenotype, colonic polyposis, was not the result of the same mutation, this genetic difference not being detected *in vivo,* but rather *in vitro.*

From this *in vitro* research, we concluded that abnormalities in *in vitro* biological properties (Table 8-3) should be used to detect increased risk for colonic cancer only if family studies are done to determine that all clinically affected persons show such *in vitro* abnormalities and only if vertical transmission can be documented (Fig. 8-9). Until this method of identification has been proven 100% accurate, all family members at risk, regardless of their cell-culture status, should receive close clinical observation. The significance of increased *in vitro* tetraploidy in a clinically asymptomatic family member is that the attending physician should be informed so that the member will receive appropriate cancer surveillance.

This research demonstrates that comparative studies on biological properties of cultured skin cells from members of families with HCC syndromes with and without polyposis coli reveals *in vitro* differences that should aid in the recognition of genotypes that increase the risk of colon cancer. It has been predicted that this panel (Table 8-3) will be expanded to include other biological properties already known and others yet to be associated with cellular transformation and cancer.

Acknowledgements. This research was made possible through grant CA 15973 from the National Large Bowel Cancer Project of the National Cancer Institute Division of Cancer Research and NATO Research Grant 213.82.

REFERENCES

1. Dukes, C.E.: Familial polyposis. *Ann. Eugen.* **17:**1-14, 1952.
2. Woolf, C.M.; Richards, R.C.; and Gardner, E.J.: Occasional discrete polyps of the colon and rectum showing an inherited tendency in a kindred. *Cancer* **8:**403-408, 1955.
3. Gardner, E.J.: Discovery of the Gardner syndrome. *Birth Defects: Orig. Art. Ser.* **8:**48-51, 1972.

4. Oldfield, M.C.: The association of familial polyposis of the colon with multiple sebaceous cysts. *Br. J. Surg.* **41**:534-541, 1954.

5. Turcot, J.; Despres, J.P.; and St. Pierre, F.: Malignant tumors of the central nervous system associated with familial polyposis of the colon: Report of two cases. *Dis. Colon Rect.* **2**:465-468, 1959.

6. Kluge, T.: Familial cancer of the colon. *Acta Chir. Scand.* **127**:292-398, 1964.

7. Peltokallio, P., and Peltokallio, V.: Relationship of familial factors to carcinoma of the colon. *Dis. Colon Rect.* **9**:367-370, 1966.

8. Danes, B.S., and Alm, T.: *In vitro* studies on adenomatosis of the colon and rectum. *J. Med. Genet.* **16**:417-422, 1979.

9. Lynch, H.T.; Albano, W.A.; Danes, B.S.; Lynch, J.; and Lynch, P.M.: Precursor conditions and monitoring of high colon cancer risk patients. In: *Gastrointestinal Cancer* (Stroehlein, J.R., and Romsdahl, M.M., eds.). New York, NY: Raven Press, 1981, pp. 297-325.

10. Danes, B.S.: Increased *in vitro* tetraploidy: tissue specific within the heritable colorectal cancer syndromes with polyposis coli. *Cancer* **41**:2330-2334, 1978.

11. Danes, B.S.; Alm, T.; and Veale, A.M.O.: Modifying alleles in the heritable colorectal cancer syndromes with polyps. In: *Colorectal Cancer: Prevention, Epidemiology, and Screening* (Winawer, S.J., Schottenfeld, D., and Sherlock, P. eds.). New York, NY: Raven Press, 1980, pp. 73-81.

12. Risser, R.; and Pollack, R.: A nonselective analysis of SV40 transformation of mouse 3T3 cells. *Virology* **59**:477-489, 1974.

13. Schwarzacher, H.G., and Schnedl, W.: Endoreduplication in human fibroblast cultures. *Cytogenetics* **4**:1-18, 1965.

14. Schmid, W.: Multipolar spindles after endoreduplication. *Exp. Cell Res.* **42**:201-204, 1966.

15. Levan, A., and Hauschka, T.S.: Endomitotic reduplication mechanisms in ascites tumors of the mouse. *JNCI* **14**:1-43, 1953.

16. Ising, U., and Levan, A.: The chromosomes of two highly malignant human tumors. *Acta Pathol. Microbiol. Scand.* **40**:13-24.

17. Mark, J.; Mitelman, F.; Dencker, H.; Norryd, C.; and Tranberg, K.G.: The specificity of chromosomal abnormalities in human colonic polyps. *Acta Pathol. Microbiol. Scand.* **81**:85-90, 1973.

18. Hayflick, L., and Moorhead, P.S.: The serial cultivation of human diploid cell strains. *Exp. Cell Res.* **25**:585-621, 1961.

19. Wolman, S.R.; Hirschhorn, K.; and Todaro, G.J.: Early chromosomal changes in SV40-infected human fibroblast cultures. *Cytogenetics* **3**:45-61, 1964.

20. Danes, B.S.: The Gardner syndrome: a study in cell culture. *Cancer* **36**:2327-2333, 1975.

21. Danes, B.D.: The Gardner syndrome: increased tetraploidy in cultured skin fibroblast. *J. Med. Genet.* **13**:52-56, 1976.

22. Parshad, R., and Sanford, K.K.: Effect of horse serum, fetal calf serum, bovine serum, and fetuin on neoplastic conversion and chromosomes of mouse embryo cells *in vitro. JNCI* **41**:767-779, 1968.

23. Danes, B.S.: Occurrence of *in vitro* tetraploidy in the heritable colon cancer syndromes. *Cancer* **48**:1596-1601, 1981.

24. Danes, B.S.; Bulow, S.; and Svendsen, L.B.: Hereditary colon cancer syndromes: an *in vitro* study. *Clin. Genet.* **18**:128-136, 1980.

25. Pollack, R.; Risser, R.; Conlon, S.; Freedman, V.; Shin, S. I.; and Rifkin, D.B.: Production of plasminogen activator and colonial growth in semisolid medium are *in vitro* correlates of tumorigenecity in the immune-deficient nude mouse. In: *Proteases and Biological Control,* Vol. 2 (Reich, E.; Rifkin, D.B.; and Shaw, E., eds.). Cold Spring Harbor Conference on Cell Proliferation. New York, NY: Cold Spring Harbor Laboratory, 1975, pp. 885-899.

26. Pfeffer, L.; Lipkin, M.; Stutman, O.; and Kopelovich, L.: Growth abnormalities of cultured skin fibroblasts derived from individuals with hereditary adenomatosis of the colon and rectum. *J. Cell Physiol.* **89**:29-37, 1976.

27. Kopelovich, L.; Pfeffer, L.M.; and Bias, N.: Growth characteristics of human skin fibroblasts *in vitro:* a simple experimental approach for the identification of hereditary adenomatosis of the colon and rectum. *Cancer* **43**:218-223, 1979.

28. Danes, B.S.: Heritable colonic cancer syndromes: induction of anchorage-independence in dermal cultures derived from patients with adenomatosis of the colon and rectum. *Oncology* **37**:386-389, 1980.

29. Danes, B.S., and Alm, T.: *In vitro* evidence of genetic heterogeneity within the heritable colon cancer syndromes with polyposis coli. *Scand. J. Gastroenterol.* **16**:421-427, 1981.

30. Smith, H.S.; Scher, C.D.; and Todaro, G.J.: Induction of cell division in medium lacking serum growth factor by SV40. *Virology* **44**:359-370, 1971.

31. Holley, R.W., and Kiernan, J.A.: "Contact inhibition" of cell division in 3T3 cells. *Proc. Natl. Acad. Sci. USA* **60**:300-304, 1968.

32. Kruse, P. Jr., and Miedema, E.: Production and characterization of multiple-layered populations of animal cells. *J. Cell Biol.* **27**:273-279, 1965.

33. Levine, E.M.; Becker, Y.; Boone, C.W.; and Eagle, H.: Contact inhibition, macromolecular synthesis, and polyribosomes in cultured human diploid fibroblasts. *Proc. Natl. Acad. Sci. USA* **53**:350-356, 1965.

34. Todaro, G.J.; Green, H.; and Goldberg, B.D.: Transformation of properties of an established cell line by SV40 and polyoma virus. *Proc. Natl. Acad. Sci. USA* **51**:66-73, 1964.

35. Macpherson, I., and Montagnier, L.: Agar suspension culture for selective assay of cells transformed by polyoma virus. *Virology* **23**:291-294, 1964.

36. Stoker, M., and O'Neill, C.: Anchorage and growth regulation in normal and virus-transformed cells. *Intern. J. Cancer* **3**:683-693, 1968.

37. Freedman, V.H., and Shin, S.I.: Cellular tumorigenecity in nude mice: correlation with cell growth in semisolid medium. *Cell* **3**:355-359, 1974.

9
Colon Cancer Research on Dermal Monolayer Cultures

B. Shannon Danes, M.D., Ph.D.
and Rulon W. Rawson, M.D.

With the exception of the autosomal-dominant heritable colon cancer (HCC) syndromes, the role of genetics in colon cancer has not been delineated. If this role could be clarified, relevant clinical surveillance and genetic counseling would be available to persons at increased risk for colon cancer due to inheritance of such cancer-prone genes.

Recently, *in vitro* research on dermal monolayer cultures has offered the opportunity of identifying the *in vitro* expressions of cancer genes for some of the HCC syndromes. Comparison of *in vitro* biological properties (growth kinetics and chromosomes) have shown differences between cultures from persons with and without HCC syndromes. Cultures derived from affecteds with some HCC syndromes have alterations in biological properties associated with *in vitro* transformation, defined as the acquisition of cellular characteristics associated with a cancer cell and absent from a normal cell.[1] An attempt will be made to put such research in perspective for future use in colon cancer.

ASSAYS OF *IN VITRO* BIOLOGICAL PROPERTIES

Growth Kinetics

Growth kinetics have been assayed for six properties in four different laboratories (Table 9-1).[2-9] In each study, biopsies have been taken from patients with the clinical syndrome familial polyposis coli (FPC) and some of its variant forms.

There is no standardization of biopsying the skin; biopsies are not been divided for establishment of monolayer cultures from the same biopsy in different laboratories. Establishment of the monolayer culture from the primary biopsy from which the subcultures were derived varies. In one

Table 9-1. Panel of Biological Properties (Altered Growth kinetics and Increased *In Vitro* Tetraploidy) in Skin Cultures from Patients with Heritable-Colon-Cancer Syndromes Reported in Two Studies

HERITABLE COLON CANCER SYNDROMES STUDIED — STUDIES

BIOLOGICAL PROPERTIES	NL[4]				FPC[4]				GS[4]				TS[4]	HCC[4]
	1	2	3	4	1	2	3	4	1	2	3	4	2	2
Increased *in vitro* tetraploidy	−	−[2]	−	−	+	−	+	+	−	+	+[1]	+	−	+
Lower serum requirement for growth	−	−	−	−	+	+	+	+	−	−	+	+	−	+
Density-dependent regulation of growth in subconfluent and confluent monolayers	+	+	−	−	−	−	−	+	−	+	+	+	−	−
Increased saturation density of growth	−	−	−	−	+	−	+	+	+	−	+	+	−	−
Random arrangement in monolayers[3]	−	+	−	−	+	+	+	+	+	+		+	+	+
Anchorage-independent growth	−	−	−	−	−[1]	−	−	−	−[1]	−	−	−	−	−
Tumorigenic in athymic nude mice	−	−	−	−	−	−	−	−	−	−	−	−	−	−

[1] Anchorage sensitivity is not absolute since growth in agar might occur but at a low frequency.
[2] Approximately 3% of normals showed increased tetraploidy.
[3] Random arrangement = regions of crisscrossed arrays and multilayered pattern. [3] One GS patient studied.
[4] FPC = Familial polyposis coli
GS = Gardner's syndrome
TS = Turcot's syndrome
HCC = Heritable colon cancer without polyposis coli
NL = Normal

Studies: (1) Kopelovich;[4] Pfeffer et al.;[3] Kopelovich et al.;[5]
(2) Danes and Alm;[6] Danes et al.;[7]
(3) Rasheed and Gardner[8]
(4) Utsunomiya[9]

laboratory, primary cultures that did not show an epithelial outgrowth were excluded from the study so that both epithelial and fibroblastic cells would be present at the first subculture.[6, 10] In the other studies, no mention was made of any such cellular requirement or standardization of cell types included in the sublines.[3, 4, 8, 9]

Dermal-fibroblast cultures from affecteds and some at-risk members of FPC families have shown alterations in *in vitro* growth kinetics. After concluding his *in vitro* studies, Kopelovich[2] concluded that "the scatter of values emphasizes that each test by itself cannot be used with absolute certainty as a marker of cancer risk for this or any other population at risk. The use of all tests together, and a large sample, may help define confidence limits for determining the probable risk of cancer in any individual with a certain value" (p. 105).

Differential toxicity by the tumor promoter 12-0-tetradecnoyl phorbo-13-acetate (TPA) was reported to be the most reliable single parameter to distinguish between normal and FPC.[11] The induction of T antigen positive cells by SV_{40} has also been suggested as a marker of cancer risk in human skin-fibroblast cultures.[12] The usefulness of T antigen as an assay of cancer risk has been questioned because of the complexity of factors influencing its expression in individual cases.[13] Of the *in vitro* parameters studied for the FPC genotype (Table 9-1),[2, 3, 14] Lipkin included only one of these *in vitro* properties, actin pattern, in his risk-factor profile for FPC families as there was no overlap in the percentages of cells showing a normal actin pattern between cultures with and without the FPC genotype.[15]

Some of the other assays done did not appear to detect any alterations in *in vitro* expressions that were useful in discriminating between cells with and without certain known cancer-prone genes (With more detailed studies, some of these alterations could prove useful.) For example, cultured fibroblasts with and without the FPC genotype were equally susceptible to killing by ultraviolet irradiation.[2, 9] The resistance of cultured FPC fibroblasts to the lethal effects of ionizing radiation has been reported as increased[9] and indistinguishable from fibroblasts without the FPC gene.[2] Whereas, the cells from Gardner's syndrome (GS), considered to be a variant form of FPC, showed increased *in vitro* radiation resistance.[16]

Chromosome Studies

Chromosome damage of a relatively specific nature has been associated with the primary event responsible for neoplastic transformation of a cell. The preexistence of chromosome damage in the chromosome breakage syndromes, the increased susceptibility to neoplasia in Down's syndrome, the detection of x-ray-induced chromosome damage long before the occurrence of neoplasia, and the specificity of chromosome abnormalities associated with specific neoplasms lends credence to the concept that specific chromosome imbalance may be a primary event in tumorigenesis. This imbalance might be reflected either by loss of growth controlling genes, the duplication of genes acting in the opposite direction, or even a specific gene loss or position effect produced by chromosomal rearrangements. The expression of appropriate recessive phenotypes might result from such mitotic errors as a prerequisite for malignant transformation in a diploid cell.[17]

Chromosomal studies on dermal monolayers derived from the HCC syndromes have been reported from two laboratories. In family studies (Tables 9-2 and 9-3), Danes found increased *in vitro* tetraploidy in cultures derived from all affecteds and some family members at risk studied in some families with HCC syndromes (15 of 16 GS families, 3 Oldfield syndrome [OS] families, and 4 HCC syndrome without polyposis coli families) but not in all (1 GS family, 16 of 19 FPC families, and 2 Turcot's syndrome [TS] families).[18] One of 38 normals without a family history of solid tumors showed increased *in vitro* tetraploidy (Danes, unpublished data). Rasheed and Gardner reported that increased *in vitro* tetraploidy occurred in the one GS patient studied.[18]

From this *in vitro* research it has become evident that it cannot be predicted which, if any, alteration in an *in vitro* biological property will be demonstrated by dermal-monolayer cultures derived from different autosomal-dominant, colon cancer syndromes.[6] Each property must be assayed on cultures derived from affecteds, family members at risk for each syndrome, and persons without a family history of cancer. These studies must be done without laboratory personnel knowing the source of the biopsy tissue.

Past research has shown the value of standardizing skin biopsies (as to anatomical site, i.e., upper, inner aspect of the arm; type, i.e., split-thickness or full-thickness punch); establishment of monolayer cultures (as to cell types included in first subculture from the primary explant culture and number of subcultures before assays); and assays of biological properties. Growth kinetics should be performed on duplicate cultures and repeated to verify reproducibility of an alteration from considered normal activity. Growth kinetics of dermal-monolayer cultures from persons without a family history of solid tumors in a broad age range should be established in each laboratory. Chromosomal alterations should be assayed on cultures showing a "burst" of mitotic activity so that a sufficient number of metaphases are present (i.e., over 100 metaphases per slide). Several determinations (i.e., at 5, 10, and 15 subcultures) have yielded information on *in vitro* expression of cancer-prone genes (where the abnormality was not present *in vivo* nor was consistently present in early subcultures).[19] Transformation assays should use rigorous criteria of genetic transformation and not for epigenetic phenomena. Morphological criteria, limited growth in semisolid media, or transient growths

Table 9-2. Identification of Members with Increased *In Vitro* Tetraploidy in Skin Cultures from Families with HCC Syndromes (FPC, GS, OS, and HCC Syndrome without Polyposis Coli) in which Cultures from All Clinically Affected Members Studied Showed Increased Tetraploidy*

SYNDROME	NUMBER OF FAMILIES STUDIED	TOTAL NUMBER OF MEMBERS STUDIED	OCCURRENCE OF IN VITRO TETRAPLOIDY					
			ALL AFFECTEDS +	FAMILY MEMBERS AT RISK		OBSERVED	EXPECTED	
				+	−	+/TOTAL	+/TOTAL	
FPC	3	11	5	3	3	8/11	6/11	
GS	15	147	56	18	73	74/147	74/147	
OS	3	13	10	1	2	11/13	7/13	
HCC	4	31	5	11	15	16/31	16/31	

Source: From B.S. Danes. Occurrence of *in vitro* tetraploidy in the heritable colon cancer syndromes. *Cancer* 48:18, 1981.
*Range of tetraploidy in cultures derived from normals not at risk: 0-7%. Increased tetraploidy: + = present; − = absent.

**Table 9-3. Families with HCC Syndromes with and without
Increased In Vitro Tetraploidy in Skin Cultures
Derived from Clinically Affected Members**

SYNDROME	NUMBER FAMILIES STUDIED	IN VITRO TETRAPLOIDY OF ALL CLINICALLY AFFECTED MEMBERS STUDIED WITHIN EACH FAMILY	
		NORMAL	INCREASED
		NUMBER OF FAMILIES	
FPC	19	16	3
GS	16	1	15
HCC	4	—	4
OS	3	—	3
(FPC c cysts)			
TS	2	2	—

FPC = familial polyposis coli; GS = Gardner's syndrome; HCC = heritable colon cancer without polyposis; OS = Oldfield syndrome; TS = Turcot's syndrome

in athymic nude mice have been found not to be as reliable for transformation as continuous tumor growth in athymic nude mice.

The *in vitro* studies on dermal-monolayer cultures should follow the standardized disciplines used in microbial genetics. Each step (obtaining specimens, establishing cultures and sublines, performing assays) must be done under known, controlled conditions with the limitations inherent in each step taken into consideration.

The ideal altered biological property would be one that is gene specific. None of the differences in biological properties studied nor any grouping of them has permitted identification of a specific genotype. Rather, the differences appeared to be *in vitro* expressions of a number of cancer-prone genes. In the rare autosomal-dominant, colon cancer syndromes specificity has been difficult to establish. A sufficient number of living affecteds in single, unrelated families must be found in order to verify that all affecteds with the same syndrome show this *in vitro* alteration. Past research has demonstrated that affecteds considered to have the same syndrome on the basis of clinical stigmata did not all show the same *in vitro* alterations. For example, cells from two of three FPC patients and four of five GS patients transformed with Kirstin murine sarcoma virus at increased efficiency.[8] The occurrence of *in vitro* tetraploidy (Tables 9-1-9-3) and serum requirements for growth (Table 9-1) varied for patients similarly affected with FPC.[6] When reproducibility of the *in vitro* observation has been verified through repeat biopsies, genetic heterogeneity has been considered (more than one mutation can give the clinical stigmata described as a single syndrome). This difference is detected *in vitro* rather than *in vivo*.

This *in vitro* research has made evident the value of accurate and extensive clinical evaluations. Erroneous conclusions based on *in vitro* data could be made if only a superficial knowledge of the clinical expressions within a family are known. Clinical testing should include a thorough evaluation of not only those systems showing overt clinical pathology but also those commonly showing gene expression. For example, Utsunomiya found that if radiological examinations of the oral region were done on all FPC affecteds, 94% showed localized radiopaque lesions, one of the extracolonic lesions used to distinguish GS from FPC.[9] Many of the extracolonic lesions could go undetected during a routine medical examination. Since the extracolonic benign lesions and solid tumors occurring in HCC syndromes sometimes show consistency within and between generations and show inconsistency in other kindreds, the occurrence of such extracolonic lesions should be determined for an entire kindred.

With the establishment of the clinical diagnosis and the detection of an alteration in an *in vitro* property in an affected, the next step should be a thorough study of the family and its kindred. A pedigree containing both clinical involvement and the occurrence of an altered *in vitro* property, increased *in vitro* tetraploidy (Fig. 9-1), illustrates such an approach. A general principle should be that no alteration can be considered to be an *in vitro* genetic expression unless all affecteds in the kindred show the same alteration in the biological property assayed and unless the alteration's vertical transmission can be documented.

Interpretation of the *in vitro* findings, although well intentioned, has often been generalized (i.e., the interpretation that alteration in a biological property means gene expression). The alteration might or might not be associated with the mutation within the family. For example, it might be an alteration occurring at a high frequency in the general population; therefore, this frequency should be known. For example, the occurrence of increased *in vitro* tetraploidy in dermal monolayers derived from normal persons without a family history of solid tumors has been determined to be approximately 3%.[18] This might be another mutation transmitted in the family; every human carries four to six mutations that are often recognized only from an affected offspring. Since interactions between cancer-prone genes and environmental factors have been considered to be required before clinical cancer (with the exception of the autosomal-dominant cancer syndromes), their presence probably goes undetected in the majority. Thus, pedigree data of kindreds rather than of single families should be established before assigning any genetic significance to *in vitro* data.

So far, the *in vitro* research done on the HCC syndromes has been directed

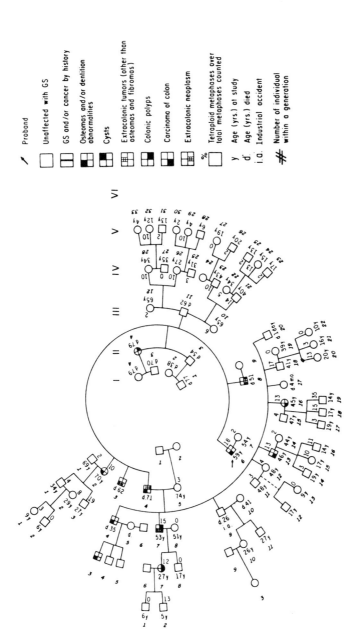

Figure 9-1. Pedigree of a Gardner's syndrome kindred showing clinical stigmata and occurrence of increased *in vitro* tetraploidy.

at detection of alterations in biological properties associated with transformation and not at identification of *in vitro* biomarkers for cancer-prone genes. A genetic marker has been defined as a protein or other phenotype determined by a single locus with two or more alleles present in the general population.[20] A cellular property has been excluded if it undergoes quantitative changes for physiological rather than genetic reasons. None of the alterations in growth kinetics studied met this definition. For example, the source of serum influenced the serum requirement for growth (Table 9-1), and susceptibility to viral transformation was affected by donor and culture age.[21]

As colonic cancer does not usually occur in members of families with HCC syndromes until or after the third decade of life,[22] recognition of specific genotypes that increase the risk of colon cancer would make possible identification of members at increased risk of cancer before clinical expression. If there is a genetic component in the majority of colon cancers that occur after the fourth decade of life, the identification of such cancer-prone genes would make feasible the delivery of relevant cancer surveillance to a group who, without such *in vitro* tests, would be unaware of their increased genetic risk for colon cancer.

Until the *in vitro* detection of such cancer-prone genes has been proven to be 100% accurate, every person known to be at increased genetic risk for colon cancer, regardless of his cell-culture status, should receive close clinical observation. For the future, the use of dermal-monolayer cultures appears to offer an approach to detecting cancer-prone genes and studying their roles in human carcinogenesis. But caution and judgment must be used in undertaking both the identification of alterations in *in vitro* biological properties due to cancer-prone gene expression and the ultimate application of this approach to preventive oncological surveillance and genetic counseling.

Acknowledgements.   This research was made possible through a grant CA 15973 from The National Large Bowel Cancer Project of the National Cancer Institute Division of Cancer Research and NIH-NCI CA 27831.

REFERENCES

1. Macpherson, I., and Montagnier, L.: Agar suspension culture for the selective assay of cells transformed by polyoma virus. *Virology* **23:**291-294, 1964.
2. Kopelovich, L.: Hereditary adenomatosis of the colon and rectum: Recent studies on the nature of cancer promotion and cancer prognosis *in vitro*. In: *Colorectal Cancer: Prevention, Epidemiology, and Screening* (Winawer, S.; Schottenfeld, D.; and Sherlock, P., eds.) New York, NY: Raven Press, 1980, pp. 97-108.

3. Pfeffer, L.; Lipkin, M; Stutman, O.; and Kopelovich, L.: Growth abnormalities of cultured human skin fibroblasts derived from individuals with hereditary adenomatosis of the colon and rectum. *J. Cell Physiol.* **89:**29-38, 1976.

4. Kopelovich, L.: Phenotypic markers in human skin fibroblasts as possible diagnostic indices of hereditary adenomatosis of the colon and rectum. *Cancer* **40:**2534-2541, 1977.

5. Kopelovich, L.; Pfeffer, L.M.; and Bias, N.: Growth characteristics of human skin fibroblasts *in vitro:* A simple experimental approach for the identification of hereditary adenomatosis of the colon and rectum. *Cancer* **43:**218-223, 1979.

6. Danes, B.S., and Alm, T.: *In vitro* evidence of genetic heterogeneity within the heritable colon cancer syndromes with polyposis coli. *Scand. J. Gastroenterol.* **16:**421-427, 1981.

7. Danes, B.S.; Bulow, S.; and Svendsen, L.B.: Hereditary colon cancer syndromes: An *in vitro* study. *Clin. Genet.* **18:**128-136, 1980.

8. Rasheed, S., and Gardner, M.B.: Growth properties and susceptibility to viral transformation of skin fibroblasts from individuals at high genetic risk for colorectal cancer. *JNCI* **66:**43-49, 1981.

9. Utsunomiya, J.: Present status of adenomatosis coli in Japan. In: *Pathophysiology of Carcinogenesis in Digestive Organs* Farber, E.; Kawachi, T.; Nagayo, T.; Sugano, H.; Sugimura, T.; and Weisburger, J.H., eds.). Baltimore, MD: University Park Press, 1977, pp. 305-321.

10. Danes, B.S.: Increased *in vitro tetraploidy: Tissue specific within the heritable colorectal cancer syndromes with polyposis coli. Cancer* **41:**2330-2334, 1978.

11. Kopelovich, L.: The use of a tumor promoter as a single parameter approach for the detection of individuals predisposed to colorectal cancer. *Proc. Am. Assn. Cancer Res.* **21:**192, 1980.

12. Kopelovich, L., and Sirlin, S.: Human skin fibroblasts from individuals genetically predisposed to cancer are sensitive to an SV40-induced T-antigen display and transformation. *Cancer* **45:**1108-1111, 1980.

13. Blattner, W.A.; Lubiniecki, A.S.; Mulvihill, J.J.; Lalley, P.; and Fraumeni, J.F., Jr.: Genetics of SV40 T-antigen expression: studies of twins, heritable syndromes and cancer families. *Intern. J. Cancer* **22:**231-238, 1978.

14. Kopelovich, L.; Lipkin, M.; Blattner, W.A.; Fraumeni, J.F., Jr.; Lynch, H.T.; and Pollack, R.E.: Organization of actin-containing cables in cultured skin fibroblasts from individuals at high risk of colon cancer. *Intern. J. Cancer* **26:**301-307, 1980.

15. Lipkin, M.: Risk factor profile in the identification of increased susceptibility to cancer of the large intestine. In: *Workshop on Large Bowel Cancer.* Dallas, TX: National Large Bowel Cancer Project, 1981, pp. 73-79.

16. Kopelovich, L; Drozdoff, V.; and Zeitz, L.: Transformation of human mutant cells by γ-irradiation. *Proc. Am. Assn. Cancer Res.* **22:**63, 1981.

17. Ohno, S.: Aneuploidy as a possible means employed by malignant cells to express recessive genes. In: *Chromosomes and Cancer* (German, J., ed.). New York, NY: John Wiley, 1974, pp. 77-94.

18. Danes, B.S.: Occurrence of *in vitro* tetraploidy in the heritable colon cancer syndromes. *Cancer* **48:**1596-1601, 1981.

19.   Danes, B.S.; Alm, T.; and Veale, A.M.O.: Modifying alleles in the heritable colorectal cancer syndromes with polyps. In: *Colorectal Cancer: Prevention, Epidemiology, and Screening* (Winawer, S.; Schottenfeld, D.; and Sherlock, P., eds.). New York, NY: Raven Press, 1980, pp. 73-81.

20.   King, M.C., and Petrakis, N.L.: Genetic markers and cancer. In: *Genetics of Human Cancer* (Mulvihill, J.J.; Miller, R.W.; and Fraumeni, J.F., Jr., eds.). New York, NY: Raven Press, 1977, pp. 281-289.

21.   Todaro, G.J.: Variable susceptibility of human cell strains to SV40 transformation. *NIH NCI Mongr.* **29:**271-275, 1968.

22.   Bussey, H.J.R.: *Familial polyposis coli; family studies, histopathology, differential diagnosis, and results of treatment.* Baltimore, MD: The Johns Hopkins University Press, 1975, p. 104.

10
Immunological Parameters as Possible Biomarkers for Disclosure of Cancer-Prone Genotypes in Familial Cancers

Guy S. Schuelke, Ph.D., Henry T. Lynch, M.D.,
and Edward A. Chaperon, Ph.D.

A prodigious body of literature has accumulated on immune abnormalities in cancer patients.[1,2] But even though there is a paucity of solid immunological information on hereditary cancer in general, there is also an increasing number of discrete, heritable, immunodeficiency states that have been observed to have multiple cancer associations. In certain immunodeficiency syndromes, patients surviving associated cancers of childhood have gone on to develop adenocarcinoma of the colon. For example, patients with Bloom's syndrome, a cancer-associated genodermatosis with well know immunological aberrations, have developed colorectal cancer.[3]

RATIONALE FOR STUDYING CANCER-PRONE FAMILIES

Members of cancer-prone families comprise a small but readily identifiable fraction of patients seen routinely in the clinic.[4,5] This subgroup constitutes a largely untapped, though theoretically valuable, resource for cancer immunology research. As other chapters have pointed out, recognition of high-risk families in the course of straight-forward interviews could easily lead the investigator to subjects who are at increased cancer risk and who may harbor significant immunologic aberrations. Specific patients may be studied long before the onset of malignancy. Occult as well as clinically evident carcinoma may perturb the patient's immune system but can, nevertheless, be informative when evaluated in a longitudinally monitored patient.

Before considering specific immunological studies, it is necessary to discuss possible mechanisms relating immune changes to cancer predisposing genotypes. Initially, one may consider an immune characteristic as a stable, genetically determined trait demonstrable on immunological maturity. In a given case, such a trait may be an integral component of a cancer-predisposing genotype. Defects in immunodeficiency states are clearly related to malignancy, though they are typically of hematopoietic lineage. Although the search for profound, primary, immune perturbations continues in colonic and other solid tumors, subtler immune findings now appear to be more attractive possibilities. Recently defined *in vitro* assays of unproven *in vivo* relevance include natural-killer (NK) and antibody-dependent cellular cytotoxicity (ADCC) activities. Subtle immune changes may not be sufficient to predispose persons to such readily identified clinical symptomatology as is often seen with the classical immunodeficiency syndromes. Any cancer-predictive immune findings could hypothetically be genetically determined and of central importance in cancer etiology. As mentioned previously, an immune parameter may be an event purely secondary (epigenetic) to cancer development. Finally, there is always the possibility that an immunological trait may segregate in a kindred without any casual relevance to the occurring cancers, yet be closely linked chromosomally to other carcinogenic loci.

By way of analogy, in one study, tumor-antigen-specific immunological reactivity was present in persons occupationally exposed to urinary bladder carcinogens before overt expression of clinical cancer.[6] Moreover, the increases in reactivity were related to the degree of carcinogen exposure and early malignant changes in the urothelium. Such an immunological test, while having no screening value in the general population, could have great usefulness in selected subjects at extraordinary cancer risk by virtue of a readily identified trait, namely that of occupational exposure. Frequent immunological screening of subjects likely to have immune changes related to early cancer could be of special value in those people unwilling or unable to submit to intensive physical surveillance.

IMMUNOLOGICAL INVESTIGATIONS IN CANCER-PRONE KINDREDS

Table 10-1 summarizes immunological findings in subjects with a possible genetic predisposition to various types of cancer.[7-63] Every attempt has been made to present the authors' data and interpretations as comprehensively as space limitations permit. All references to family members are expressed in relation to the propositus. Proposed inheritance patterns are included only where the authors stated such information. The table is organized according to major immunological findings with particular attention to quantitative immunoglobulin findings. A criterion for inclusion of studies was that the immune study be performed on subjects from kindreds not having clearly recognized biomarkers otherwise associated with carriage of cancer predisposing genes. When reported, associated findings such as chromosomal analysis, human leukocyte antigen (HLA), carcinoembryonic antigen

Table 10-1. Summary of Pertinent Literature Dealing with Immunological Findings in Persons with a Possible Genetically Determined Cancer Predisposition

REFERENCE AUTHOR, TUMOR SPECTRUM, INHERITANCE	IMMUNOGLOBULINS	LYMPHOCYTE-PROLIFERATION STUDIES	OTHER	CLINICAL AND MISCELLANEOUS
Massimo et al.[7] Hodgkin's disease in 1 family member	↓ or absent IgA or IgM in subjects from 3 generations	Several family members anergic to PHA stimulation	RFs, antiliver, and antikidney antibodies in several relatives	Father of 2 Down's syndrome patients appeared normal with a 46XY/47XY (trisomy-21) mosaicism
Seligman et al.[8] Waldenström's macroglobulinemia; 65 families and patients with 216 close relatives	1. 8 1st-degree relatives, IgM spike—6, no symptoms (G and A normal in 3, ↑ in 2, ↓ in 1) 2. ↑ or ↓ Ig in 42% of relatives without paraprotein 3. No G or A paraproteins		1. ↑RF in 1st-degree relatives <60 yr 2. Blood counts normal in asymptomatics with IgM paraprotein 3. Paraproteins biochemically and immunologically distinct	1. ANAs (+) in 28 relatives (↑ over control) 2. Less antithyroid and gastric Ab vs. control 3. No ↑ infections 4. 1 w/low % abnormal-chromosome findings
Twomey et al.[9] Acute, undifferentiated leukemia; brain tumor; breast carcinoma; heredphoretic titers	1. Propositus and both sisters ↓ IgA and M 2. 7 other abnormal electrophoretic titers 3. Paternal aunt and 1 sister slight ↓IgG 4. 3 slight ↑ in IgA and a cousin ↓ IgA 5. ↓ IgM in 9 of 16	Many cytogenetic preparations low in mitotic figures and 2 paternal sibs failed to grow (3X attempt)	1. Both daughters low in Ig were (+) in DTH 2. Normal Ab to polio 3. No serum-virus-like particles in EM	1. No ↑ infections 2. Dysgammaglobulinemia not associated with telangiectasia 3. Normal hematologies 4. 2 phenotypic normals had altered cytogenetics

↑ = Increased levels of substance or activity under consideration
↓ = Decreased levels of substance or activity under consideration
= Number

κ = Kappa immunoglobulin light chains
λ = Lambda immunoglobulin light chains

(continued)

Table 10-1. *(Continued)*

REFERENCE AUTHOR, TUMOR SPECTRUM, INHERITANCE	IMMUNOGLOBULINS	LYMPHOCYTE-PROLIFERATION STUDIES	OTHER	CLINICAL AND MISCELLANEOUS
Fraumeni et al.[10] Chronic lymphocytic leukemia	↓ G and M in proband and 1 normal sib; ↓A and M in leukemic sib; G in 1 sib; ↓M in 1 sib	↓ PHA in G and M-deficient sib, and in leukemic sib	1. All (+) DTH for at least 1 recall antigen 2. All sibs Coomb's (−)	1. No SLE in sibs 2. Parental consanguinity—recessive? 3. Arthritis in sib ↓ in G, M, and PHA
Freeman et al.[11] Lymphosarcoma in sibs	↓IgA, G, and M in propositus; probably since prior ↑ infections	PHA for cytogenetics judged normal preceded tumor	1. Propositus DTH ↓ to recall and DNCB 2. Cytogenetic abnormalities	1. Abnormal erythroid maturation 2. Sister's thymus aplastic and she had lymphosarcoma
Potolsky et al.[12] Chronic lymphocytic leukemia; lymphocytic lymphoma; reticulum cell sarcoma (? cell type); breast cancer; other uncertain cancers	All ↓ IgG; 1 ↓ IgM; 1 ↓ IgA w/slight ↓ G; 1 ↓ IgA with ↑ anti-B isoagglutinin associated with ↓ PHA	↓ PHA in the 1 ↓ A, G, and M and absence of germinal centers	All ↓ DTH in 23 antigens; 1 ↓ anti-B isoagglutinin also ↓ germinal centers); no RF, ANAs, or Coomb's (+); virus studies including EM of serum and lymphocytes) negative	1. 12 total—4 survived cancer for testing; 3 arthritis, 1 atopic 2. Normal karyotypes 3. 1 subsequently developed lymphosarcoma
Ertel and Hamoudi et al.[13, 14] Multiple primary cancers in proband; lymphosarcoma in brother; other relatives w/cancer	1. Female proband with ↓ IgA and normal PHA 2. Absent IgA in brother 3. ↓ IgM in father	Proband: normal PHA		1. Sister: adenocarcinoma large bowel, age 12 2. Brother: cancer at age 15 3. Hereditary spherocytosis

190

Reference / Disease	Proband findings	Cytogenetic findings	Immunologic findings	Other findings
Abels and Reed[15] Multiple primary malignancies (Fanconi-like syndrome) *Autosomal Recessive*	Proband ↓↓ IgA with ↑ IgG	Cytogenetic cultures did not grow (6X)	Recall DTH negative while proband in fairly good health	1. Proband: no thymus and infections 2. No ↑ photosensitivity 3. Brother treated for pancytopenia and was immunologically normal
Creagan and Fraumeni[16] Adenocarcinoma of stomach and colon	1. ↓ IgA (both κ and λ) and 1 with ↓ proliferation and DTH anergy 2. 2 ↓ IgG and slight ↓ IgA 3. ↑ AFP in 1 of #2 above and parietal antibodies in other 2	1. ↓ PHA or SLO in 6 unaffected relatives 2. SLO ↓ in stomach patient and 4 relatives with ↓ proliferation	1. Antiparietal antibodies in 6 of 16; statistically significant in younger age group 2. No intrinsic factor or mitochondrial antibodies 3. ↑ Ab to EBV in 4 of 16 4. ↑ AFP in the 1 ↓ in IgA	1. Chromosomes normal 2. 1 pernicious anemia 3. Lymphocytopenia in 2 stomach-cancer patients and 5 relatives
Fraumeni[17] Waldenström's macroglobulinemia in propositus; lymphosarcoma in 4 other sibs, 1 of whom had a child with HD	Other family members w/ polyclonal ↑ IgM that were subclinical		Other family members w/ impaired CMI	
Maldonado et al.[42] HD			Affected brothers w/HLA—A1 and B5	
Jones[43] Familial retinoblastoma *AD (incomplete penetrance)*			No simple correlation between HLA or MLR antigens and presence or absence of retinoblastoma gene	Normal chromosomes

↑ = Increased levels of substance or activity under consideration
↓ = Decreased levels of substance or activity under consideration
= Number

κ = Kappa immunoglobulin light chains
λ = Lambda immunoglobulin light chains

(continued)

191

Table 10-1. *(Continued)*

REFERENCE AUTHOR, TUMOR SPECTRUM, INHERITANCE	IMMUNOGLOBULINS	LYMPHOCYTE-PROLIFERATION STUDIES	OTHER	CLINICAL AND MISCELLANEOUS
Buehler et al.[44] HD: lymphosarcoma; thymoma; retinoblastoma; neuroblastoma; rhabdomyosarcoma *AD with low penetrance?*			10% family members homozygous for HLA— much inbreeding	Normal chromosomes
Lynch et al.[45] CFS *AD*			Suggested association with HLA-A2, B12	
Lawler[46] Acute lymphoblastic leukemia			Normal HLA haplotype segregation	
Larson et al.[47] HD as in Ref. #43			No HLA antigen or haplotype common to cancer patients	
Takasugi et al.[48] Malignant melanoma			Suggested segregation with "blank" HLA specificities	
Bowers et al.[49] HD and nonlymphoid malignancies			Propositi shared maternal B7 and lacked Dw2	HD in sisters within 3 mo. of 25th birthdays
Lynch et al.[50] Breast cancer			HLA antigens or haplotypes not unique to cancer-prone lines	

Katano et al.[36] Colon adeno-carcinoma	Normal	↑% clinically cancer-free relatives w/↓ PHA response	1. Probable association w/HLA A9-Bw35 haplotype in the family 2. % T and B lymphocytes CH_{50} and CEA within normal limits	All cancer affecteds were male
Hersey et al.[37] Patient and 1 or more close relatives with malignant melanoma	Most PHA responses normal		1. Most T and B cells normal % 2. Familial patients had lower NK activity than nonfamilial patients 3. ↓ NK correlated in close relatives only 4. ↑ frequency HLA A2; no apparent linkage with disease or low NK	1. 13 families total—18 patients and 53 relatives 2. In some cases, NK inheritance appeared AD 3. Low incidence Rh− subjects who have lower NK activity than Rh+. Explain ↓ NK in these families?
Sullivan et al.[38] (as Ref. #25)			Decreased NK activity in 10 of 12 males affected; % T and B normal	2 normal NK−1 w/lymphoma and common variable immunodeficiency
Fudenberg et al.[39] Osteogenic sarcoma; leukemia; undefined			↓ active T rosettes in maternal and paternal family members	Proband had precocious aging, ↓ active and total rosettes; developed osteogenic sarcoma

↑ = Increased levels of substance or activity under consideration
↓ = Decreased levels of substance or activity under consideration
= Number
κ = Kappa immunoglobulin light chains
λ = Lambda immunoglobulin light chains

(continued)

Table 10-1. *(Continued)*

REFERENCE AUTHOR, TUMOR SPECTRUM, INHERITANCE	IMMUNOGLOBULINS	LYMPHOCYTE-PROLIFERATION STUDIES	OTHER	CLINICAL AND MISCELLANEOUS
Mendius et al.[40] HD; 10 patients and 131 relatives (different families) *No Family History in 4 of 10 Patients*	↑ IgA in 3, ↑ IgM in 5, and ↓ IgG in 2 (not significantly different than controls)		1. 35.5% had antibody to lymphocytes vs. control of 8.6% 2. Few antibodies to RNA and DNA in either subjects or controls	1. Suggestion of spouse effect, but consangunity clearly important in antibody development 2. 2 families greatly ↑ # lymphotoxins; inheritance pattern not evident
Forbes and Morris[41] HD			Normal segregation of HD associated ALL and W5 Ags	
Salimonu et al.[32] Familial HD	1. ↑ IgM in CVID disease patients' relatives 2. 20x ↑ IgD in HD. May be environmental factor or genetic and environmental combined			
Schuelke et al.[33] Prominant ovarian cancer; multiple other solid tumors; one non-Hodgkin's lymphoma *AD*	1. ↓ IgA in 14 of 45 bloodline relatives 2. ↑ IgM in 3 not associated with ↓ IgA 3. ↓ IgG associated with ↓ IgA in 1 heavy smoker 4. ↓ IgA in 2 of 4 living cancer affecteds	1. ↓ innate proliferation to one or more of Con-A, PHA, or PWM in 18 people 2. Autologous serum ↓ responses in 12 subjects; 3 of these were also ↓ in innate responses	1. Normal % T cells and total T cells 2. Serum NK inhibitory activity in 13 people 3. ADCC inhibitory activity 4. Sera suppression	1. 49 bloodline people and 9 spouses investigated 2. Clustering of multiple significant findings in some people—even decades before expected clinical cancer in this family

5. Female predominance in ↓ IgA	3. Female predominance in serum suppression	detected in 3 people (2 cancer affecteds and 1 spouse with benign breast disease) 5. DTH responses unremarkable	3. No obvious associations w/ABO, HLA, or Rh 4. No ↑ allergies or infections 5. Interactive environmental factors not widely identified 6. Clinical autoimmune findings not widespread and not correlated with immune findings 7. No obvious correlation of immune findings and *in vitro* endoreduplication
McBride and Fennelly[34] HD in 3 sisters	1. ↓ IgA in one HD 2. Paraprotein in mother	↓ PHA in all family members that fluctuated w/time	↓ DTH in mother and 4 of 5 sibs	1. Normal cytogenetics 2. HLA-A1, B8 in 2 HD sibs
Berlinger and Good[35] CFS *AD*	MLC suppressor cells in cancer affecteds and unaffected relatives		Differentiate CFS, Gardner's syndrome, and hereditary polyposis?

↑ = Increased levels of substance or activity under consideration
↓ = Decreased levels of substance or activity under consideration
= Number
κ = Kappa immunoglobulin light chains
λ = Lambda immunoglobulin light chains

(continued)

195

Table 10-1. *(Continued)*

REFERENCE AUTHOR, TUMOR SPECTRUM, INHERITANCE	IMMUNOGLOBULINS	LYMPHOCYTE- PROLIFERATION STUDIES	OTHER	CLINICAL AND MISCELLANEOUS
Blattner et al.[28] Waldenström's macroglobulinemia in father and 3 of 4 children	2 κ and 2 λ chains associated w/paraprotein		All people with macroglobulinemia or autoantibody were HLA, A-2, B-8, DRW-3	1. Daughter and her 30-year-old son w/Hashimoto's thyroiditis and antithyroid Ab 2. +ANAs in 2 affected sons, 3 grandchildren + RF with ↑ IgM in 2 of the 3 3. One grandchild + antithyroid w/polyclonal ↑ IgA 4. One grandchild w/antimyocardial Ab
Blattner et al.[29] Chronic lymphocytic leukemia; lymphocytic lymphoma; squamous-cell carcinoma; prostate carcinoma; skin cancer *Dominant?*	↓ IgM in CLL; ↓ IgG in normal sib; polyclonal ↑ IgA and M in 1 well relative; polyclonal ↑ IgM in 3 well relatives	1. PHA, Con-A, PWM, SPL, and MLC tested 2. ↓ PHA in CLL and 4 clinically well people 3. ↓ SPL in CLL 4. Proband's son ↓ PHA; taking phenytoin 5. ↓ MLC in CLL and 3 normals 6. ↓ PHA and MLC in 1 well younger person w/o altered Igs	1. % T ↓ in CLL patient 2. Proband's 1st-degree relatives with his inferred HLA haplotypes were ↓ PHA response 3. 2 nieces w/o haplotype were also ↓ PHA response	1. Proband's sister w/ leukemia did not have ↑ infections 2. Complete blood counts normal except in leukemics

196

Dean et al.[30] 4 families with cutaneous malignant melanoma and precursor nevus syndrome	Normal except 2 melanoma patients with ↑ IgA	1. Tested PHA, Con-A, PWM, SPL, PPD, mumps, and SK-SD 2. 16 of 60 ↓ to 1 or more mitogen (not significant) 3. PHA and PWM ↓ most frequently 4. 23 of 60 ↓ MLC (significant) 5. ↓ MLC and B-lymphocytes in some spouses and blood relatives w/o cancer or nevi	1. ANA, isohemagglutnin, and RF tested (not significant) 2. Skin tests to recall antigens normal	No correlation between ↓ T cells and ↓ PHA or MLC
Evans and Burn[31] Mother w/HD and child w/progressive ↓ Ig (common variable immunodeficiency)	Child: initially normal IgG with ↓ IgM and A; later, ↓ IgG also	Child ↓ in PHA and PWM	1. Child NBT positive 2. Child normal T% and B% 3. DTH normal to recall antigens and DNCB 4. ↓ germinal centers	1. Child: HLA-A1, 3; B5, 7 2. Child recovered from chickenpox and mumps 3. Recurrent respiratory problems
Dworsky et al.[24] HD included in 5 families with 2 or more lymphoreticular neoplasms in 1st- and 2nd degree relatives	↑IgM in lymphoma family group vs. control; IgG normal; IgA ↓ by 30% (not significant)	↓Con-A in lymphoma families vs. control; PHA and PWM not changed	1. ↓DTH to Candida in lymphoma family group 2. Ab to EBV-VCA correlated inversely with PHA and Con-A responses in lymphoma families	

↑ = Increased levels of substance or activity under consideration
↓ = Decreased levels of substance or activity under consideration
= Number
κ = Kappa immunoglobulin light chains
λ = Lambda immunoglobulin light chains

(continued)

Table 10-1. *(Continued)*

REFERENCE AUTHOR, TUMOR SPECTRUM, INHERITANCE	IMMUNOGLOBULINS	LYMPHOCYTE-PROLIFERATION STUDIES	OTHER	CLINICAL AND MISCELLANEOUS
Lynch et al.[25] Malignant melanoma; HD and lung cancer *AD*	1. Mother and 4 children with ↓ IgA; 1 child also ↑ IgG. IgA findings were maintained in a 5-year follow-up study. 2. 5 other ↑ IgG 3. IgM normal in all subjects tested		↑ AFP in 12 of 13 tested; ↑ CEA in 4 of 15 tested	
Blattner et al.[26] Acute lymphocytic leukemia	↑IgG in father and oldest sib with RA; κ:λ ratios normal; otherwise A, G, and M normal	Normal Con-A, PHA, PWM, and SPL in cancer-free subjects	1. % T ↓ in one leukemic sib 2. Leukemic sibs identical for HLA-A, B, and MLC locus. Homozygous at B loci—one from each parent 3. Several RFs 4. Father: antistriated muscle Ab 5. Sister: antithyroid and antimicrosomal Ab 6. No anergy to PPD, mumps, SK-SD	Parents had RA and sibs presented w/leukemia within 3 weeks of each other
Purtilo et al.[27] Lymphomas; immunoblastic sarcoma; plasmacytoma *X-Linked Recessive*	↓ IgA and ↑ IgM in some affecteds	Normal PHA and PWM responsive	1. Spontaneous *in-vitro* lymphocyte proliferation 2. Herpes-like virus in EM 3. EBV nuclear antigen present	↑ infections and immediate hypersensitivities to allergens in affecteds

198

Study				
Fraumeni et al.[18] HD: lymphocytic and histiocytic lymphomas; Waldenström's macroglobulinemia; lung adenocarcinoma	1. 3 of 4 w/↓PHA also ↑ polyclonal IgM 2. Other immunoglobulins normal 3. ↑ IgM persistent on repeat study	↓PHA in 4 of 9 healthy persons; one also ↓ to Streptolysin 0	2 with ↓PHA had ↑Ab to EBV	1. No ↑ infections 2. Autoimmune diseases in relatives 3. 1 woman with abnormal immune findings developed lung carcinoma and her grandson developed leukemia 4. Deficient immune response to EBV and other viruses
Blattner et al.[19] Chronic lymphocytic leukemia in father and 4 of 5 children	1. Serum Igs normal in unaffected sib 2. Normal lymphocyte surface Igs in unaffected	Normal response in unaffected	Normal ADCC and mitogen-induced cytotoxicity in unaffected	Affected sibs abnormal in immune studies
Bjorkholm et al.[20] Six healthy surviving twins whose partners died of HD		↓Con A in all twins; ↓PPD proliferation in 3 twins	↓DTH responses; no change in T or B lymphocyte subpopulations	
Law et al.[21] Carcinoma of colon and uterus; lymphoproliferative malignancy	IgA, G, and M normal	1. 8 of 15 ↓ MLC 2. Also tested PHA, Con-A, PWM, and SPL; 9 of 15 ↓ to 1 or more mitogens	1. ↓ % T in 5 tumor patients and 5 family members 2. + DHT in 3 colon patients and 9 of 13 affecteds 3. 1 cancer patient unreactive to recall DTH	1. Hematocrit and WBCs normal 2. Chromosomal findings in 6

↑ = Increased levels of substance or activity under consideration   κ = Kappa immunoglobulin light chains
↓ = Decreased levels of substance or activity under consideration   λ = Lambda immunoglobulin light chains
= Number

(continued)

Table 10-1. *(Continued)*

REFERENCE AUTHOR, TUMOR SPECTRUM, INHERITANCE	IMMUNOGLOBULINS	LYMPHOCYTE-PROLIFERATION STUDIES	OTHER	CLINICAL AND MISCELLANEOUS
Purtilo et al.[22] Histiocytic lymphoma, glioblastoma multiforme; poorly differentiated carcinoma 5 *Males; Maternal Mutation?*	↓ IgA in 2	PHA and PWM normal in 1 tested	% T normal in one tested; 2 were lymphopenic; lymphocytes abnormal in EM studies	1. Idiopathic thrombocytopenia purpura 2. ADA and other enzymes normal
Bjorkhom et al.[23] Consanguinous and non-consanguinous relatives of 12 HD patients		7 of 15 relatives of the 6 HD patients w/↓ Con-A were also ↓ for Con-A vs. 0 of 12 relatives of Con-A-responsive HD patients; also ↓ PWM in PPD in the ↓ Con-A responders	No differences in lymphocyte subpopulations	↓ response in some spouses suggests environmental influence
Marshall et al.[51] HD as in Ref. #43			Hypothesize association with HLA at population level w/a link w/B18 as a "carrier state"	
Rosner et al.[52]			Suggest association w/B13 in a family	
Greene et al.[53] HD in 13 families			↑ Bw35 and Bw37 among probands	
Nunez-Roldan et al.[54] Torres et al.[55]			3 patients each had maternal A1-B5 and paternal A26-B18	3 sibs diagnosed with HD at same time

Farid et al.[56] MEN-I (especially prolactinomas)		Suggest haplotype association consistent w/dominant-linkage model
Sivak et al.[57] Adenocarcinoma of colon *AD*		Suggest possibility of linkage with histo-compatibility complex
George et al.[58] Medullary thyroid carcinoma		1. Patients responded with mononuclear leukocyte migration inhibition on challenge w/cancer Ag 2. Spouses and ↑ risk members: no response to antigen
Rocklin et al.[59] Medullary thyroid carcinoma *AD*	SK-SD proliferation similar to normal	1. Patients and ↑ risk family members (6 of 12) respond to tumor antigen in macrophage-migration inhibition or proliferative-response tests 2. SK-SD macrophage migration similar to normal + immune findings in absence of + calcitonin findings

↑ = Increased levels of substance or activity under consideration
↓ = Decreased levels of substance or activity under consideration
= Number
κ = Kappa immunoglobulin light chains
λ = Lambda immunoglobulin light chains

(continued)

201

Table 10-1. *(Continued)*

REFERENCE AUTHOR, TUMOR SPECTRUM, INHERITANCE	IMMUNOGLOBULINS	LYMPHOCYTE-PROLIFERATION STUDIES	OTHER	CLINICAL AND MISCELLANEOUS
Vandenbark et al.[60] Malignant melanoma			1. Family members including spouses: ↑ LAI responses to melanoma extract 2. Relatives of 10-year survivors responded stronger than <5-year exposure to affected	1. 3 families w/40 members studied 2. Conclude that transmissible material immunizes
Felberg et al.[61] Presumed sporadic retinoblastoma			CEA significantly ↑ in patients' relatives; spouse effect also present (personal communication	
Levine et al.[62] 21 families w/lymphomas and multiple other cancers; Two 1st-degree relatives had cancer		1. Antibodies to EBV capsid and EA antigens were studied 2. Significant ↑ in family members vs. controls. Most significant <20 years old 3. Antibodies higher in families w/carcinoma and soft tissue sarcomas		

202

| Meisner et al.[63] Leukemia, lymphoma, osteogenic sarcoma, meningeal sarcoma, adenocarcinoma of cecum (proband: age 16) *Three-Locus-Model Hypothesis* | PHA for cytogenetics judged normal | 1. ↑ EBV antibodies in all family members except proband 2. Normal DTH to recall Ags and DNCB 3. Abs to common Ags normal |

↑ = Increased levels of substance or activity under consideration
↓ = Decreased levels of substance or activity under consideration
= Number
κ = Kappa immunoglobulin light chains
λ = Lambda immunoglobulin light chains

Note: A list of abbreviations used in this table is given on following page.

Abbreviations used in Table 10-1:

Ab = Antibody
ADA = Adenosine deaminase
ADCC = Antibody-dependent cellular cytotoxicity
AFP = Alpha fetoprotein
Ag = Antigen
ANA = Antinuclear antibody
CEA = Carcinoembryonic antigen
CFS = Cancer family syndrome
CMI = Cell-mediated immunity
Con-A = Mitogen *Concanavalin A;* Used to stimulate polyclonal lymphocyte blastogenesis
DNCB = Dinitrochlorobenzene
DTH = Delayed-type hypersensitivity (skin test)
EBV, VCA, EA = Epstein Barr virus, EBV capsid antigen, EBV early antigen
EM = Electron microscopy
HLA = Human-leukocyte antigens
HD = Hodgkin's disease
IgA, D, G, M = Immunoglobulins of A, D, G, and M isotypes
LAI = Leukocyte-adherence inhibition
MLC, or MLR = Mixed leukocyte culture, mixed leukocyte reaction
NBT = Nitroblue-tetrazolium tests
NK = Natural-killer cell or activity
PHA = Mitogen phytohemagglutinin; used to stimulate polyclonal lymphocyte blastogenesis
PPD = Purified-protein derivative
PWM = Pokeweed mitogen; used to stimulate polyclonal lymphocyte blastogenesis
RF,RA = Rheumatoid factor, rheumatoid arthritis
Sib/sibs = Sibling, siblings
SK-SD = Streptokinase-streptodornase antigen
SLE = Systemic lupus erythematosus
SLO = Streptolysin-O
SPL = Staphylococcus phage lysate
T or B = T- or B-lymphocytes; rosettes refer to detection by rosetting assay
w/, w/o = With, without
WBC = White blood cells
+ = Positive
− = Negative

(CEA), and alpha-fetoprotein (AFP) are included.[64, 65] Reports of familial cancers associated with recognized, genetically determined immunodeficiency diseases have not been repeated. In some cases, this distinction may be artifactual in that immune deficiency states are probably under-reported when not accompanied by sufficient clinical symptomatology to prompt immunological evaluations.[66]

Quantitative Serum Immunoglobulins

Serum immunoglobulins A, G, and M (IgA, IgG, IgM) have for some time been routinely quantitated. Twenty-eight reports in Table 1 investigated these immune parameters [7-19, 21, 22, 24-34] and of these, 23 found abnormalities.

Most suggestive of a simple cancer association are increased immunoglobulin levels in kindreds with a propensity for lymphocytic malignancy.[8, 17, 18, 24, 29] Other immunoglobulin findings[9, 15, 25-27, 29, 30, 32, 33, 40] defy attempts at a single unifying explanation. In some cases, increases may be a compensatory mechanism associated with a decrease in another immunoglobulin class; associated with autoimmunity; or reflections of chronic antigen exposure. Investigation of IgD levels in future investigations may also prove fruitful in light of the report of elevated IgD concentrations in subjects from a Hodgkin's disease-prone kindred.[32]

Decreased immunoglobulin concentrations have also been commonly observed.[7-16, 22, 25, 27, 29, 31, 33] In some cases, low immunoglobulin levels were the predominant or only immune abnormality. Immunoglobulin A was depressed in 15 reports, IgG in 8, and IgM in 7. In some families, IgA deficiency appears to be an autosomal-dominant trait.[7, 25, 33] Lowered immunoglobulin levels were present in some families with decreased *in vitro* lymphocyte proliferation or autoimmunity.[7-10, 12, 15, 16, 18, 29, 31, 33]

Lymphoproliferative Responses

A widely investigated assay of immune function has been lymphocyte proliferation in response to antigens or plant mitogens.[4, 7, 9-16, 18-24, 26, 27, 29, 31, 33-37, 59] Several families had depressed mitogen responsiveness in a sufficient number of relatives as to suggest a relationship with cancer-predisposing genotypes.[4, 7, 9, 16, 18, 21, 29, 30, 33, 35, 36] Studies of putative environmental influences[28] and depressed mixed-lymphocyte suppressor cells[33] should also be useful in deciding if depressed lymphoproliferation represent innate abnormalities in stimulation-cell-division responses or a modulation of division by extrinsic factors. The need for cautious interpretations of cancer proneness in this context is accented by the finding of depressed mixed-leukocyte response in precursor, nevi-free relatives and spouses from malignant melanoma-prone families.[28]

Natural-Killing and Antibody-Dependent Cellular Cytotoxicity

At least three studies have dealt with NK activity in genetically susceptible cancer patients and their relatives. Hersey[37] and Sullivan[38] demonstrated deficient activity in relatives of malignant melanoma patients and in patients manifesting the X-linked, recessive lymphoproliferative syndrome. Our laboratory has found sera from an ovarian cancer-prone kindred to suppress NK or ADCC activities by normal donor lymphocytes.[33] Observed dissociation of NK and ADCC activity appear functionally similar to that in mouse tumor systems[67] and in human ovarian-carcinoma ascites fluid.[68] Yet, normal ADCC effector cell activity has been seen in a leukemia-prone family.[19] Assaying a subject's effector cell activities both in the presence and absence of autologous serum might yield a better understanding of *in vivo* functional capabilities.

T Lymphocytes

One report indicates that decreased, active T rosettes should be considered a potential immune marker in familial cancer.[39] The apparent lack of an association between depressed proliferative responses and abnormal T cell levels[30, 33] in some cases constitutes an observation different from the description of a family with relatively widespread depression of both.[21]

Antilymphocyte Antibodies

Autoantibody activity against human lymphocytes in relatives of Hodgkin's disease patients[40] may be involved with immune abnormalities in this disease. How these antibodies relate to the finding of depressed *Concanavalin A* (Con-A) and other mitogen responses in relatives of Hodgkin's patients is uncertain.[20, 23] Tenable explanations for these findings include both genetic and environmental influences. Prospective evaluations in families with Hodgkin's disease could prove interesting even though immune findings may not distribute in a manner consistent with a simple inheritance pattern.

Human Leukocyte Antigen

A relationship between HLA antigens and familial cancer would provide a ready biomarker. In some studies, such an association has been suggested, [36, 41, 42, 45, 49, 51-53] while in other studies, less encouraging observations have been noted.[43, 46, 48, 50, 57] Continued investigations seem warranted in the interest of disclosing loci that segregate within family units. Evaluation of past work, including review of cross-reactive antigens,[69] might clarify suggested associations. Immunological investigations in addition to HLA study may also prove enlightening. In addition to a possible HLA association, Katano et al. have found depressed phytohemagglutinin (PHA) responsiveness in one colon cancer-prone kindred.[36]

Tumor-Antigen Sensitization

In four studies investigating tumor-related antigen sensitization, lymphocytes from the affected family subjects were responsive to specific tumor-antigen preparations.[21, 58-60] Only one study failed to show specific responsiveness in relatives.[58] Such responsiveness may correlate with extent of exposure to cancer-affected persons.[60] Superficially similar sensititzations have also been noted in families with presumably sporadic cancer.[70, 71]

Fetal Antigens

Two antigenic substances, AFP and CEA, can be demonstrated in fetal tissues and in certain adult tumors. Serum levels of both these antigens are elevated in some cancer patients.[65] Elevated CEA levels have been seen in unaffected, high-risk members of families with colon cancer. Apparent connubiality of CEA elevation in such families[25, 61] requires further elucidation. Increased AFP levels were present in most family members in one study[25] and were associated with abnormal, quantitative immunoglobulin levels in some subjects.[16, 25] In the melanoma-prone family reported by Lynch et al.,[25] IgA levels remained low through a six-year follow-up study.

Viruses

Levine et al.[62] and Meismer et al.[63] concentrated research on Epstein-Barr virus antibodies, demonstrating increased antibody titers in lymphoma- and leukemia-prone families. This suggests either a role in oncogenesis or an immune defect allowing continued viral-antigen expression.[72] The strongest evidence of a role for deficient immune response to the virus is the X-linked, recessively inherited lymphoproliferative syndrome.[27] However, the inverse relationship between antiviral antibodies and mitogen responsiveness[16, 18] in such families must be conservatively interpreted inasmuch as the relationships may simply suggest antigen persistence and expression in a host with altered immune response.[72]

Other Findings

From results obtained to date, it seems important to continue documenting histories of microbial infection[8-10, 15, 27, 29, 31, 33] in order to gain a better insight into the extent of immune abnormalities. Documentation of infection may help determine whether the immune changes preceded clinical cancer in those instances where prospective immune evaluation is not obtainable.[11, 15, 25] Chromosomal studies[7, 9, 11, 21] and attention to possible spouse effects[25, 29, 50, 61] may be significant in some families.

IMMUNE FINDINGS RELATIVE TO COLORECTAL CANCER

Although still incompletely investigated, several suggestive observations relative to immune parameters have been made in kindreds expressing colorectal cancer. Probably the most widely investigated immune parameter in such kindreds has been the search for an association between HLA antigens and cancer susceptibility.[36, 45, 50, 57] Early work by Lynch et al. on a large, midwestern, cancer family syndrome caucasion (CFS) kindred suggested a possible association between cancer and the HLA haplotype A2-B12.[45] Investigation of a smaller kindred from Japan with site-specific colorectal cancer suggested an association with the A9-Bw35 haplotype.[36] Linkage of the cancer predisposing genes with various HLA haplotypes in different kindreds would be one possible hypothesis. Much more extensive evaluation of HLA in colon cancer-prone kindreds is clearly indicated before the significance of such observations can be determined.[57]

The report by Berlinger and Good of macrophages suppressing the mixed leukocyte culture (MLC) responses in both cancer-affected and clinically-well persons from CFS kindreds[35] is among the more exciting of the immune-function studies. Despite the relatively small number of subjects tested, these results suggest that suppressor activity may precede clinical cancer in some kindreds, a finding which, if validated in prospective studies, might have great etiologic significance. The mechanism by which the macrophages mediate this suppression is probably through prostaglandins (personal communication, Dr. Norman T. Berlinger). Extension of these studies to members of families with the adenomatosis coli and Gardner's syndromes is needed to further investigate the genetically determined, cancer-predisposing conditions in which this type of suppressor cell may be present.[35] In this regard, it is interesting that depressed MLC responsiveness was the most common finding in members of four kindreds with malignant melanoma,[30] although the reason for the depressed responses was not investigated. Depressed MLC responses in some spouses in the melanoma families demonstrates the need to consider the possibility that MLC suppressor cells in colon cancer-prone kindreds might show a connubiality similar to that postulated for CEA elevation in spouses of high-risk subjects.[25]

Lymphocyte blast transformation in response to mitogen stimulation can be abnormally low in kindreds with colon cancer. Reported kindreds include one with site-specific colon cancer,[35] one with colon, uterine, and lymphoid malignancies,[21] and one with gastric and colon cancer.[16] A relationship between low mitogen responses and cancer susceptibility is suggested by the finding in all three families that approximately 50% of the clinically cancer-free persons had depressed mitogen responsiveness. Yet to be elucidated is the possible significance of kindreds with genetically determined colon cancer susceptibility but normal blastogenic responses (personal communication, Dr. D. C. Arthur).

Most assays of serum immunoglobulins have either been normal[36] or not investigated in reported colon cancer-prone kindreds. One report did find one apparently healthy family member with selectively low serum IgA.[16] One kindred with a proclivity for ovarian cancer also included one case of colon cancer. Selectively low IgA was distributed in members in a manner suggestive of a possible relationship to a cancer-predisposing genotype.[33] Immunoglobulins were quantitated by radial immunodiffusion using serum from persons in three colon cancer-prone kindreds under study by our group (Fig. 10-1A, B, C; clinical information on these three pedigrees is presented in the Appendix). Only the kindred presented in Figure 10-1 had persons with low serum IgA levels (subjects IV-8, IV-16, V-4, V-11, and V-13) (p exceeding close to zero by the binomial-proportion test by normal approximation with correction for continuity, personal communication, Dr. S. C. Cheng). The only other immunoglobulin level outside the normal range was serum IgM in III-2, III-11, IV-1, and V-4. These findings, in conjunction with our observation of consistently low IgA in members of a malignant melanoma-prone kindred, indicate that abnormal immunoglobulin levels may be a prominent immune finding in kindreds with colon and other solid tumors.

Our laboratory has identified serum factors suppressing ADCC or NK in sera from members of the ovarian-cancer-prone kindred just mentioned.[33] The three kindreds with colon cancer also had more than the expected 1 in 50 control subjects' incidence of such suppressor activities. Spouses in the kindreds also showed one or both suppressive activities.

Another example of potentially useful immunological research is our ongoing collaborative research with Dr. Henry F. Sears of the Fox Chase Cancer Center in Philadelphia. At the Center, monoclonal-antibody studies are performed on sera samples from colon cancer-prone kindreds, and preliminary results are currently being further evaluated. More research with newly evolving immunological assays on subjects with a genetic susceptibility to colon and other cancers is needed to put all of these preliminary observations into perspective.

SYNTHESIS, CONCLUSIONS, AND RECOMMENDATIONS

Most colon cancer-prone families do not demonstrate profound immunologic perturbations similar to those often seen in the classical immunodeficiencies. Instead, the diversity of immunological observations suggests

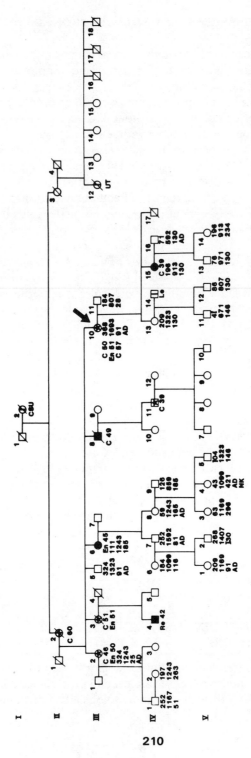

Figure 10-1A.   Pedigree of a CFS kindred presenting the results of quantitative serum IgA, IgG, and IgM determinations and the ability of sera to inhibit either ADCC or NK effector functions. The numbers are, from top to bottom, the mg/dl of serum IgA, IgG, and IgM that were observed.

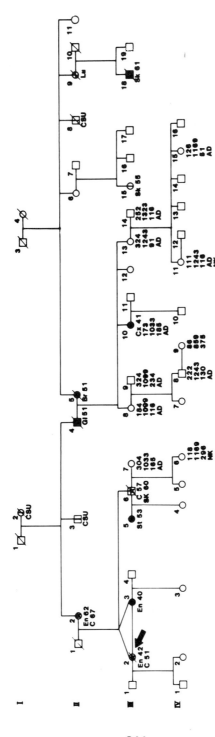

Figure 10-1B. Pedigree of a CFS kindred presenting the results of quantitative serum IgA, IgG, and IgM determinations and the ability of sera to inhibit either ADCC or NK effector functions. The numbers are, from top to bottom, the mg/dl of serum IgA, IgG, and IgM that were observed. For figure key see Fig. 10-1C.

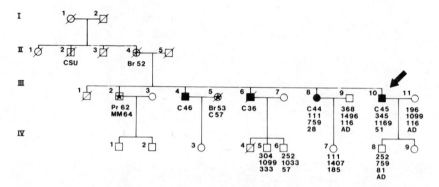

Figure 10-1C.   Pedigree of a CFS kindred presenting the results of quantitative serum IgA, IgG, and IgM determinations and the ability of sera to inhibit either ADCC or NK effector functions. The numbers are, from top to bottom, the mg/dl of serum IgA, IgG, and IgM that were observed.

☐¹ ◯²	Code Number Male or Female Unaffected	Br Breast
■ ●	Cancer Verified by Pathology	C Colon CSU Cancer Site Unknown
✪ ✪	Multiple Primary Cancers by Family History	Cx Cervix En Endometrium Gl Glioma Le Leukemia
⊟ ⊕	Cancer by Family History	Lu Lung MM Malignant Melanoma
➤	Proband	Pr Prostate Re Rectum
✚	Individuals who had Serum Immunoglobulins Determined	Sk Skin St Stomach Ut Uterus

Ov 50   Cancer Site and Age at Diagnosis

d 49   Age at Death

63   Current Age

IgA concentration 95% range 85-385 mg/dl
IgG concentration 95% range 564-1765 mg/dl
IgM concentration 95% range 53-375 mg/dl

AD   Serum significantly suppressed
      antibody dependent cellular
      cytotoxicity by normal donor
      effector cells

NK   Serum significantly suppressed
      natural killer activity by normal
      donor effector cells

multiple and, in certain circumstances, subtle immune changes that may or may not be related with the familial cancer genotype. Perhaps then, complex interactions with environmental factors[16, 25, 30, 61] are involved in phenotypic cancer expression. Strongly supportive of this integrative, multifactorial hypothesis is the X-linked, recessive lymphoproliferative syndrome wherein profound unresponsiveness to the Epstein-Barr virus[27] and depressed NK activity[38] could contribute to the cancer phenotype. Kindreds with cancer-prone and cancer-free branches, as presented in the Appendix, might prove valuable in dissecting genetically determined immune parameters from environmental factors common to high- and low-risk branches of the subject kindreds.

This research could provide a clinically useful biomarker for cancer-prone-genotype identification as well as for the elucidation of theoretical insights into the relationships between human cancer and immune functions. To date, no single unifying hypothesis has emerged even though some studies have produced highly provocative results. Therefore, it is mandatory that future studies continue to fully report the cancer spectrum within pedigrees as well as both "positive" and "negative" immune findings. Significant observations relative to the potentially tumor-limiting NK or ADCC functions[73] highlight the importance of applying emerging immunological theories and technologies to familial cancer.

A word of caution should be interjected into this discussion. Specifically, since the immune system is composed of a finite number of cell types, it is to be expected that a genetic defect in a particular segment of the immune system could be mimicked by interacting, modulatory, exogeneous, environmental factors. This is referred to as a phenocopy in formal genetic terminology. It is, therefore, of paramount importance to identify noncancer conditions and pertinent environmental factors that might produce immune changes that could confound cancer-related immune changes. A few examples of potentially interactive influences include mononucleosis,[74, 75] aspirin use,[76] cephalosporins,[77] cigarette smoking,[78] alcohol intake,[79] black-walnut ingestion,[80] circadian rhythms,[81] and age-dependent immune hyporesponsiveness.[82]

Blood samples should be obtained from psychologically unstressed subjects[83] and extensive histories should be obtained to permit evaluation of possible sources of false, positive findings. Unfortunately, few familial cancer reports to date indicate that such considerations have been given systematic attention.[29, 33]

In light of the diverse immune findings presented in Table 10-1, we must recommend that as many immune parameters be evaluated as is logistically possible. We urge that newer assays such as T cell subpopulation rosettes, cell-sorter evaluations of lymphocyte subpopulations, and antigen searches with monoclonal antibodies be included in the total immunological evaluation.

Samples should also be obtained for cytogenetic,[84] cellular physiology,[85-87] and enzymatic analysis.[88] Such a multifactoral evaluation provides maximum opportunity to find biomarkers in families and to detect any associations between multiple laboratory findings.

Our final recommendation is that every effort must be made to assure good investigator–subject relationships so that longitudinal cancer development can be followed and laboratory reevaluations can be performed as new immunological information and assays become available. The genetic basis of these cancers should provide a relatively more homogeneous population than random cancer occurrences presently being investigated in areas such as therapy with monoclonal antibodies[89] or characterization of tumor-produced immunosuppressive factors.[90] Thus, long-range therapeutic, screening, and management implications may be the reward of meticulous attention to immunology in cancer-prone families.

REFERENCES

1. Vance, J.C.: Immune system evaluation in genetic immunodeficiency diseases associated with malignancies. In: *Cancer-Associated Genodermatoses* (Lynch, H.T., and Fusaro, R.M., eds.), New York, NY: Van Nostrand Reinhold, 1982, pp. 321-332.

2. Marshall, R.H.; Hazzie, C.; Linder, A.E.; and Maklansky, D.: Small bowel in immunoglobulin deficiency syndromes. *AJR* 122:227, 1974.

3. German, J.; Bloom, D.; and Passarge, E.: Bloom's syndrome. V. Surveillance for cancer in affected families. *Clin. Genet.* 12:162-168, 1977.

4. Lynch, H.T.; Follett, K.L.; Lynch, P.M.; Albano, W.A.; Mailliard, J.L.; and Pierson, R.L.: Family history in an oncology clinic. Implications for cancer genetics. *JAMA* 242: 1268-1272, 1979.

5. Albano, W.A.; Lynch, H.T.; Recabaren, J.A.; Organ, C.H.; Mailliard, J.A.; Black, L.E.; Follette, K.L.; and Lynch, J.: Familial cancer in an oncology clinic. *Cancer* 47:2113-2118, 1981.

6. Taylor, G.; Kumar, S.; Brenchley, P.; Wilson, P.; Costello, B.; and Shaw, G.H.: Immunosurveillance in premalignant occupational bladder disease. *Intern. J. Cancer* 23:487-493, 1979.

7. Massimo, L.; Barrone, C.; Vianello, M.G.; and Dagna-Bricarelli, F.: Familial immune defects. *Lancet* 1:108, 1967.

8. Seligmann, M.; Danon, F.; Mihaesco, C.; and Fudenberg, H.H.: Immunoglobulin abnormalities in families of patients with Waldenstrom's macroglobulinemia. *Am. J. Med.* 43:66-83, 1967.

9. Twomey, J.J.; Levin, W.C.; Melnick, M.B.; Trobaugh, F.E.; and Allgood, J.W.: Laboratory studies on a family with a father and son affected by acute leukemia. *Blood* 29:920-930, 1967.

10. Fraumeni, J.F.; Vogel, C.L.; and DeVita, V.T.: Familial chronic lymphocytic leukemia. *Ann. Int. Med.* 71:279-284, 1969.

11. Freeman, A.I.; Sinks, L.F.; and Cohen, M.M.: Lymphosarcoma in siblings associated with cytogenetic abnormalities, immune deficiency, and abnormal erythropoiesis. *J. Ped.* **77:**996-1003, 1970.

12. Potolsky, A.I.; Heath, C.W.; Buckley, C.E.; and Rowlands, D.T.: Lymphoreticular malignancies and immunologic abnormalities in a sibship. *Am. J. Med.* **50:**42-48, 1971.

13. Ertel, I.J.; Hamoudi, A.B.; Kontras, S.B.; Clatworthy, W.; and Newton, W.A.: Multiple primary cancers associated with reticulum cell sarcoma. *Ped. Res.* **6:**369, 1972.

14. Hamoudi, A.B.; Ertel, I.; Newton, W.A.; Reiner, C.B.; and Clatworthy, H.W.: Multiple neoplasms in an adolescent child associated with IgA deficiency. *Cancer* **33:**1134-1144, 1974.

15. Abels, D., and Reed, W.B.: Fanconi-like syndrome. Immunologic deficiency, pancytopenia, and cutaneous malignancies. *Arch. Dermatol.* **107:**419-423, 1973.

16. Creagan, E.T., and Fraumeni, J.F.: Familial gastric cancer and immunologic abnormalities. *Cancer* **32:**1325-1331, 1973.

17. Fraumeni, J.F.: Family studies in Hodgkin's disease. *Cancer Res.* **34:**1164-1165, 1974.

18. Fraumeni, J.F.; Wertelecki, W.; Blattner, W.A.; Jensen, R.D.; and Leventhal, B.G.: Varied manifestations of a familial lymphoproliferative disorder. *Am. J. Med.* **59:**145-151, 1975.

19. Blattner, W.A.; Strober, W.; Muchmore, A.V.; Blease, R.M.; Broder, S.; and Fraumeni, J.F., Jr.: Familial chronic lymphocytic leukemia. *Ann. Int. Med.* **84:**554-557, 1976.

20. Bjorkholm, M.; Holm, G.; DeFaire, U.; and Mellstedt, H.: Immunological defects in healthy twin siblings to patients with Hodgkin's disease. *Scand. J. Haem.* **19:**396-404, 1977.

21. Law, I.P.; Hollinshead, A.C.; Whang-Peng, J.; Dean, J.H.; Oldman, R.K.; Herberman, R.B.; and Rhode, M.C.: Familial occurrence of colon and uterine carcinoma and of lymphoproliferative malignancies II. Chromosomal and immunologic abnormalities. *Cancer* **39:**1229-1236, 1977.

22. Purtilo, D.T.; Riordan, J.A.; Deflorio, D.; Yang, J.P.S.; Sun, P.; and Vawter, G.: Immunological disorders and malignancies in five young brothers. *Arch. Dis. Child* **52:**310-313, 1977.

23. Bjorkholm, M.; Holm, G.; and Mellstedt, H.: Immunological family studies in Hodgkin's disease: is the immunodeficiency horizontally transmitted? *Scand. J. Haem.* **20:**297-305, 1978.

24. Dworsky, R.; Baptista, J.; Parker, J.; Chandor, S.; Noble, G.; Herrmann, K.; Henle, W.; and Henderson, B.: Immune function in healthy relatives of patients with malignant disease. *JNCI* **60:**27-30, 1978.

25. Lynch, H.T.; Guirgis, H.A.; Harris, R.E.; Frichot, B.C.; Lynch, J.; Vandevoorde, J.; and Lynch, P.: Familial clustering of plasma carcinoembryonic antigen (CEA) in the cancer family syndrome. *Scand. J. Immunol.* (Suppl. 8) **8:**465-470, 1978.

26. Blattner, W.A.; Naiman, J.L.; Mann, D.L.; Wimer, R.S.; Dean, J.H.; and Fraumeni, J.F.: Immunogenetic determinants of familial acute lymphocytic leukemia. *Ann. Int. Med.* **89:**173-176, 1978.

27. Purtilo, D.T.; Hutt, L.; Bhawan, J.; Yang, J.P.S.; Cassel, C.; Allegra, S.; and Rosen, F.S.: Immunodeficiency to the Epstein-Barr virus in the X-linked recessive lymphoproliferative syndrome. *Clin. Immunol. Immunopathol.* **9:**147-156, 1978.

28. Blattner, W.A.; Garber, J.; Mann, D.L.; Fisher, A.W.; Bauman, A.W.; and Fraumeni, J.F., Jr.: Macroglobulinemia and autoimmune disease in a family abstr C-505. *ASCO* **20:**413, 1979.

29. Blattner, W.A.; Dean, J.H.; and Fraumeni, J.F., Jr.: Familial lymphoproliferative malignancy: Clinical and laboratory followup. *Ann. Int. Med.* **90:**943-944, 1979.

30. Dean, J.H.; Greene, M.H.; Reimer, R.R.; LeSane, F.V.; McKeen, E.A.; Mulvihill, J.J.; Blattner, W.A.; Herberman, R.B.; and Fraumeni, J.F., Jr.: Immunologic abnormalities in melanoma-prone families. *JNCI* **63:**1139-1145, 1979.

31. Evans, D.I.K., and Burn, J.L.: Progressive hypogammaglobulinamia in a child born to a mother with Hodgkin's disease. *Arch. Dis. Child* **54:**313-315, 1979.

32. Salimonu, L.S.; Bryant, D.G.; Buehler, S.K.; Chandra, R.K.; Crumley, J.; and Marshall, W.H.: Immunoglobulins in familial Hodgkin's disease and immunodeficiency in Newfoundland. *Intern. Arch. Allergy Appl. Immunol.* **63:**52-63, 1980.

33. Schuelke, G.S.; Lynch, H.T.; Lynch, J.F.; Chaperon, E.A.; Recabaren, J.A.; Grabner, B.; and Albano, W.A.: Cellular immune function study in an ovarian cancer prone kindred. *Br. J. Cancer* **46:**687-693, 1982.

34. McBride, A., and Fennelly, J.J.: Immunological depletion contributing to familial Hodgkin's disease. *Eur. J. Cancer* **13:**549-554, 1977.

35. Berlinger, N.T., and Good, R.A.: Suppressor cells in healthy relatives of patients with hereditary colon cancer. *Cancer* **45:**1112-1116, 1980.

36. Katano, M.; Fujiwara, H.; Toyoda, K.; and Torisu, M.: Immunogenetic studies of familial large bowel cancer. *Gann* **71:**583-588, 1980.

37. Hersey, P.; Edwards, A.; Honeyman, M.; and McCarthy, W.H.: Low natural-killer-cell activity in familial melanoma patients and their relatives. *Br. J. Cancer* **40:**113-122, 1979.

38. Sullivan, J.L.; Byron, K.S.; Brewster, F.E.; and Purtilo, D.T.: Deficient natural killer cell activity in X-linked lymphoproliferative syndrome. *Science* **210:**543-545, 1980.

39. Fudenberg, H.H.; Schuman, S.H.; Goust, J.M.; and Jorgenson, R.: T cells, precocious aging, and familial neoplasia. *Gerontology* **24:**266-275, 1978.

40. Mendius, J.R.; DeHoratius, R.J.; Messner, R.P.; and Williams, R.C.: Family distribution of lymphocytotoxins in Hodgkin's disease. *Ann. Int. Med.* **84:**151-156, 1976.

41. Forbes, J.F., and Morris, P.J.: Analysis of HL-A antigens in patients with Hodgkin's disease and their families. *J. Clin. Invest.* **51:**1156-1163, 1972.

42. Maldonado, J.E.; Taswell, H.F.; and Kiely, J.M.: Familial Hodgkin's disease. *Lancet* **2:**1259, 1972.

43. Jones, A.L.: Immunogenetics of retinoblastoma. *Trans. Ophthalmol. Soc. UK* **94:**945-952, 1974.

44. Buehler, S.K.; Fodor, G.; Marshall, W.H.; Firme, F.; Frase, G.R.; and Vaze, P.: Common variable immunodeficiency, Hodgkin's disease, and other malignancies in a Newfoundland family. *Lancet* **1:**195-197, 1975.

45. Lynch, H.T.; Thomas, R.J.; Terasaki, P.I.; Ting, A., Guirgis, H.A.; Kaplan, A.R.; Magee, H.; Lynch, J.; Kraft, C.; and Chaperon, E.: HLA in cancer family "N." *Cancer* **36:**1315-1320, 1975.

46. Lawler, S.D.: The HL-A system and neoplasia. In: *Cancer Genetics* (Lynch, H.T., ed.). Springfield, IL.: Charles C Thomas Co., 1976, pp. 87-100.

47. Larsen, B.; Barnard, J.M.; Buehler, S.K.; and Marshall, W.H.: HLA haplotypes in a genetic isolate in Newfoundland: A population showing 8% homozygosity and a familial aggregate of lymphoma and immunodeficiency cases. *Tis Antigens* **8:**207-215, 1976.

48. Takasugi, M.; Krain, L.; and Terasaki, P.: Histocompatibility in cancer. In: *Cancer Genetics* (Lynch, H.T., ed.). Springfield IL.: Charles C. Thomas Co., 1976, pp. 76-86.

49. Bowers, T.K.; Moldow, C.F.; Bloomfield, C.D.; and Yunis, E.J.: Familial Hodgkin's disease and the major histocompatibility complex. *Vox Sang* **33:**273-277, 1977.

50. Lynch, H.T.; Terasaki, P.I.; Guirgis, H.A.; Sherard, B.D., et al.: HLA in breast cancer-prone families and the cancer family syndrome. *Prog. Clin. Biol. Res.* **16:**149-163, 1977.

51. Marshall, W.H.; Barnard, J.M.; Buehler, S.K.; Crumley, J.; and Larsen, B.: HLA in familial Hodgkin's disease. Results and a new hypothesis. *Intern. J. Cancer* **19:**450-455, 1977.

52. Rosner, D.; Cohen, E.; Gregory, S.G.; Khurana, U.; and Cox, C.: Breast cancer and the HLA relationship in a high risk family. *Prog. Clin. Biol. Res.* **16:**169-174, 1977.

53. Greene, M.H.; McKeen, E.A.; Li, F.P.; Blattner, W.A.; and Fraumeni, J.F., Jr.: HLA antigens in familial Hodgkin's disease. *Intern. J. Cancer* **23:**777-780, 1979.

54. Nunez-Roldan, A.; Martinez-Guibelalde, P.; Gomez-Garcia, P.; Gomez-Pereira, C.; Nunez-Ollero, G.; and Torres-Gomez, A.: Possible HLA role in a family with Hodgkin's disease. *Tis Antigens* **13:**377-378, 1979.

55. Torres, A.; Martinez, F.; Gomez, P.; Gomez, C.; Garcia, J. M.; and Nunez-Roldan, A.: Simultaneous Hodgkin's disease in three siblings with identical HLA genotype. *Cancer* **46:**838-843., 1980.

56. Farid, N.R.; Buehler, S.; Russell, N.A.; Maroun, F.B.; Allerdice, P.; and Smyth, H.S.: Prolactomas in familial multiple endocrine neoplasia syndrome type I. Relationship to HLA and carcinoid tumors. *Am. J. Med.* **69:**874-880, 1980.

57. Sivak, M.V., Jr.; Sivak, D.S.; Braun, W.A.; and Sullivan, B.H., Jr.: A linkage study of HLA and inherited adenocarcinoma of the colon. *Cancer* **48:**76-81, 1981.

58. George, J.M.; Williams, M.A.; Almoney, R.; and Sizemore, G.: Medullary carcinoma of the thyroid: Cellular immune response to tumor antigen in a heritable human cancer. *Cancer* **36:**1658-1661, 1975.

59. Rocklin, R.E.; Gagel, R.; Feldman, Z.; and Tashjian, A.H., Jr.: Cellular immune responses in familial medullary thyroid carcinoma. *N. Eng. J. Med.* **296:**835-838, 1977.

60. Vandenbark, A.A.; Greene, M.H.; Burger, D.R.; Vetto, R.M.; and Reimer, R.R.: Immune response to melanoma extracts in three melanoma-prone families. *JNCI* **63:**1147-1151, 1979.

61. Felberg, N.T.; Michelson, J.B.; and Shields, J.A.: CEA family syndrome: abnormal carcinoembryonic antigen (CEA) levels in asymptomatic retinoblastoma family members. *Cancer* **37**:1397-1402, 1976.

62. Levine, P.H.; Fraumeni, J.F.; Reisher, J.L.; and Waggoner, D.E.: Antibodies to Epstein-Barr virus-associated antigens in relatives of cancer patients. *JNCI* **52**:1037-1040, 1974.

63. Meisner, L.F.; Gilbert, E.; Ris, H.W.; and Haverty, G.: Genetic mechanisms in cancer predisposition: report of a cancer family. *Cancer* **43**:679-689, 1979.

64. Winchester, R.J., and Kunkel, H.G.: The human Ia system. *Adv. Immunol.* **28**:221-292, 1979.

65. Shuster, J.; Freedman, S.O.; and Gold, P.: Fetal antigens in clinical medicine. In: *Laboratory Diagnosis of Immunologic Disorders* (Yas, G.N.; Stites, D.P.; and Brecher, G., eds.). New York, NY: Grune & Stratton, 1975, pp. 239-258.

66. Spector, B.D.; Perry, G.S.; and Kersey, J.H.: Genetically determined immunodeficiency diseases (GDID) and malignancy: report from the immunodeficiency cancer registry. *Clin. Immunol. Immunopathol.* **11**:12-29, 1978.

67. Nair, P.N.M.; Fernandes, G.; Onoe, K.; Day, N.K.; and Good, R.A.: Inhibition of effector cell functions in natural killer cell activity (NK) and antibody-dependent cellular cytotoxicity (ADCC) in mice by normal and cancer sera. *Intern. J. Cancer* **25**:667-677, 1980.

68. Badger, A.M.; Oh, S.K.; and Moolten, F.R.: Differential effects of an immunosuppressive fraction from ascites fluid of patients with ovarian cancer on spontaneous and antibody-dependent cytotoxicity. *Cancer Res.* **41**:1133-1139, 1981.

69. Schwartz, B.D.; Luehrman, L.K.; Lee, J.; and Rodey, G.E.: A public antigenic determinant in the HLA-B5 cross-reacting group: a basis for cross-reactivity and possible link with Becket's disease. *Hum. Immunol.* **1**:37-54, 1980.

70. Byers, V.S.; Levin, A.S.; Hackett, A.J.; and Fudenberg, H.H.: Tumor-specific cell-mediated immunity in household contacts of cancer patients. *J. Clin. Invest.* **55**:500-513, 1975.

71. Graham-Pole, J.; Ross, C.E.; Ogg, L.J.; Cochran, A.J.: Sensitization of neuroblastoma patients and related and unrelated contacts to neuroblastoma extracts. *Lancet* **1**:1376-1379, 1976.

72. Henle, W., and Henle, G.: Seroepidemiology of the virus. In: *The Epstein-Barr Virus* (Epstein, M.A., and Achong, B.G., eds.). New York, NY: Springer-Verlag, 1979, pp. 61-78.

73. Marx, J.L.: Natural killer cells help defend the body. *Science* **210**:624-626, 1980.

74. Haynes, B.F.; Schooley, R.T.; Grouse, J.E.; Payling-Wright, C.R.; Dolin, R.; and Fauci, A.S.: Characterization of thymus-derived lymphocyte subsets in acute Epstein-Barr virus-induced infectious mononucleosis. *J. Immunol.* **122**:699-702, 1979.

75. Carney, W.P.; Rubin, R.H.; Hoffman, R.A.; Hansen, W.P.; Healey, K.; and Hirsch, M.S.: Analysis of T lymphocyte subsets in cytomegalovirus mononucleosis. *J. Immunol.* **126**:2114-2116, 1981.

76. Crout, J.E.; Hepburn, B.; and Ritts, R.E.: Suppression of lymphocyte transformation after aspirin ingestion. *N. Eng. J. Med.* **292**:222-223, 1975.

77. Chaperon, E.A., and Sanders, W.E.: Suppression of lymphocyte responses by cephalosporins. *Infect. Immun.* **19:**378-384, 1978.

78. Ferson, M.; Edwards, A.; Lind, A.; Milton, G.W.; and Hersey, P.: Low natural killer cell activity and immunoglobulin levels associated with smoking in human subjects. *Intern. J. Cancer* **23:**603-609, 1979.

79. Saxena, Q.B.; Mezey, E.; and Adler, W.H.: Regulation of natural killer activity in vivo. II. The effect of alcohol consumption on human peripheral blood natural killer activity. *Intern. J. Cancer* **26:**413-417, 1980.

80. Oppenheim, J.J.; Sandberg, A.L.; Altman, L.C.; Hook, W.A.; and Daugherty, S.F.: Relationship of mitogen and tannins in walnuts to suppression of lymphocyte transformation after ingestion of walnuts. In: *Lymphocyte Recognition and Effector Mechanisms* (Lindahl-Kiessling, K., and Osoba, D., eds.). Proceedings of the Eighth Leucocyte Culture Conference. New York, NY: Academic Press, 1974, pp. 79-84.

81. Abo, T.; Kawate, T.; Itoh, K.; and Kumagai, K.: Studies on the bioperiodicity of the immune response. I. Circadian rhythms of human T, B, and K cell traffic in the peripheral blood. *J. Immunol.* **126:**1360-1363, 1981.

82. Makinodan, T., and Kay, M.M.B.: Age influence on the immune system. *Adv. Immunol.* **29:**287-330, 1980.

83. Stein, M.; Keller, S.; and Schleifer, S.: Role of the hypothalamus in mediating stress effects on the immune system. In: *Mind and Cancer Prognosis* (Stoll, B.A., ed.). New York, NY: Wiley & Sons, 1979, pp. 85-101.

84. Danes, B.S.: Increased tetraploidy: cell-specific for the Gardner gene in the cultured cell. *Cancer* **38:**1983-1988, 1976.

85. Kopelovich, L.; Bias, N.E.; and Helson, L.: Tumour promoter alone induces neoplastic transformation of fibroblasts from humans genetically predisposed to cancer. *Nature* **282:**619-621, 1979.

86. Kopelovich, L.; Lipkin, M.; Blattner, W.A.; Fraumeni, J.F.; Lynch, H.T.; and Pollack, R.E.: Organization of actin-containing cables in cultured skin fibroblasts from individuals at high risk of colon cancer. *Intern. J. Cancer* **26:**301-307, 1980.

87. Rasheed, S., and Gardner, M.B.: Growth properties and susceptibility to viral transformation of skin fibroblasts from individuals at high genetic risk for colorectal cancer. *JNCI* **66:**43-49, 1981.

88. King, M.C.; Elston, R.C.; Lynch, H.T.; and Petrakis, N.L.: Allele increasing susceptibility to human breast cancer may be linked to the glutamate-pyruvate transaminase locus. *Science* **208:**406-408, 1980.

89. Ritz, J., and Schlossman, S.F.: Utilization of monoclonal antibodies in the treatment of leukemia and lymphoma. *Blood* **59:**1-11, 1982.

90. Roth, J.A.; Grimm, E.A.; Gupta, R.K.; and Ames, R.S.: Immunoregulatory factors derived from human tumors. I. Immunologic and biochemical characterization of factors that suppress lymphocytic proliferative and cytotoxic responses *in vitro. J. Immunol.* **128:**1955-1962, 1982.

11
Hereditary Colon Cancer and DNA Repair

John A. Johnson, Ph.D.

Any attempt to assess the possible association of abnormal deoxyribonucleic acid (DNA) repair and hereditary colon cancer is compromised by the fact that little published information is available. One must instead rely primarily on data concerning measures of DNA repair in other systems. Characteristics such as growth kinetics, cell survival after treatment with DNA-damaging agents, ability to repair damaged viral DNA, chromosomal abnormalities and instabilities, and ease of transformation must be considered as possible indicators of altered DNA repair.

As noted by Lynch et al. (Chap. 1), hereditary colon cancers constitute a significant fraction of the total colon cancers reported. Furthermore, many instances of "sporadic" colon cancer may be mislabeled because of incomplete family histories. Kussin et al. pointed out that cases thought to be sporadic may actually be familial if careful family histories are obtained.[1] This comment is reminiscent of that of Elder et al.[2] with regard to "sporadic" cases of dysplastic nevus syndrome.[2] At any rate, hereditary colonic disorders such as familial polyposis coli (FPC) afford a wealth of surgical tissue-containing tumors (polyps) representing a spectrum of stages in the progression of a mucosal cell to a frank malignancy.[3] Also, if the genetic flaw is expressed in skin fibroblasts, present techniques for analyzing DNA repair allow a variety of informative investigations. The use of fibroblasts also permits the establishment of cell lines that may be stored in cell repositories[4] and be made available to other investigators. Epidermal cells may be most appropriate for DNA-repair studies, and new techniques permit long-term maintenance of keratinocyte cultures.

GROWTH OF COLONIC
MUCOSAL CELLS

Normal Growth

Growth patterns and kinetics of normal[5-8] and neoplastic[9-11] colonic mucosal cells have been previously reviewed by Deschner (Chap. 6) and Lipkin (Chap. 7). I will extend these discussions by presenting a general outline of the growth of epithelial tissue in order to emphasize metabolic similarities between epidermis and intestinal epithelium. Recognition of these shared properties justifies consideration of the wealth of available information concerning DNA repair and skin cancer, with the goal of developing constructive concepts about the etiology and treatment of colon cancer.

In a topological sense, an animal may be viewed as a doughnut stretched along its axis of circular symmetry, with the skin constituting the outer surface and the gastrointestinal tract representing the hole. Thus, one may view the body surfaces as a contiguous sheet of epithelial tissue, from the squamous, stratified structures of the epidermal, oral, and esophageal layers to the mucous-producing, nonstratified structures of the gastric and intestinal linings. One may expect that these tissues share many metabolic and physiologic properties, with major differences arising through evolutionary selection to serve the specialized functions of each tissue. Thus, squamous tissues are ideally adapted to performing their important role of providing a renewable barrier against the environment.

For example, as a basal cell in the lowest cell layer of the epidermis divides, another cell leaves that layer to enter the overlying one. Under normal conditions, when a cell leaves the basal layer, it becomes a nondividing keratinocyte, and undergoes orderly, programmed differentiation as it migrates toward the skin surface. Eventually, the cell becomes a tough, flattened element of the stratum corneum. As cell aggregates of the stratum corneum become weathered and slough off, they are replaced by an equal number of newly differentiated cells. In contrast, intestinal epithelial cells occur as thin, nonstratified linings, in accord with their important functions of absorption and secretion. The occurrence of crypts lined with epithelial cells greatly increases the surface area for passage of nutrients and secretory products. The dividing cells of these tissues occur in the lower portion of the crypts, and as mitosis occurs, cells migrate laterally along the epithelial border. This lateral movement brings the cells toward the top of the crypt, and as they approach the intestinal lumen, they lose their ability to synthesize DNA. When cells arrive at the mucosal surface, they are fully differentiated and ready to slough off.

Thus, although the spatial growth patterns of epidermis and colonic mucosa are very different, they share the property of continuous proliferation balanced by sloughing of aged cells. This common growth pattern is no evolutionary accident; both tissues are well adapted to withstand the onslaught of noxious agents. In accordance with its fundamental protective role, the epidermis produces an expendable, impermeable barrier. In performing its functions of absorption and secretion, the colon is exposed to a wide variety of exogeneous and endogeneous agents, and it is likely that this tissue also serves a protective function. Such a role may be accomplished by selective exclusion of harmful substances or their sequestration in surface cells that are on the verge of sloughing. The rapid turnover of epidermis (about 4 wk), intestinal mucosa (about 1 wk), and their avascular structures, is a potent factor in the protection of underlying tissues from noxious agents. The continuous loss of aged cells (the ones most likely to have undergone mutation) must also constitute an important defense against cancer. Another adaptation that serves the epithelial tissues well in their role as bulwarks against the environment is their marvelous healing capacity.

Growth of Colonic Neoplasms

Epidermal and colonic cells both undergo a spectrum of transformations, from benign growths (e.g., psoriasis or hyperplastic polyps) to precancerous states (e.g., actinic keratosis or adenomas) to frank malignancy (e.g., squamous cell carcinoma or adenocarcinoma). Obviously, growth of a neoplasm requires an imbalance in the rates of production and loss of cells. This imbalance can arise in several ways. If the rate of cell loss remains constant, decreased cell generation time or increased growth fraction (i.e., number of dividing cells) will result in accumulation of tissue. Either of the latter factors, accompanied by a reduction in cell loss, will trigger rapid tissue growth. Psoriasis, a classic example of nonmalignant proliferation, represents an instance of increased growth fraction and reduced sloughing of surface cells. In this context, it is pertinent to review Lipkin's concept of the two phases of proliferation in colonic epithelial cells that lead to colonic cancer.[12] In a Phase-1 lesion, DNA synthesis is not turned off as cells mature (i.e., the growth fraction expands), but the number of mucosal cells does not increase. In Phase 2, prolongation of DNA synthesis persists, and increased numbers of cells accumulate. One may visualize a third phase in which neoplastic cells have acquired the ability to invade underlying tissue, thereby constituting malignancy. In this context, psoriatic lesions and other benign neoplasms may be considered to be arrested in Phase 2, with the possibility of reverting to Phase 1 or the normal state.

MECHANISMS OF DNA REPAIR

Agents that damage DNA exert a wide variety of actions such as chemical alteration of pyrimidines, conversion of cytosine to uracil, loss of purines and pyrimidines, cross-linking with endogenous proteins, formation of monoadducts and diadducts (strand cross-links), photodimerization of pyrimidines, and strand breaks. A limited number of repair processes are required to correct this wide spectrum of damage. Most of the information available about DNA repair in mammalian cells concerns removal of ultraviolet (UV) induced pyrimidine dimers and repair of strand breaks caused by γ radiation. In fact, many DNA-damaging agents may be classified as either UV-like or radiomimetic. Techniques for measuring DNA repair rely on the detection of incorporation of tritiated thymidine (^{3}H-TdR), the disappearance of damage sites, or the rejoining of strand breaks. It should be stressed that these procedures provide information about *quantity* of DNA repair but not about *fidelity* of repair. With regard to the use of ^{3}H-TdR to monitor UV-induced DNA repair, note that the major type of UV damage, formation of pyrimidine dimers, cannot be completely assessed with a single radiotracer. This was discussed in detail elsewhere,[3] but it bears repeating that it may be important to monitor the appearance and disappearance of dimers containing cytosine as well as those containing thymine. One can enumerate at least four dimer species: T-T, C-T, T-C and C-C (because of directionality in the DNA chain, C-T and T-C may look different to repair enzymes). Thus, when the reader encounters the phrase *thymine dimers* or *pyrimidine dimers* in reference to incorporation of ^{3}H-TdR, he should interpret it as *thymine-containing dimers* and recognize that little information is provided concerning dimer species.

Other analytical techniques are based on cell viability—survival of cells after treatment, the ability to reactivate damaged viral nucleic acid, and so forth. It is assumed that these live-cell parameters will reflect defective DNA repair. To some extent, the results of these methods may relate to fidelity of repair.

Three broad classes of DNA repair have been documented: repair *in situ* (repair or replacement of altered bases without strand cleavage); excision repair (removal of a damaged segment and replacement with the appropriate nucleotides); and postreplication repair (bypassing of damaged sites during replication, leaving gaps in the daughter strand that are filled later).

DNA Repair Processes

Repair *in situ.* Two mechanisms provide direct repair of altered bases without affecting the DNA strand:

Base Excision. The N-glycosidic bonds between altered bases and ribose moieties of DNA may be cleaved by specific enzymes called DNA glycosylases. Deutsch and Linn described a purine insertase that catalyzes the insertion of the appropriate purine into apurinic DNA.[13] For reasons cited elsewhere,[3] the insertion step is probably error prone.

Photoreactivation. This process specifically repairs cyclobutane-type pyrimidine dimers, the major photoproduct of ultraviolet radiation (UVR). Photoreactivating enzyme, in the presence of visible light, catalyzes monomerization of the dimer. Photoreactivation should be error free, but cytosine-containing dimers may undergo alteration before monomerization occurs. Adjacent pyrimidines photodimerize across their 5, 6 double bonds to form a cyclobutane ring. Saturation of this bond in cytosine labilizes its amino group. If this group is lost from a dimer, photomonomerization will leave uracil in the place of cytosine. Because of the universal use of ^{3}H-TdR to monitor pyrimidine dimer production and repair, little information is available about cytosine-containing dimers in mammalian cells. In my opinion, this is a serious oversight.

Excision Repair. This versatile process repairs pyrimidine dimers, base damage, strand breaks, and monoadducts and diadducts. Cleaver et al. suggested terminology according to the technique employed to monitor insertion of a new DNA segment.[14] *Unscheduled DNA synthesis* (UDS) refers to detection of ^{3}H-TdR incorporation by radioautography; *radiation-stimulated synthesis* refers to determination of the radioactivity of isolated DNA; and *dimer excision* denotes isolation of DNA, hydrolysis and separation of unrepaired photoproducts.

Excision repair requires four steps: (1) incision of the DNA strand near the damage site by a specific endonuclease; (2) excision of a number of nucleotides, including the damaged portion, by an exonuclease; (3) attachment of missing nucleotides to the incomplete strand by a DNA polymerase; and (4) joining of the free end of the new segment to the DNA strand, by a polynucleotide ligase. Since the intact sister strand is employed as a template in Step 3, the process is relatively error free.

Postreplication Repair. This process provides for synthesis of complete daughter strands in the presence of unrepaired damage sites in the parental DNA. In *gapped synthesis,* daughter strand segments between damage sites are synthesized and the gaps are filled later. This mechanism can be studied by monitoring the rate of rejoining of short daughter strands. Another process, *branch migration,* involves cessation of replication at a damage site, while replication continues on the opposite (undamaged) DNA strand. When the daughter chain of this strand is elongated sufficiently, it folds back and serves as a template for synthesis of the other daughter strand beyond the damage site of its parental template. Normal replication then resumes. Because of the complicated nature of postreplication repair, it is more error prone than excision repair.

Cell Viability and DNA Repair

Several techniques are available to assess the ability of cells to recover their viability after damage to their DNA. *Colony forming ability* (CFA) is the ability of cultured cells to proliferate after they are subjected to an experimental insult. If the agent damages DNA, CFA will reflect repair capability. Host-cell reactivation (HCR) is assessed by measuring how well a damaged virus grows in the cell; host-cell repair of the viral DNA must occur before the virus can multiply. Cell fusion may be employed to determine whether cell lines with reduced UDS have the same repair defect. Two cell lines are fused, irradiated with UVR, and incubated with ^{3}H-TdR. Radioautographs are prepared, and *heterodikaryons* (cells containing one nucleus from each cell type) are examined. Tritium activity in the nuclei is detectable as silver grains (spots) in the radioautograph. If the grain counts for the nuclei are the same as that of cells with normal DNA repair, the two cell lines are said to belong to different complementation groups. The nuclei have different repair defects and are able to complement or "cure" each other when present in the same cell.

DEFECTIVE DNA REPAIR AND CANCER

Hereditary Skin Cancer

Xeroderma Pigmentosum.   Skin fibroblasts from patients with XP have been exhaustively studied by numerous investigators. Two types of XP fibroblasts have been known since shortly after Cleaver's original discovery of defective DNA repair in 1968.[15] *Classical XP* denotes cells with reduced excision repair of UV-induced damage, whereas *XP variant* denotes cells with normal excision repair but decreased postreplication repair (PRR). It is tempting to speculate that, since excision-deficient cells must rely heavily on an error prone repair process (PRR), patients with classical XP develop more skin tumors at an earlier age than those with XP variant. However, many XP-variant patients exhibit the same clinical symptoms as those with classical XP, that is, hyperpigmentation and early onset of multiple tumors. On the other hand, late onset of skin cancer does occur in XP variant, and

Hofmann et al. reported a family, referred to as pigmented xerodermoid (PX), in which clinical symptoms did not occur until the second or third decade.[16] Of further interest, contrary to the general concept of normal incidence of noncutaneous cancer in XP patients, internal carcinomas occurred in affected *and* unaffected members of the PX family.

Studies of DNA Repair. Since classical XP fibroblasts have defective excision repair, they exhibit reduced UDS after UV irradiation, and are therefore amenable to complementation studies. Examination of heterodikaryons of fused-cell mixtures has revealed seven complementation groups, labeled A through G.[17] There is a question, however, of whether the single member of XP group B represents a unique complementation group. This patient had concurrent Cockayne syndrome, and the influence of that genetic flaw, superimposed on a possible XP-variant repair defect, has not been examined.[3] Since XP-variant cells exhibit only subtle defects in excision repair,[15] they are not amenable to complementation analysis by the conventional technique. Recently, Jaspers et al. reported a technique for estimating PRR in heterodikaryons, thus permitting analysis of variant cells.[18] They observed that nuclei of classical XP (A, C, and D) cells restored PRR to normal levels in nuclei of six variant strains, whereas pairwise fusion of variant cells did not result in complementation. This "classic" investigation provided two important conclusions: (1) that although classical XP cells of groups A, C, and D have somewhat reduced PRR,[19] they have sufficient capacity to restore the process to normal in XP-variant nuclei; and (2) that XP-variant strains do not exhibit the heterogeneity (i.e., complementation groups) of classical XP. Jaspers et al. also resolved a question that had apparently not been previously addressed: are XP-variant nuclei capable of restoring excision repair to normal in nuclei of classical XP cells? The answer is yes, at least for restoration of UDS in nuclei of groups A, C, and D. As was stressed earlier,[3] it is of at least academic importance to test complementing ability of XP-variant nuclei against all classical XP groups.

Cell viability. Andrews et al. conducted extensive studies of cell survival and CFA after UV irradiation (classical A, C, D, E and variant).[20, 21] They observed that the CFA of cell strains was inversely related to the degree of neurological abnormalities in the patients donating the cells. Andrews et al. proposed that reduced post-UV survival of fibroblasts may reflect a similar sensitivity of neurons to other carcinogens, thus leading to neuronal death and abnormalities.

Host-cell reactivation has been employed as a sensitive measure of defective DNA repair in XP fibroblasts. Day measured repair of UV-damaged adenovirus 2 by XP cells, groups A-D, and by cells from four heterozygous parents of patients.[22] Heterozygous XP cells (XPH) had repair capacities equivalent to that of normal fibroblasts, whereas XP cells had greatly reduced capacity. In contrast, Rainbow reported that XPH cells exhibited repair levels for damaged adenovirus 2 DNA that were intermediate between normal and XP cells.[23] Several techniques have detected differences between XPH and normal cells,[3] but are either too cumbersome or not definitive enough to serve as screening tests for heterozygosity. It is imperative that Rainbow's technique be evaluated with additional XPH strains, and that other investigators demonstrate that the procedure is reproducible.

Ataxia Telangiectasia. Patients with AT exhibit extreme sensitivity to ionizing radiation and elevated risk of lymphoreticular cancer. Depending on the investigator's clinical orientation, the disorder may be viewed as an immunodeficiency disease, a genodermatosis, or a chromosome instability syndrome. The latter designation arises from the fact that mitogen-stimulated lymphocytes and skin fibroblasts from AT patients exhibit spontaneous and γ-induced chromosomal aberrations.

Studies of DNA Repair. Although AT fibroblasts are capable of repairing several types of γ-induced DNA damage (e.g., single-strand break, missing bases, thymine glycol), some lines have defective excision repair.[24] Thus, fibroblasts may be classified according to their ability to repair DNA damaged by γ radiation. Two complementation groups have been detected in repair-deficient lines.[24] Repair-proficient cells are analogous to XP variant.

In contrast to the strong γ-induced inhibition of DNA synthesis in normal lymphoblastoid lines, AT cells were not as strongly affected.[25] This phenomenon was exploited by Jaspers et al. to develop a rapid diagnostic test for AT.[26] Unfortunately, the response of lymphocytes from obligate heterozygotes (parents of AT patients) was indistinguishable from that of normal cells.

Cell Viability. Since observation of chromosomal aberrations is a much more sensitive indicator of DNA damage than biochemical assay,[27] the former technique may provide information not otherwise obtainable. Shaham et al. reported that a diffusible clastogenic agent may be involved in AT. Cocultivation of plasma and lymphocytes from AT patients with cells from normal persons caused increased chromosomal damage in the normal cells.[28] Furthermore, conditioned medium from AT fibroblast cultures increased chromosomal breakage in normal lymphocytes. Shaham et al. made practical use of this information in the prenatal diagnosis of AT.[29] A clastogenic factor was detected in the amniotic fluid, and cultured amniotic cells had increased chromosomal breakage.

Chen et al. monitored viability of γ-irradiated lymphoblastoid lines by means of trypan blue exclusion.[30] Resistance of cells derived from AT heterozygotes was intermediate between that of normal and homozygous cells and clearly distinguishable from both. As stressed by Chen et al., additional AT families must be studied.

Fanconi's Anemia.   Patients with FA have congenital and chromosomal abnormalities, aplastic anemia, and a high incidence of leukemia and solid tumors. The latter are mainly hepatocellular carcinomas and squamous-cell carcinomas.[31] The question of whether heterozygotes are at increased risk for bladder, stomach, and breast cancer is unresolved.[32]

Studies of DNA Repair.   Various aspects of DNA repair in FA cells have been studied,[3] and a major area of interest is the repair of cross-links. Fibroblasts of FA patients are susceptible to chromosomal breakage and cell death after treatment with cross-linking agents such as mitomycin C (MMC). Different capabilities of FA cell lines to remove cross-links suggest the possible existence of complementation groups.[33] Frazelle et al. reported that post-treatment with adenine lessened the cytotoxic effect of MMC on FA fibroblasts.[34] On the basis of this and other observations, Michael Swift has administered adenine to patients with AT (personal communication). Although the study is still preliminary, encouraging results have been obtained.

Cell Viability.   Definitive experiments based on enumeration of chromosomal aberrations have been performed. Spontaneous chromosomal breakage in phytohemagglutinin (PHA)-stimulated FA lymphocytes was reduced by cocultivating them with normal cells.[35] Yoshida reported suppression of spontaneous MMC-induced chromosome aberrations when FA fibroblasts were fused with normal cells, and suggested that the technique may be employed to demonstrate genetic heterogeneity in FA.[36] And indeed, Zakrzewski and Sperling distinguished two FA complementation groups by fusing SV-40-transformed FA fibroblasts with FA cell lines.[37]

Auerbach and Wolman employed a difunctional alkylating agent, diepoxybutane (DEB), to distinguish FA heterozygous fibroblasts from normal.[38] The cross-linking agent induced an approximately five-fold increase in chromosome breaks in heterozygous cells, whereas normal fibroblasts were unaffected. Auerbach et al. described prenatal and postnatal diagnosis of FA and detection of heterozygotes with lymphocytes, amniotic cells, and fibroblasts.[39] Interestingly, heterozygous lymphocytes exhibited a several-fold increase in chromosome breaks after treatment with DEB. However, cells from some heterozygotes and normals had similar responses to DEB. Despite the fact that this technique may not be completely definitive, it would be worthwhile to examine inheritance patterns of the FA gene within extensive kindreds. In view of the apparent genetic heterogeneity in this disorder,[39] lymphocytes of some kindreds may exhibit clear-cut, gene-dosage responses to DEB.

Cutaneous Malignant Melanoma (CMM).   Cutaneous melanomas occur as familial or sporadic tumors, or rarely as metastases from internal melanomas. Familial CMM exhibits the usual aspects of hereditary cancer, that is, early onset of tumors that are often multiple. An unusual variant, familial atypical multiple mole melanoma (FAMMM) syndrome, has been described by Lynch et al.[40, 41] Patients with FAMMM syndrome may have unusual resilience; a patient of Lynch's has had 9 primary CMMs over an interval of 18 years.[40]

Much of the biochemical information in the literature has been obtained with animal tumors. By far, the emphasis has been on isolation and characterization of melanoma-specific antigens, with the goal of developing methods for diagnosis and therapy. Although there are many reports concerning human melanoma, investigators usually do not distinguish between hereditary and sporadic disease.

Studies of DNA Repair.   Some time ago, Whitehead and Little undertook an ambitious project to develop and characterize cell lines from most types of human primary melanoma and from metastases.[42] Kidson et al. employed several of these lines to obtain important biochemical data about human melanoma. For example, Chalmers et al. observed that several melanoma lines were very resistant to UVR. Of further interest, UV resistance was not correlated with melanin content; an amelanotic line also had high resistance.[43] The high UV resistance of melanoma lines was not due to decreased production of thymine dimers, nor to increased rates of dimer excision. Instead, it was suggested that resistance may depend on the ability of melanoma cells to continue DNA replication after high doses of UVR.[44] (Irradiation of normal fibroblasts is followed by an interval of greatly reduced replication). This ability to maintain post-UV replication was attributed to a highly efficient PRR system, and if efficiency of PRR involves nucleotide insertion rather than recombination, increased error frequency could be responsible for the high malignancy of melanoma. Hill and Setlow demonstrated the importance of PRR in the recovery of murine melanoma lines from UV-induced damage.[45]

An important exception to the observation of Chalmers et al. that melanoma lines are resistant to UVR[43] was described by Lavin et al.[46] An amelanotic line exhibited increased sensitivity that could not be attributed to increased production of thymine dimers or to defects in excision repair or PRR. Lavin et al. suggested that defective repair of a quantitatively minor, but biologically important, type of DNA damage may be responsible for cellular sensitivity to UV radiation. This concept strikes a responsive chord with me.[3] Unfortunately, the clinical histories are not available for the donors of the melanoma specimens from which these cell lines were derived. It would be of interest to know if the UV-sensitive line arose from a patient with FAMMM syndrome. This speculation arises from the report that fibroblasts from patients with dysplastic-nevus (i.e., FAMMM) syndrome are hypersensitive to UV radiation.[47]

Cell Viability.   Day et al. measured HCR by means of the ability of tumor cell lines to reactivate adenovirus 5 DNA after it was damaged by a methylating agent, N-methyl-N'-nitro-N-nitrosoguanidine (MNNG).[48] They observed that one of four melanoma lines had reduced HCR; an additional indication of defective repair was decreased cell survival in the presence of MNNG.

The preceding discussions illustrate the value of conducting investigations of DNA repair in hereditary cancer. Such studies provide information concerning genetic heterogeneity, etiology of disease states, identification of carriers of mutant genes, and possible modes of therapy. For an excellent current review of disorders involving DNA metabolism, see Cleaver.[15]

Hereditary Colon Cancer Syndromes

Of the various cancer family syndromes (CFSs), those involving colon cancer have been examined in sufficient detail to permit some tentative comments concerning DNA repair. Several genetic disorders may be listed under hereditary intestinal polyposis, with some disagreement as to whether each is a separate entity. Familial polyposis coli (FPC), also known as adenomatosis of the colon and rectum (ACR), is associated solely with colonic lesions. Other disorders involve extracolonic neoplasms as well, for example, Gardner's syndrome (GS), Peutz-Jeghers syndrome (PJS), Oldfield syndrome (OS), and Turcot's syndrome (TS). Hereditary colon cancer (HCC) is characterized by adenocarcinomas without polyposis coli.

Studies with Skin Fibroblasts.   As may be expected, much of the information concerning DNA repair and colon cancer was obtained with convenient fibroblast cultures. Even then, few investigations dealt directly with DNA repair.

Biochemical Studies.   Sasaki reported decreased survival of fibroblasts from patients with FPC, GS, and PJS after treatment with MMC.[49] Skin fibroblasts from two GS patients exhibited increased sensitivity to UVR, X-rays, and MMC but had normal UV-induced UDS.[50] Barfknecht and Little reported that fibroblasts from FPC, GS, and TS patients exhibited differential sensitivities to several alkylating agents, suggesting that the disorders may have different mechanisms of hypersensitivity.[51] Fibroblasts from a patient with FPC were reported to have normal radiosensitivity.[52]

Transformation Studies. Rasheed and Gardner demonstrated that skin fibroblasts from four of five GS patients and from two of three FPC patients had increased susceptibility to transformation by Kirsten murine sarcoma virus.[53] Of practical importance, cells from some of the young, unaffected relatives also had increased susceptibility. As noted by Rasheed and Gardner, follow-up of these and other family members will demonstrate whether efficiency of viral transformation is a marker for the colon cancer gene. Pfeffer and Kopelovich reported similar results with the same virus.[54] Fibroblasts from persons with FPC and GS exhibited increased expression of T antigen after infection with SV-40 virus but did not produce tumors in athymic mice.[55] The fact that cells from an asymptomatic member of a GS family displayed elevated T antigen expression suggests that this response may also be a marker for the polyposis gene.

Kopelovich et al. demonstrated that a tumor promoter, 12-*O*-tetradecanoyl phorbol-13-acetate (TPA) altered the characteristics of fibroblasts from FPC patients to the extent that cells injected into the anterior chamber of the eye of an athymic mouse produced a tumor. This experiment suggests that either the presence of the FPC gene represents an initiated state or the tumor produced by TPA-treated cells is an intermediate neoplasm, perhaps analogous to colonic polyps. In support of the latter interpretation, one should note that the neoplasms grew in the anterior chamber of the eye, an immunoprivileged site. Treatment of fibroblasts from FPC patients with *N*-methyl-*N'*-nitro-*N*-nitrosoguanidine (MNNG) caused morphological transformation, but the cells did not produce tumors after subcutaneous administration to nude mice.[57] Kopelovich described a unique action of TPA that distinguishes fibroblasts of persons prone to colorectal cancer from those of normal persons.[58] Both cell types exhibit reduced cloning efficiency at low concentrations of TPA, but normal cells are much more sensitive. Fibroblasts from a patient with FPC and from an asymptomatic gene carrier identified by other criteria exhibited about 30% survival under conditions where normal cells did not survive. Of further interest, cells from a patient with CFS and from a gene carrier also survived treatment with TPA. Kopelovich also reported that, with the various techniques employed by him and his colleagues, fibroblasts from GS families behaved like those from FPC groups. Thus, response to TPA may be a marker for the colorectal gene in general, and it was suggested that the technique may identify other types of familial cancer as well. Kopelovich also reported that, in order to develop a more rapid technique for identification of gene carriers, lymphocytes from persons at risk will be tested.

Increased In Vitro *Tetraploidy.* This topic is reviewed in detail by Danes et al. (Chap. 8) and Danes (Chap. 9). Briefly, cultures were obtained from split-thickness skin explants, brought through several subpassages, and examined for percent tetraploidy. It is important to ensure that, at the first passage, epithelial (presumably epidermal) cells as well as fibroblasts are transferred. Increased *in vitro* tetraploidy has been observed in several colon cancer syndromes, but it was not observed in 16 of 19 FPC families.[59] Danes reported tissue specificity in two FPC patients.[60] Increased *in vitro* tetraploidy did not develop in cultures derived from epidermis, dermis, mesentery, and colonic wall, but it was observed in cultures of unaffected colonic mucosa and polyps. A similar pattern was observed in tissue cultures from patients with GS, except that epidermal preparations also developed increased tetraploidy. Thus, the specificity of *in vitro* tetraploidy was directed toward tissues with the potential for malignant transformation (patients with GS are at increased risk for skin cancer).

Of the many intriguing aspects of *in vitro* tetraploidy, it would be illuminating to investigate DNA repair in skin cultures. For example, comparison of extent of DNA repair of cells from primary explant cultures with that of subcultures that have developed increased tetraploidy, would be informative. It may be even more informative to employ techniques for culturing pure keratinocytes.[61, 62] By cloning primary cultures, perhaps in conjunction with exposure to DNA-damaging agents, one could monitor the appearance of tetraploidy and determine whether tetraploidy confers a growth advantage. Application of these techniques to skin specimens from patients with hereditary colon cancer syndromes might provide answers to these fundamental questions:

Is development of tetraploidy a frequent event that rarely confers a growth advantage?

Does tetraploidy occur infrequently but usually result in a growth advantage?

Does induction of DNA damage alter the time course of appearance of tetraploidy?

If primary cultured cells have impaired DNA repair, do tetraploid cells inherit the defect?

Do cells with normal DNA repair develop an altered repair capacity when they become tetraploid?

An even more basic question is amenable to resolution by cloning techniques. This arises from consideration of whether increased *in vitro* tetraploidy arises from induction of new tetraploid cell lines or from growth of the original tetraploid fraction. The former interpretation seems plausible and is the basis for the questions posed above. Yet, since several cell passages are required to demonstrate increased tetraploidy, the tetraploid cells of the primary explant would need only a slight growth advantage to constitute a significant portion of the final subculture. For example, if the cells grew at 1.3 times the rate of diploid cells, an initial ratio of 2% would increase to 28% after 10 doublings.

Dexter et al. described a development that may have implications for the evaluation of *in vitro* tetraploidy.[63] They produced two sublines from a human colon carcinoma that differed in morphology and cloning efficiency and produced distinct tumors in athymic mice. One line had a normal karyotype, but the other exhibited increased hyperploidy centered around the tetraploid number. The authors cited several reasons for their belief that the tumor was heterogeneous at the time of surgical removal. This conclusion, coupled with different sensitivities of the sublines to chemotherapeutic agents, may explain why such agents may cause partial remission in patients with colon cancer but do not control the disorder.

Studies with Mucosal and Tumor Cells.   Although colon tumor lines have been established by various investigators, few reports relating to DNA repair are available. One of five colon carcinoma lines and a tumor line from a person with adenocarcinoma of the colon had impaired ability to repair MNNG-damaged adenovirus.[48, 64] In accord with clinical observations that radiotherapy is not effective for treatment of colon cancer, a cell line from a human adenocarcinoma had normal resistance to X-rays.[65] Erickson et al. noted that 5-fluorouracil (5-FU), a standard chemotherapeutic agent for colon cancer, has a response rate of about 20% and affords little increase in patient survival.[66] They investigated the action of another agent, 1-(2-Chloroethyl)-3-(4-methylcyclohexyl)-1-nitrosourea (MeCCNU), which has a clinical response rate similar to that of 5-FU. A colon carcinoma line that exhibited *in vivo* and *in vitro* resistance to MeCCNU effected complete repair of MeCCNU-induced DNA cross-links, whereas a cell line sensitive to the agent had little or no ability to repair cross-links.

Kanagalingam and Balis described an extensive investigation of DNA repair in rat intestinal mucosa cells.[67] They observed that *in vivo* exposure to known colon carcinogens caused considerable reduction in the *in vivo* ability of colonic surface cells to repair DNA damaged by alkylating agents. In accordance with the age-related incidence of colon cancer, surface and crypt cells of aged rats had greatly reduced DNA repair capacity. Thus, these observations suggest that chronic exposure of colonic cells to carcinogens, perhaps coupled with a loss of DNA repair capacity with age, operate to render colon cancer a "disease of old age." Alternatively, one may propose that a genetic flaw in DNA repair, potentiated by chronic exposure to carcinogens, would result in earlier onset of colon cancers. A study relevant to the etiology of human colon cancer was reported by Kalus.[68] He grew explants of 22 adenomas on fibrin foam and observed the development of carcinoma *in situ* in 15 of the cultures. Some of the malignant foci exhibited invasive tendencies by growing into the fibrin foam. These results suggest that adenomas have a potential for malignancy.

Transforming Genes (Oncogenes).   Detection of a transforming gene in a tumor line is the first step in the isolation and characterization of a DNA sequence involved in carcinogenesis. Murray et al. demonstrated that chromatin from a human colon carcinoma line (SW-480) could transform mouse fibroblasts.[69] By use of DNA sequence probes, they established that the transforming factor was different from those of a bladder carcinoma and a leukemia cell line. Fogh et al. have been developing and characterizing tumor cell lines for several years. They recently described 127 lines that produce tumors in nude (athymic) mice.[70] Perucho et al. described five human tumor lines capable of transforming mouse fibroblasts.[71] Three lines, two from lung cancers and one from a colon carcinoma, appeared to transfer the same human gene. Both of the colon carcinoma lines just mentioned produced tumors in athymic mice;[70, 72] the histology of the neoplasms produced by SW-480 was the same as that of the human tumor.[70] Unfortunately, perusal of the source references for the two lines did not reveal whether the tumor donors had hereditary colon cancer.

Clonal Origin of Colon Cancer.   A convenient method to assess the clonal or multicellular origin of a tumor is to examine glucose-6-phosphate dehydrogenase (G6PD) isozyme patterns in appropriate black female patients.[73] This technique is based on the knowledge that G6PD is coded on the X chromosome, that a variant (G6PD A) occurs in high frequency in blacks, and that random inactivation of the X chromosome occurs in females. Therefore, a female heterozygous for G6PD A will be a mosaic of two cell types—one producing G6PD A, and the other, the usual form (B). If a tumor arising in such a person contains a single G6PD type, it is assumed to have arisen from a single cell; appearance of both enzyme types in the tumor suggests a multicellular origin. Since G6PD is a dimer (A_2 and B_2), a hybrid (AB) would arise if both X chromosomes were active. This circumstance has not been observed in the numerous tumors examined to date, but the study of FPC and its variants may be rewarding. Since the only effective treatment for colon cancer in these disorders is resection of the colon, numerous neoplasms—in various stages from benign polyps to malignant tumors—are available. Although the incidence of colon cancer is now comparable in black and white Americans,[4] there appears to be no data concerning the clonal origin of tumors in FPC.[74] Beutler et al. reported that a colon carcinoma had a multicellular origin, whereas several liver metastases had either G6PD A or B.[75] This presents the interesting concept that metastatic offshoots of a primary tumor are often monoclonal, which is consistent with the premise that a metastatic cell undergoes considerable selection before it can survive at a site distant from the original neoplasm. Adolphson et al. demonstrated the monoclonal origin of a colonic villous adenoma from a female heterozygous for G6PD.[76] After separation from nonadenoma cells, the mucosal cells exhibited only G6PD A. With regard to *in vitro* tetraploidy, if clones of tetraploid keratinocytes from appropriate patients can be obtained, examining their G6PD patterns would be very interesting.

Is a Genetic Flaw in DNA Repair Involved in Hereditary Colon Cancer?

In an earlier section, I drew on my knowledge of skin metabolism and on insight gained in preparing a review of genodermatoses[3] to discuss the growth of colonic mucosal cells. I have already noted that the common growth pattern of mucosal and epidermal cells, that is, continuous proliferation balanced by loss of mature cells, is an evolutionary adaptation that enables the tissues to cope with their hostile environments. I also noted that continuous tissue turnover must be a potent defense against carcinogenesis and that this must be especially true for the colon. A logical extension of these premises is that the tissues have also developed efficient DNA repair systems, and I stress that these mechanisms may be to some extent tissue specific. For example, the epidermal repair systems of humans (and, perhaps, of other nonfurry animals) may be uniquely adapted for correction of DNA damage caused by a single ubiquitous carcinogen that other tissues receive little or no exposure to: ultraviolet radiation. This concept will be presented in detail elsewhere.[77] For the present discussion, let me simply state that I am becoming increasingly convinced of the validity of this hypothesis and would like to cite the following experiment of nature in its support.

Patients with XP develop multiple skin neoplasms at an early age and often die young of cutaneous malignant melanoma. Yet, in spite of the well-documented fact that defective DNA repair occurs in noncutaneous tissues of XP patients,[3] there are few reports of noncutaneous cancer in such patients. After an extensive review of the literature, Kraemer reported[13] cases of noncutaneous, nonocular cancer in XP patients.[78] Seven of these tumors were squamous cell carcinomas or unspecified tumors of the oral cavity; none involved the gastrointestinal tract. Kraemer presented several reasons why the incidence of internal cancers in XP patients may be underreported, but the fact that patients often died young in the past provides reasonable explanation for the lack of reports of internal cancers. If this reason is valid, the present circumstances of early diagnosis of XP and institution of lifetime avoidance of UVR will ensure that patients live long enough to develop noncutaneous cancers. Nevertheless, it may be productive to consider the implications of the premise that efficiency of DNA repair systems may be tissue specific for those tissues that are exposed to a unique carcinogen (epidermis) or a unique array of carcinogens (colonic mucosa).

Colonic mucosal cells are continuously assaulted by a battery of exogenous and endogenous agents to an extent not encountered by other tissues. Lying at the end of the gastrointestinal tract, the colon endures full exposure to harmful endogenous compounds and bacterial metabolites. Furthermore, the ability of the colon to concentrate its contents tenfold[8] exposes the tissue to high concentrations of noxious agents. It is reasonable, then, to consider that, in addition to other defenses against cancer (e.g., rapid cell turnover to minimize exposure interval, sequestration of carcinogens in aged surface cells), the colonic mucosal cell may have acquired uniquely efficient DNA repair systems. Also, depending on whether the colon of man is exposed to unique, ubiquitous carcinogens, repair capability may be specific to the extent that it is directed toward DNA damage caused by those agents.

The above considerations suggest that intensive investigation of DNA repair of colonic epithelial cells will be productive. Surgical material from patients with polyposis syndromes provides a spectrum of experimental tissue, from normal-appearing mucosa through several stages leading to malignant carcinoma. *In vitro* studies with cell cultures, analogous to the *in vivo* experiments conducted by Kanagalingam and Balis in rats,[67] may be especially informative. A unique problem in the investigation of colonic cells, in the context of detecting unique repair properties, is the selection of appropriate DNA-damaging agents. My inclination would be alkylation agents, as employed by Kanagalingam and Balis.[67] Those knowledgeable in the area of dietary factors and colon cancer may suggest more appropriate candidates.

While assembling information for this communication, I perused many reports that do not directly relate to DNA repair and colon cancer. This activity led to some concepts that, though speculative and perhaps naive, may provide starting points for productive follow-up by colon cancer experts.

Dietary Factors in Colon Cancer

Recognizing the enormous complexity of this topic and the extensive studies already performed by competent investigators, I suggest that a break-through in control and treatment of colon cancer may arise from consideration of information that is presently available. For example, Murray et al. reported a significantly higher incidence of nuclear dehydrogenating *Clostridium* in the feces of colorectal cancer patients than in control patients.[79] On the other hand, in comparing fecal constituents of a low-risk (Finnish) population and a high-risk (North American) one, Reddy et al. observed that fecal *Lactobacillus* -occurred in all members of the low-risk group and in 73% of the high-risk subjects.[80] One may then ask the following questions: Does *Clostridium* thrive in the colon in the absence of *Lactobacillus,* and does the former produce colon carcinogens? Are the persons in the high-risk group of Reddy et al. who do not have fecal *Lactobacillus* (27%) the ones at risk for colon cancer? And, can one reduce the risk of colon cancer by permanently *altering the gut flora in favor of Lactobacillus?*

I have a personal, unscientific bias for this last concept, based on an observation made many years ago. In an uncontrolled experiment, my wife rapidly cured herself of multiple, large aphthous ulcers by ingesting an inoculum of *Lactobacillus.* This salutary action on deranged metabolism of oral epithelium, effected by establishing *Lactobacillus* in the gut flora, left a lasting impression, and I have often wondered if this therapy might have more general applicability. Information concerning the enormity of extrapolating this concept to prophylaxis of colon cancer may be in the literature: Are populations or persons who regularly ingest yogurt at low risk for cancer?

While I was organizing the foregoing ruminations, an exciting report appeared.[81] The structure of a mutagen appearing in human feces was reported as an unsaturated lauryl ether of glycerol. The compound is produced by five *Bacteroides* species that occur in human colon, and it decomposes in the presence of trace amounts of acid. If this mutagen proves to be a colon carcinogen, *Lactobacillus* inoculum may play a two-fold prophylactic role. It may swamp out *Bacteroides* in the colon, and even if *Bacteroides* survives, the lactic acid produced by *Lactobacillus* will lower the pH of the colon to the extent that the carcinogen may decompose as rapidly as it is released.

Another report may be pertinent to these discussions. In their initial study, DeCosse et al. observed that administration of megadoses of vitamin C to polyposis patients accomplished reduction in number and size of rectal polyps in some patients.[82] A more rigorous double-blind study is now in progress. In my opinion, large doses of vitamin C must affect gut flora, and I would not be surprised if facultative anaerobes such as *Lactobacillus* were selected.

Therapeutic Use of 5-FU

In mulling over possible analogies between XP and hereditary colon cancer, I considered the fact that 5-FU is effective for removal of actinic keratoses and squamous cell carcinomas, whereas it is not as effective in treatment of colon cancer. The reasons for the therapeutic discrepancy is obvious: topical application to skin neoplasms produces high local 5-FU levels without serious systemic effect, but administration of sufficient agent to attain chemotherapeutic concentrations at the colonic mucosa is accompanied by systemic toxicity. These thoughts lead to the question: can one deliver 5-FU to the colon in a manner similar to topical skin application? The answer is so apparent, it must have been considered by oncologists, but perhaps it was not diligently pursued. One might prepare an alkali-stable, acid-sensitive derivative of 5-FU (carbonyl addition compound?) and encapsulate it to ensure undisturbed passage through the stomach. The capsule would be of such a nature as to dissolve in the alkaline milieu of the small intestine, and the 5-FU derivative would pass unchanged to the colon. The colon could be prepared for reception of the derivatized chemotherapeutic agent by prior inoculation with *Lactobacillus*. A more elegant technique would be to prepare an acid- and base-resistant derivative that could be selectively cleaved by a ubiquitous colon bacterium.

REFERENCES

1. Kussin, S.Z.; Lipkin, M.; and Winawer, S.J.: State of the art. Inherited colon cancer: Clinical implications. *Am. J. Gastroenterol.* **72:**448-457, 1979.
2. Elder, D.E.; Greene, M.H.; Bondi, E.E.; and Clark, W.H.: Acquired melanocytic nevi and melanoma. In: *Pathology of Malignant Melanoma* (Ackerman, A.B., ed.). New York, NY: Masson Publishing USA, Inc., 1981, pp. 185-215.
3. Correa, P.: Epidemiology of polyps and cancer. *Major Probl. Pathol.* **10:**126-152, 1978.
4. Johnson, J.A.: Biochemical aspects of cancer-associated genodermatoses. In: *Cancer-Associated Genodermatoses* (Lynch, H.T., and Fusaro, R.M., eds.). New York, NY: Van Nostrand Reinhold, 1982, pp. 440-540.
5. Sanford, P.A.: *Digestive System Physiology.* Baltimore, MD: University Park Press, 1982, pp. 124-145.
6. Phillips, S.F., and Devroede, G.J.: Functions of the large intestine. *Intern. Rev. Physiol.* **19:**263-290, 1979.
7. Eastwood, G.L.: Gastrointestinal epithelial renewal. *Gastroenterology* **72:**962-975, 1977.
8. Carey, W.D.: Colon physiology. *Cleveland Clin. Qtr.* **44:**73-81, 1977.
9. Lane, N.; Fenoglio, C.M.; Kaye, G.I.; and Pascal, R.P.: Defining the precursor tissue of ordinary large bowel carcinoma: Implications for cancer prevention. In: *Gastrointestinal Tract Cancer* (Lipkin, M., and Good, R.A., eds.). New York, NY: Plenum Medical Book Co., 1978, pp. 295-324.
10. Morson, B.C. (ed.): The pathogenesis of colorectal cancer. In: *Major Problems in Pathology.* Vol. 10. Philadelphia, PA: W.B. Saunders, 1978.

11. Lesher, S., and Bauman, J.: Cell kinetic studies of the intestinal epithelium: Maintenance of the intestinal epithelium in normal and irradiated animals. *NCI Mongr.* **30:**185-198, 1969.

12. Lipkin, M.: Phase 1 and phase 2 proliferative lesions of colonic epithelial cells in diseases leading to colonic cancer. *Cancer* **34:**878-888, 1974.

13. Deutsch, W.A., and Linn, S.: DNA binding activity from cultured human fibroblasts that is specific for partially depurinated DNA and that inserts purines into apurinic sites. *Proc. Natl. Acad. Sci. USA* **76:**141-144, 1979.

14. Cleaver, J.E.; Bootsma, D.; and Friedberg, E.: Human diseases with genetically altered DNA repair processes. *Genetics* **79:**215-225, 1975.

15. Cleaver, J.E.: Defective repair replication of DNA in xeroderma pigmentosum. *Nature* **218:**652-656, 1968.

16. Hofmann, H.; Jung, E.G.; and Schnyder, U.W.: Pigmented xerodermoid: First report of a family. *Bull. Cancer (Paris)* **65:**347-350, 1978.

17. Cleaver, J.E.: DNA damage, repair systems and human hypersensitive diseases. In: *Cancer and the Environment* (Demopoulos, H.B., and Mehlman, M.A., eds.). Park Forest So., IL: Pathotex Publications, 1980, pp. 53-58.

18. Jaspers, N.G.J.; Jansen-Van de Kuilen, G.; and Bootsma, D.: Complementation analysis of xeroderma pigmentosum variants. *Exp. Cell Res.* **136:**81-90, 1981.

19. Lehman, A.R.; Kirk-Bell, S.; Arlett, C.F.; Harcourt, S.A.; deWeerd-Kastelein, E.A.; Keijzer, W.; and Hall-Smith, P.: Repair of ultraviolet light damage in a variety of human fibroblast cell strains. *Cancer Res.* **37:**904-910, 1977.

20. Andrews, A.D.; Barrett, S.F.; and Robbins, J.H.: Relation of DNA repair processes to pathological aging of the nervous system in xeroderma pigmentosum. *Lancet* **1:**1318-1320, 1976.

21. Andrews, A.D.; Barrett, S.F.; and Robbins, J.H.: Xeroderma pigmentosum neurological abnormalities correlate with colony-forming ability after ultraviolet radiation. *Proc. Natl. Acad. Sci. USA* **75:**1984-1988, 1978.

22. Day, R.S., III: Studies on repair of adenovirus 2 by human fibroblasts using normal, xeroderma pigmentosum, and xeroderma pigmentosum heterozygous strains. *Cancer Res.* **34:** 1965-1970, 1974.

23. Rainbow, A.J.: Reduced capacity to repair irradiated adenovirus in fibroblasts from xeroderma pigmentosum heterozygotes. *Cancer Res.* **40:**3945-3949, 1980.

24. Paterson, M.C.; Smith, B.P.; Knight, P.A.; and Anderson, A.K.: Ataxia telangiectasia: An inherited human disease involving radiosensitivity, malignancy and defective DNA repair. In: *Research in Photobiology* (Castellani, A., ed.). New York, NY: Plenum Press, 1977, pp. 207-218.

25. Edwards, M.J. and Taylor, A.M.R.: Unusual levels of (ADP-ribose)$_n$ and DNA synthesis in ataxia telangiectasia cells following X-ray irradiation. *Nature* **287:**745-747, 1980.

26. Jaspers, N.G.J.; Scheres, J.M.J.C.; de Wit, J.; and Bootsma, D.: Rapid diagnostic test for ataxia telangiectasia. *Lancet* **2:**473, 1981.

27. Sheridan, R.B., III, and Huang, P.C.: Ataxia telangiectasia: Further considerations of the evidence for single strand break repair. *Mutat. Res.* **61:**415-417, 1979.

28. Shaham, M.; Becker, Y.; and Cohen, M.M.: A diffusable clastogenic factor in ataxia telangiectasia. *Cytogenet. Cell Genet.* **27:**155-161, 1980.

29. Shaham, M.; Voss, R.; Becker, Y.; Yarkoni, S.; Ornoy, A.; and Kohn, G.: Brief clinical and laboratory observations. Prenatal diagnosis of ataxia telangiectasia. *J. Ped.* **100:**134-137, 1982.

30. Chen, P.C.; Lavin, M.F.; and Kidson, C.: Identification of ataxia telangiectasia heterozygotes, a cancer prone population. *Nature* **274:**484-486, 1978.

31. Ortonne, J.P.; Jeune, R.; Coiffet, J.; and Thivolet, J.: Squamous cell carcinomas in Fanconi's anemia. *Arch. Dermatol.* **117:**443-444, 1981.

32. Swift, M.; Caldwell, R.J.; and Chase, C.: Reassessment of cancer predisposition of Fanconi anemia heterozygotes. *J. Natl. Cancer Inst.* **65:**863-867, 1980.

33. Fujiwara, Y.; Tatsumi, M.; and Sasaki, M.S.: Cross-link repair in human cells and its possible defect in Fanconi's anemia cells. *J. Mol. Biol.* **113:**635-649, 1977.

34. Frazelle, J.H.; Harris, J.S.; and Swift, M.: Response of Fanconi anemia fibroblasts to adenine and purine analogues. *Mutat. Res.* **80:**373-380, 1981.

35. Nordenson, I.; Bjorksten, B.; and Lundh, B.: Prevention of chromosomal breakage in Fanconi's anemia by concultivation with normal cells. *Hum. Genet.* **56:**169-171, 1980.

36. Yoshida, M.C.: Suppression of spontaneous and mitomycin C-induced chromosome aberrations in Fanconi's anemia by cell fusion with normal human fibroblasts. *Hum. Genet.* **55:** 223-226, 1980.

37. Zakrzewski, S., and Sperling, K.: Genetic heterogeneity of Fanconi's anemia demonstrated by somatic cell hybrids. *Hum. Genet.* **56:**81-84, 1980.

38. Auerbach, A.D., and Wolman, S.R.: Carcinogen-induced chromosome breakage in Fanconi's anaemia heterozygous cells. *Nature* **271:**69-71, 1978.

39. Auerbach, A.D.; Adler, B.; and Chaganti, R.S.K.: Prenatal and postnatal diagnosis and carrier detection of Fanconi anemia by a cytogenetic method. *Pediatrics* **67:**128-135, 1981.

40. Lynch, H.T.; Fusaro, R.M.; Pester, J.; Oosterhuis, J.A.; Went, L.N.; Rumke, P.; Neering, H.; and Lynch, J.F.: Tumour spectrum in the FAMMM syndrome. *Br. J. Cancer* **44:**553-560, 1981.

41. Lynch, H. T.; Fusaro, R.M.; and Pester, J.A.: Genetic heterogeneity and malignant melanoma. In: *Cancer-Associated Genodermatoses* (Lynch, H.T., and Fusaro, R.M., eds.). New York, NY: Van Nostrand Reinhold, 1982, pp. 394-439.

42. Whitehead, R.H., and Little, J.H.: Tissue culture studies on human malignant melanoma. In: *Mechanisms in Pigmentation.* (McGovern, V.J., and Russell, P., eds.). New York, NY: Karger, 1973, pp. 382-389.

43. Chalmers, A.H.; Lavin, M.; Atisoontornkul, S.; Mansbridge, J.; and Kidson, C.: Resistance of human melanoma cells to ultraviolet radiation. *Cancer Res.* **36:**1930-1934, 1976.

44. Lavin, M.; Chalmers, A.H.; and Kidson, C.: DNA repair and UV resistance in human melanoma. In: *Molecular Mechanisms for DNA Repair. Part B.* (Hanawalt, P.C., and Setlow, R.B., eds.). New York, NY: Plenum Press, 1974, pp. 817-819.

45. Hill, H.Z., and Setlow, R.B.: Postreplication repair in three murine melanomas,

a mammary carcinoma, and a normal mouse lung fibroblast line. *Cancer Res.* **40:**1867-1872, 1980.

46. Lavin, M.F.; Good, M.; Counsilman, C.; and Kidson, C.: Sensitivity and resistance of human melanoma cells to ultraviolet radiation. *Aust. J. Exp. Biol. Med. Sci.* **59:**515, 1981.

47. Dysplastic moles linked to melanoma. *Med. World News* **23:**25, 1982.

48. Day, R.S., III; Ziolkowski, C.H.J.; Scudiero, D.A.; Meyer, S.A.; and Mattern, M.R.: Human tumor cell strains defective in the repair of alkylation damage. *Carcinogen* **1:**21-32, 1980.

49. Sasaki, M.A.: Fanconi's anemia: A condition possibly associated with a defective DNA repair. In: *DNA Repair Mechanisms* (Hanawalt, P.C.; Friedberg, E.D.; and Fox, C.F., eds.). New York, NY: Academic Press, 1978, pp. 675-684.

50. Little, J.B.; Nove, J.; and Weichselbaum, R.R.: Abnormal sensitivity of diploid skin fibroblasts from a family with Gardner's syndrome to the lethal effects of X-irradiation, ultraviolet light and mitomycin-C. *Mutat. Res.* **70:**241-250, 1980.

51. Barfknecht, T.R., and Little, J.B.: Abnormal sensitivity of skin fibroblasts from familial polyposis patients to DNA alkylating agents. *Cancer Res.* **42:**1249-1254, 1982.

52. Weichselbaum, R.R.; Nove, J.; and Little, J.B.: X-ray sensitivity of fifty-three human diploid fibroblast cell strains from patients with characterized genetic disorders. *Cancer Res.* **40:**920-925, 1980.

53. Rasheed, S., and Gardner, M.B.: Growth properties and susceptibility to viral transformation of skin fibroblasts from individuals at high genetic risk for colorectal cancer. *J. Natl. Cancer Inst.* **66:**43-49, 1981.

54. Pfeffer, L.M., and Kopelovich, L.: Differential genetic susceptibility of cultured human skin fibroblasts to transformation by Kirsten murine sarcoma virus. *Cell* **10:**313-320, 1977.

55. Kopelovich, L., and Sirlin, S.: Human skin fibroblasts from individuals genetically predisposed to cancer are sensitive to an SV40-induced T antigen display and transformation. *Cancer* **45:**1108-1111, 1980.

56. Kopelovich, L.; Bias, N.E.; and Helson, L.: Tumour promoter alone induces neoplastic transformation of fibroblasts from humans genetically predisposed to cancer. *Nature* **282:**619-621, 1979.

57. Rhim, J.S.; Huebner, R.J.; Arnstein, P.; and Kopelovich, L.: Chemical transformation of cultured human skin fibroblasts derived from individuals with hereditary adenomatosis of the colon and rectum. *Intern. J. Cancer* **26:**565-569, 1980.

58. Kopelovich, L.: The use of a tumor promoter as a single parameter approach for the detection of individuals genetically predisposed to colorectal cancer. *Cancer Lett.* **12:**67-74, 1981.

59. Danes, B.S.: Occurrence of *in vitro* tetraploidy in the heritable colon cancer syndromes. *Cancer* **48:**1596-1601, 1981.

60. Danes, B.S.: Increased *in vitro* tetraploidy: Tissue specific within the heritable colorectal cancer syndromes with polyposis coli. *Cancer* **41:**2330-2334, 1978.

61. Kitano, Y.: Keratinization of human epidermal cells in culture. *Intern. J. Dermatol.* **18:**787-796, 1979.

62. Watt, F.M., and Green, H.: Stratification and terminal differentiation of cultured epidermal cells. *Nature* **295:**434-436, 1982.

63. Dexter, D.L.; Spremulli, E.N.; Fligiel, Z.; Barbosa, J.A.; Vogel, R.; VanVoorhees, A.; and Calabresi, P.: Heterogeneity of cancer cells from a single human colon carcinoma. *Am. J. Med.* **71:**949-956, 1981.

64. Day, R.S., III; Ziolkowski, C.H.J.; Scudiero, D.A.; Meyer, S.A.; Lubiniecki, A.S.; Girardi, A.J.; Galloway, S.M.; and Bynum, G.D.: Defective repair of alkylated DNA by human tumour and SV40-transformed human cell strains. *Nature* **288:**724-727, 1980.

65. Drewinko, B.; Yang, L-Y.; and Romsdahl, M.M.: Radiation response of cultured human carcinoembryonic antigen-producing colon adenocarcinoma cells. *Intern. J. Radiation Oncol. Biol. Physiol.* **2:**1109-1114, 1977.

66. Erickson, L.C.; Osieka, R.; and Kohn, K.W.: Differential repair of 1-(2-chloroethyl)-3-(4-methylcyclohexyl)-1-nitrosourea-induced DNA damage in two human colon tumor cell lines. *Cancer Res.* **38:**802-808, 1978.

67. Kanagalingam, K., and Balis, M.E.: *In vivo* repair of rat intestinal DNA damage by alkylating agents. *Cancer* **36:**2364-2372, 1975.

68. Kalus, M.: Carcinoma and adenomatous polyps of the colon and rectum in biopsy and organ tissue culture. *Cancer* **30:**972-982, 1972.

69. Murray, M.J.; Shilo, B-Z.; Shih, C.; Cowing, D.; Hsu, H.W.; and Weinberg, R.A.: Three different human tumor cell lines contain different oncogenes. *Cell* **25:**355-361, 1981.

70. Fogh, J.; Fogh, J.M.; and Orfeo, T.: One hundred twenty-seven cultured human tumor cell lines producing tumors in nude mice. *J. Natl. Cancer Inst.* **59:**221-226, 1977.

71. Perucho, M.; Goldfarb, M.; Shimuzu, K.; Lama, C.; Fogh, J.; and Wigler, M.: Human tumor-derived cell lines contain common and different transforming genes. *Cell* **27:**467-476, 1981.

72. Fogh, J., and Trempe, G.: New human tumor cell lines. In: *Human Tumor Cells In Vitro* (Fogh, J., ed.) New York, NY: Plenum Press, 1975, pp. 115-159.

73. Fialkow, P.J.: Clonal origin of human tumors. *Ann. Rev. Med.* **30:**135-143, 1979.

74. Murphy, E.A., and Krush, A.J.: Familial polyposis coli. *Prog. Med. Genet.* **4:**59-101, 1980.

75. Beutler, E.; Collins, Z.; and Irwin, L.E.: Value of genetic variants of glucose-6-phosphate dehydrogenase in tracing the origin of malignant tumors. *New Engl. J. Med.* **276:**389-391, 1967.

76. Adolphson, C.C.; Prchal, J.T.; and Carroll, A.J.: Colonic villous adenoma. Monoclonal origin. *J. Am. Med. Assn.* **247:**829-830, 1982.

77. Johnson, J.A.: Defective DNA repair as a biomarker for hereditary cancer. In preparation.

78. Kraemer, K.H.: Oculo-cutaneous and internal neoplasms in xeroderma pigmentosum: Implications for theories of carcinogenesis. In: *Carcinogenesis: Fundamental Mechanisms and Environmental Effects* (Pullman, B.; Ts'o, P.; and Gelboin, H., eds.). Boston, MA: Reidel, 1980, pp. 503-507.

79. Murray, W.R.; Blackwood, A.; Trotter, J.M.; Calman, K.C.; and MacKay, C.: Faecal bile acids and *Clostridia* in the aetiology of colorectal cancer. *Br. J. Cancer* **41**:923-928, 1980.

80. Reddy, B.S.; Hedges, A.R.; Laakso, K.; and Wynder, E.L.: Metabolic epidemiology of large bowel cancer. *Cancer* **42**:2832-2838, 1978.

81. Mutagen implicated in human colon cancer. *Chem. Eng. News* **60**:22-23, 1982.

82. DeCosse, J.J.; Bussey, H.J.R.; Thompson, J.P.S.; Eyers, A.A.; Ritchie, S.M.; and Morson, B.C.: Ascorbic acid in polyposis coli. In: *Colorectal Cancer: Prevention, Epidemiology, and Screening* (Winawer, S.; Schottenfeld, D.; and Sherlock, P., eds.). New York, NY: Raven Press. 1980, pp. 59-64.

12
Biological and Clinical Nuances in Hereditary Colon Cancer

Henry T. Lynch, M.D. and
Patrick M. Lynch, J.D., M.D.

The purpose of this chapter is two-fold: to review recent contributions to the literature on both polyposis and nonpolyposis hereditary colon cancer (HCC) that have not been addressed elsewhere in this book and to comment on crucial issues that have been discussed, but that the reader should assess independently.

THE FAMILIAL POLYPOSIS SYNDROMES

Although familial polyposis coli (FPC) is the most well known genetic disease predisposing to intestinal cancer, and perhaps the most well known of any hereditary precancerous disease, the current controversies that surround it merit discussion in the context of its historical development.

The first description of FPC was by Cripps in 1882;[1] its cancer association was established by Handford in 1890.[2] Research into the etiology and control of this disease was facilitated by the establishment of the St. Mark's Hospital (London) registry of families with FPC by Lockhart-Mummery in 1925.[3] Families comprising this registry have been described by others.[4-6] Dukes recognized variability in the clinical expression of adenomatous polyps in FPC families, but he emphasized a narrow set of criteria for the disease's classical presentation: by age 20 onset of isolated, adenomatous polyps, usually in the rectum and sigmoid colon, followed by a fairly rapid increase in number to cover most or all of the colon by age 30. If untreated (by colectomy) colonic cancer almost invariably follows generally by age 40 or 45.[7] Because this phenotype has been regarded as a clearly defined entity, FPC has frequently been cited as a model for the study of hereditary, cancer-predisposing disease.[4]

With increasing interest in FPC, attention gradually became focused on kindreds with extracolonic features. This, in turn, led to the supposition that distinct clinical entities exist.[8] Gardner and Richards, in describing the triad of polyposis coli, osteomas, and sebaceous cysts (Gardner's syndrome [GS]), were among the first to recognize the multifaceted clinical associations in this syndrome.[9] The genetic basis for several other polypoid disorders with extracolonic manifestations has been explored by many investigators, though debate continues over whether GS and FPC are distinguishable genetic entities.[10-12]

Variable Adenoma Expression

Familial aggregation of solitary polyps and colon cancer has been observed.[13, 14] The aggregation of solitary polyps was considered to be a distinct genetic entity rather than the result of incomplete penetrance of the polyposis gene, a supposition reinforced by the absence of diffuse polyposis coli in any patients from the family originally reported by Woolf et al.[14]

Maintaining a clear distinction between FPC and solitary, colorectal polyp syndrome[8] has been difficult in other families because of the observation of patients with diffuse polyposis coli (classical FPC) and those with only solitary polyps whose colon cancer predisposition appears to be equally high.

Two families (C-205 and C-210, Figs. 12-1 and 12-2) from our registry were studied in accordance with standard medical–genetic protocols.[15] Particular emphasis was given to descriptions of the number and anatomical distribution of adenomatous polyps in the colon and other areas of the gastrointestinal tract, as well as their association with carcinoma of the colon and other anatomic sites. In spite of the rate of medical record retrieval in these families, a number of the medical and pathology documents contained either limited or imprecise descriptions. For example, the records contained descriptions such as "hugh polyps" for which no precise measurements were given, polyps located at the "lower section" of the colon, or polyps described as "multiple" but lacking more accurate quantification. Consequently, classification of patients as having either isolated or diffuse polyps at a given time has, in some cases, been tentative and arbitrary, reflecting the incomplete and occasionally imprecise descriptions in available medical records.

Ages of onset for isolated and diffuse polyps was similar. Both pedigrees show extreme variability in the age when polyps were initially detected. Family C-205 had a mean onset of 28 years with a range of 5 to 72 years. Family C-210 had a mean onset of 24 years with a range of 14 to 53 years. In each pedigree, the occurrence of colorectal polyps spans at least three generations.

Figure 12-3 contrasts the cumulative age-of-onset distribution of initial colon polyps in the two subject pedigrees with that of diffuse polyps in FPC. The age-of-onset curve for FPC is based on figures for 281 pathologically

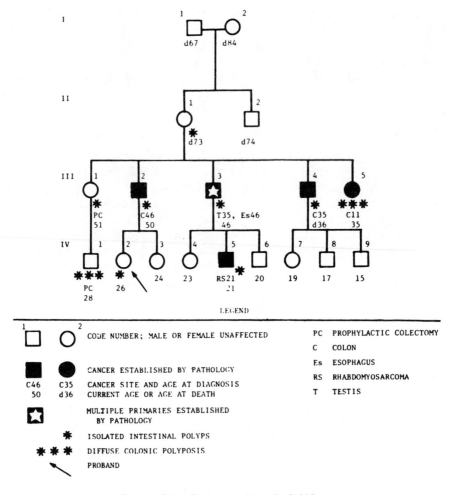

Figure 12-1. Pedigree of family C-205.

confirmed cases. The curves reflect earlier diagnosis of isolated polyps in FPC by a span of about 10 years, consistent with generally accepted notions regarding the temporal progression from isolated polyps of the distal colon to diffuse polyps in the entire large bowel. Affected members of the subject pedigrees show extreme variability in time intervals between diagnosis of isolated polyps and later symptoms of either diffuse polyps or cancer. In certain patients less than 2 years elapses (see Fig. 12-1, patient IV-1) to those who will probably never develop diffuse polyposis (see Fig. 12-2; patient III-3 developed one adenoma 21 yr ago).

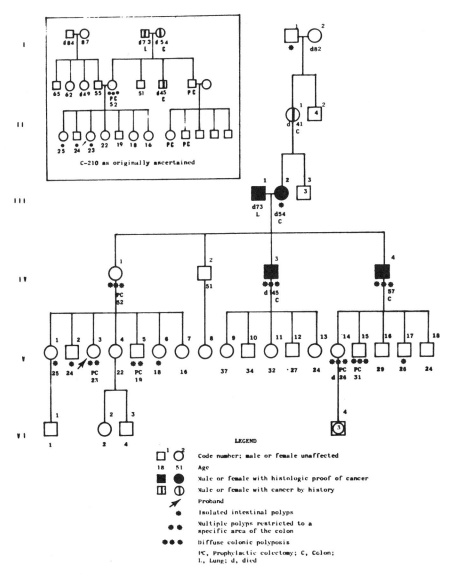

Figure 12-2. Pedigree of family C-210.

Other families have been reported with marked variation in phenotype. Lindberg and Kock report a family in which expression of colonic polyps ranged from few to diffuse in 5 of 11 members of an informative sibship.[16] Of note were 39-year-old male identical twins, one of whom underwent subtotal

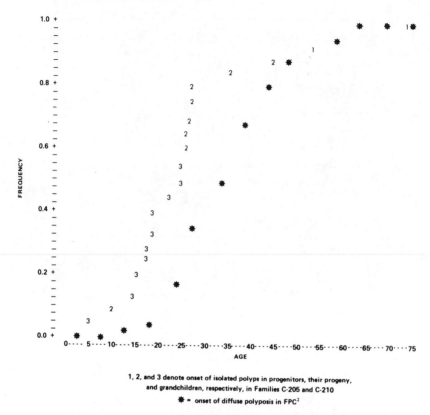

1, 2, and 3 denote onset of isolated polyps in progenitors, their progeny,
and grandchildren, respectively, in Families C-205 and C-210

＊ = onset of diffuse polyposis in FPC[2]

Figure 12-3. Age of onset of isolated polyps in families C-205 and C-210 (pooled) and of diffuse polyps in patients with FPC. *(From H.T. Lynch, P.M. Lynch, K.L. Follett, and R.E. Harris. Familial polyposis coli: heterogeneous polyp expression in two kindreds. J. Med. Genet. 16:3, 1979.)*

colectomy with ileorectal anastamosis (IRA) because of multiple polyps in the colon and rectum. Polyps were subsequently found to be primarily clustered in the ascending colon and sigmoid. Cancer was present in the cecum. The identical twin showed only several small polyps in the rectum, one of which contained cancer on histologic examination. Proctocolectomy revealed the rectal cancer and a second cancer involving the cecum. Numerous small polyps were also found in the cecum, with only a few polyps present in the sigmoid.

One sister in this family underwent abdominal-perineal resection for carcinoma of the rectum. Two polyps were observed in the operative specimen.

This patient subsequently underwent a colectomy on suspicion of FPC. A 2 cm × 2 cm polypoid tumor was found in the cecum, which microscopically was an adenoma with cellular atypia. No further adenomata were present. A 35-year-old brother underwent barium enema and two polyps were found in the sigmoid. Following a sigmoid resection, microscopic examination revealed only cellular atypia in the adenomatous polyps. A 45-year-old sister was found to have two polyps in the sigmoid on barium enema; no further treatment was provided. Barium enemas on the remaining members of this sibship did not reveal any evidence of polyps.

The father of these patients died of gastric carcinoma at age 61. Barium enema had not revealed any evidence of colonic polyps. The father's 74-year-old sister had a 3 cm polyp in the distal sigmoid and histology showed no evidence of malignancy; however, she subsequently presented with unresectable cancer in the same anatomic area, though barium enema did not reveal any other evidence of polyps. Finally, the father's 47-year-old brother underwent a gastrectomy for cancer of the stomach; no polyps were observed.

The kindred showed no evidence of mucosal pigmentation consistent with the Peutz-Jeghers syndrome (PJS), nor were there any cutaneous findings suggestive of GS. Variation in the phenotypic presentation of polyps in the kindred described raises a question as to the minimal criteria required to establish an FPC diagnosis; namely, whether there is some arbitrary minimum number of polyps or a particular anatomic site. As recently as 1970, it was stated that in polyposis coli, "experience suggests that there are never fewer than about 200 polyps," (Morson and Bussey [17], p. 31) though 100 may be a more generally accepted figure.

The preceding discussion suggests that accurate classification of each member is particularly critical in families whose members have both known diffuse polyposis and only isolated colonic polyps. Reliance on an arbitrary minimum number may cause the physician to dismiss the significance of isolated polyps, which may, in fact, represent limited expression of FPC in carriers of the deleterious gene. Conversely, more than 5% of the adult American population has one or more solitary polyps.[18, 19] Therefore, a dogmatic assumption that isolated polyps in a first-degree relative of an FPC proband represent reduced penetrance of the polyposis coli gene must be avoided and so must the assumption of "sporadic occurrence." Implicitly then, in the absence of reliable biological markers or distinguishing physical signs of the geotypic status (as in GS), it may not be possible to discriminate between patients with reduced penetrance of the FPC gene who are at high colon-cancer risk and patients who are free of the deleterious gene but have sporadic polyps. Patients whose genetic cancer risk is uncertain may one day be reliably distinguished by the use of one or more biomarkers currently under investigation.

Extra Colonic Signs

While "uncomplicated" FPC was at one time erroneously thought to be a rare and yet straightforward diagnosis, the earliest reports of GS demonstrated that the disorder would ultimately be recognized as a rather pleiomorphic one. In 1953, Gardner and Richards presented the first well-documented report of a family showing the cardinal features of the syndrome, namely, dermal cysts, intestinal polyps, and osteomas.[9] The family had previously been reported (in 1950 and 1951) as an example of FPC, and in a separate study, as showing hereditary multiple osteomas (1951). The 1953 report, however, related the several features in the common syndrome. Then, at about the same time, Oldfield reported a British family manifesting multiple sebaceous cysts and polyposis of the colon, having many years previously described the cystic features only.[20] Remarkably, the initial report of the sebaceous lesions included no reference to any colorectal cancers in the family.

The scores of more recent case reports containing detailed clinical and laboratory investigations have added greatly to our understanding of the syndrome. However, one preliminary point regarding nomenclature should be made. Because Gardner's and Oldfield's reports appeared to stress different clinical features of the syndrome, some have labeled the triad of polyposis, cysts, and osteomas with the eponym "Gardner's syndrome," while families having only polyposis and cysts have been referred to as having "Oldfield's syndrome" (OS). The distinction is an unnatural one for two reasons: there is no histologic difference between the sebaceous cysts of Oldfield and the epidermal cysts of Gardner, and because of the variability that exists in phenotypic expression, particularly with respect to occult osteomatous changes,[21] it is probable that, in any sufficiently large family, meticulous radiologic survey would uncover subtle syndrome characteristics, including osteomas. Failure to identify the full range of phenotype in a given kindred appears more consistent with the pleiotropic effects of a single gene than with the existence of two or more distinct genotypes.

Complex Tumor Expression in FPC

Cancer of extracolonic sites in so-called uncomplicated, multiple-adenomatous FPC, as well as in those with extracolonic signs, have been given increasing attention. In a recent review, Harned and Williams report a patient with FPC and a positive family history of colorectal cancer.[22] This patient lacked any stigmata of GS, presenting for evaluation of a suspected common-bile-duct stricture. Air-contrast barium enema revealed diffuse polyposis. A subtotal colectomy with ileoproctostomy was performed. Histopathology confirmed the presence of multiple adenomatous polyps of the colorectum. Subsequently, a Whipple procedure was performed for a well-differentiated periampullary adenocarcinoma. Two year follow-up showed no evidence of recurrent cancer.

We reviewed the controversy regarding the distinction between FPC and GS. Specific extracolonic lesions, including gastric and duodenal polyps, were noted to occur in at least 8% of patients with FPC as well as GS.[23, 24] The increased incidence of periampullary cancer in both FPC and GS suggested that the disorders were not distinct but rather a continuous expression of a single pleiotropic gene. Twenty-one documented cases of periampullary neoplasm were found in FPC and GS. Ten of these were malignancies of the ampulla of Vater (not otherwise specified), while seven were duodenal carcinomas and four were pancreatic cancers. In 14 patients, extracolonic signs consistent with GS were observed. The average age for development of periampullary cancer in these patients was 45 years with a range of 18 to 63 years. It was concluded that patients with FPC, with or without extracolonic signs, have a greater risk of developing periampullary cancer, particularly when duodenal polyps are present. Patients with FPC were admonished to have a thorough radiologic examination of the upper gastrointestinal tract at the time of initial diagnosis of FPC. Emphasis was given to the need for air-contrast studies in order to identify the gastric and duodenoal polyps. Finally, we calculated that the average time for development of periampullary cancer was about 15 years following the initial diagnosis of colonic polyps.

The problem of cancer of multiple anatomic sites in FPC may be even more extensive than indicated above.[25] Kindred C-205 (Fig. 12-1) showed not only variations in polyp phenotype but extracolonic tumors as well. One patient (III-3) with isolated colonic polyps had a seminoma at age 35 and gastroesophageal carcinoma at age 46. His son (IV-5), also with isolated colonic polyps, had a pararectal rhabdomyosarcoma. Determining whether any of these malignancies are genetically linked to the major cancer determinants in the polyposis syndromes will require follow-up of an even greater number of families.

Weinberger et al. described a patient who at age 3½ underwent a left lobectomy because of a multinodular tumor occupying most of the left lobe of the liver.[26] Histologic examination showed hepatocellular carcinoma. At age 8, the patient was found to have small (1-4 mm) cystic nodules on her face. Histologic examination revealed these to be epidermoid cysts. Follow-up of this patient at age 20 revealed multiple tubulovillous adenomas of the colon, necessitating subtotal colectomy with IRA. The unusual survival of this patient led Weinberger et al. to suggest the possibility of a polyposis-linked resistance to extracolonic malignancies.[26]

Weinberger et al., in their review of the literature, also found periampullary carcinoma to be the most common extracolonic malignancy in patients with FPC. Other tumors included papillary thyroid carcinoma, gliomas, carcinoid tumors of the small bowel, osteogenic sarcomas, cystadenocarcinoma of the ovary, transitional cell carcinoma, prostatic carcinoma, basal cell carcinoma, nevoid basal cell carcinoma, malignant melanoma, gastric carcinoma, carcinoma *in situ* of the gallbladder, adrenal carcinoma, carcinoma of the cervix, carcinoma of the uterus, chronic lymphatic leukemia, and hepatoma.

Hepatoblastoma has been observed in three other FPC kindreds.[27] Each patient had a mother and other maternal relatives affected with FPC. Survival of hepatoblastoma patients was exceptionally good.

Greenberg et al. recently described two brothers with classic features of FPC, including colonic adenocarcinoma.[28] In addition, each brother developed acute myelocytic leukemia. The parents of these brothers were first cousins, suggesting the possibility of an autosomal-recessive mode of genetic transmission. However, autosomal-dominant or X-linked transmission was also considered a possibility. The investigators suggest that this particular constellation of cancers is distinct from the usual forms of adenomatosis coli.

Juvenile Polyposis

Traditionally, juvenile polyps have been considered inflammatory or hamartomatous and lacking in malignant potential. The polyps typically have a smooth exterior, and their cut surfaces show multiple cystic spaces containing mucin, accounting for their occasionally being termed "retention polyps." They are further characterized by an increase in the supportive, connective-tissue matrix with the tubules separated by a fine reticulin. Such features are typically lacking in adenomas, which instead show a more lobulated surface, a relative decrease in goblet cells, crowding of nuclei, and hyperchromasia.[29]

Sachatello et al. subclassified juvenile polyposis into three categories: juvenile polyposis of infancy; juvenile polyposis coli; and generalized juvenile gastrointestinal polyposis.[30, 31] The distinctions are intended to emphasize that the infantile form carries a particularly unfavorable prognosis, with recurrent gastrointestinal bleeding, rectal prolapse, and intussuception. The second category of juvenile polyposis coli stresses that those patients surviving infancy may develop a diffuse colonic involvement that may be wrongly diagnosed as adenomatosis coli unless careful histologic evaluation is performed. Finally, the extracolonic presence of juvenile polyps occurring in certain patients must be considered because the distribution of polyps is not unlike that of PJS, and must be distinguished on the basis of the lack of melanin pigmentation of the oral mucosa and distal phalanges.

A growing number of case reports of multiple family members affected with juvenile polyposis coli has led to considerable speculation as to the possible relationship to the adenomatosis coli syndromes. At first blush, this should not be considered a problem due to the clear histologic differences that exist in the polyps themselves and the associated difference in premalignant potential. That such questions have arisen is important since invasive cancer has been known to supervene in patients with juvenile polyposis, with or without familiality of the condition. Several very well documented family studies[32-35] have included patients and their relatives with a definite continuum of polyp expression ranging from simple juvenile polyps through mixed forms to distinctly adenomatous forms.

Goodman et al. theorized that an unknown initiating event leads to focal areas of mucosal hyperplasia that evolve into small hyperplastic polyps.[36] These in turn become inflamed, ulcerate, and heal with development of cystic dilatation and mucus collection forming the typical juvenile polyp. In larger polyps, foci of epithelial atypia is believed to develop either because of genetic predisposition or increased susceptibility to carcinogens. In this way, tubulovillous polyps with precancerous features are thought to occur in a field of otherwise typical juvenile polyps.

BIOMARKER STUDIES

In Vitro Studies

Barfknecht and Little studied fibroblast cell cultures obtained from patients with the following hereditary FPC syndromes: FPC without extracolonic signs, TS, and GS. The cells were tested for sensitivity to the DNA-alkylating agents, methyl methanesulfonate (MMS); ethyl methanesulfonate; N-methyl-N'-nitro-N-nitrosoguanidine (MNNG); and 4-nitroquinoline 1-oxide.[37] Survival of fibroblast-cell strains in the respective syndromes was determined by clone-forming ability in relation to average survival from normal, human fibroblast strains. Fibroblasts from the FPC patient were moderately but significantly more sensitive to 4-nitroquinoline 1-oxide than normals. This FPC fibroblast strain was also significantly more sensitive to ethyl methanesulfonate. Fibroblasts from patients with TS were hypersentitive to MMS. Fibroblasts from the single patient with GS were moderately sensitive to MMS, ethyl methanesulfonate, and MNNG. The authors concluded that the differential sensitivity of putatively distinct, hereditary colon cancer syndromes may be a function of genotypic differences in the fibroblasts from these patients.

Kinsella et al. demonstrated a heterogeneous response to x-ray and far ultraviolet (UV) light irradiation in cultured skin-fibroblast lines from two unrelated kindreds with GS. In one family, all four clinically affected members had cell lines sensitive to the lethal effects of both x-ray and UV light irradiations. The x-ray damage was found to be intermediate between normal controls at one extreme, and sporadic colon cancer, and ataxia telangiectasia at the other. Similar findings were observed with respect to UV irradiation—values were intermediate between controls and patients with xeroderma pigmentosum. In contrast, two clinically affected persons with GS from the second family had skin fibroblast lines responding normally to x-ray and UV irradiation. The phenotypic expression of GS was similar in the two families. Moreover, there was no evidence in either kindred of intolerance to therapeutic irradiations such as premature skin aging or skin cancer.

Kinsella et al. reviewed the sensitivity to X-irradiation of skin fibroblasts in other dominantly inherited disorders. Regarding familial retinoblastoma, *in vitro* radiosensitivity was observed in patients with hereditary retinoblastoma, but not in those with sporadic forms. Those with hereditary retinoblastoma had a high rate of second primary cancer, usually osteogenic sarcoma. In addition, studies of radiosensitivity in D-deletion-retinoblastoma patients suggested a locus for radiosensitivity in the long arm of chromosome 13, adjacent to that for retinoblastoma.

Kinsella et al. concluded that sensitivity of cultured skin fibroblasts to X-ray and UV irradiation does not appear to be a consistent *in vitro* marker of GS. It was suggested that radiosensitivity may segregate with the GS gene in some affected families but not others. When these genes are present, they could be considered potentially useful for the identification of patients at high cancer risk. These findings are consistent with the possibility of heterogeneity in GS and could have a bearing on the data of Danes who has found increased *in vitro* tetraploidy in most but not all gene carriers of GS.[39] A 22-year-old female with classical GS stigmata showed no evidence of increased tetraploidy in cultured skin fibroblasts. This patient had one sibling with verified brain tumor. Her parents had no phenotypic features of GS nor have we been able to establish the presence of this disease in any maternal or paternal relatives, a picture suggestive of recessive TS.

Perucho et al. employed gene transfer as a tool for genetic analysis in human cancers.[40] Cultured cell lines stably incorporated and expressed foreign genes. Single-copy genes can be so transformed when total genomic DNA is the donor. Perucho et al. reported their work on DNA transfer from 21 human tumor cell lines with NIH/3T3 as a recipient. Five of the 21 tumor cell lines contained a gene or genes that were capable of transforming mouse cells. Perucho et al. observed that at least " . . . three different transforming genes are present in these lines, and three cell lines, one derived from colon and two from lung carcinomas, transfer the same or closely related human gene or genes" (p. 404).

Goldfarb et al. reviewed DNA-mediated gene transfer studies.[41] DNA from T24 human bladder carcinoma cells were capable of inducing foci of morphological transformed cells in NIH/3T3 recipients. From T24 DNA, biologically active sequences responsible for transformation were cloned. Their hybridization studies indicated " . . . that the transforming sequences contained in T24 are of human origin and closely homologous sequences are present in DNA from each of 40 different human sources that we have examined" (p. 409). The sequences were " . . . 5 kilobase pairs in size and homologous to a 1,100 base polyadenylated RNA species found in T24 and HeLa cells. Blot analysis indicates extensive restriction endonuclease polymorphism near this gene in human DNA" (p. 404).

Animal Models

The spontaneous occurrence of colonic cancer is relatively infrequent at the infrahuman level.[42] So, in order to use animal models for the study of colon cancer, investigators have had to rely on chemically induced or transplantable tumor models.

Spontaneous colonic carcinoma occurs in significant excess and is transmitted vertically in the *Saguinus oedipus oedipus,* a species of cotton-topped marmoset.[43] Multiple polyposis of the colon is not present, however, chronic ulcerative colitis occurs in excess in these animals. These two diseases may occur independently or concordantly. Of interest is the fact that in a very closely related species, *Saguinus fuscicollis illigeri,* and in the more common marmoset, *Callithrix jacchus,* colonic carcinoma does not develop. In the presence of virtually identical environmental exposures, the tumor expression in each species (susceptibility and resistance) remains the same. This clearly implicates the etiologic role of host factors.

The similarity in pathology as well as the pattern of tumor occurrence in the marmoset and in the human offers a unique model for the investigation of oncogenic processes. It should provide an opportunity to search out biochemical, physiological, virological, environmental, and genetic factors that might be etiologic in carcinogenesis. Given their phylogenetic similarity to humans, study of the marmoset could enable us to better comprehend oncogenic mechanisms in human colonic carcinoma.

Miyamoto and Takizawa studied spontaneous carcinoma of the large intestine in rats and considered this to be a model for the CFS.[44] They observed atypicality of basal cells, a phenomenon also described by Oohara et al.[45]

CANCER-ASSOCIATED GENODER-MATOSES AND COLORECTAL CANCER

A host of rare, colon-cancer-predisposing syndromes are distinguished by the presence of characteristic cutaneous signs. In all likelihood, the colon-cancer diathesis would not even be appreciated but for the associated skin findings. Several such syndromes are described by Lynch and Fusaro and are reviewed here.[46]

Cowden's Disease

This autosomal dominantly inherited disorder is characterized by multiple tricholemmomas and papillomas of the tongue and oral mucosa. Other cutaneous signs include facial papules, fibromas, keratoses of the acral portions of the limbs, angiomas, lipomas, vitiligo, and cafe-au-lait spots. In addition, these patients show virginal hypertrophy of the breasts, often with severe bilateral cystic disease.[46]

The dominant cancer association in this disease is carcinoma of the breast, often bilateral. Thyroid cancer has also been described as has malignant melanoma and squamous-cell carcinoma of the skin. These patients may have polyposis of the colon and be at risk of adenocarcinoma of the colon, though known cases are few.[46]

Turcot's Syndrome

This disorder is characterized by multiple, adenomatous, colonic polyps with secondary adenocarcinoma of the colon. In addition, patients are at high risk for malignant gliomas of the central nervous system. Cutaneous signs include occasional multiple pigmented nevi and cafe-au-lait spots.[46]

Most authorities consider this disorder to be inherited as autosomal recessive.[47, 48] However, a recent study by Lewis et al. suggests that autosomal-dominant inheritance may be a more correct interpretation.[49] Lewis et al. also suggest the possibility that certain TS patients may, in fact, manifest GS. Our personal experience is in accord with that reasoning.

Dyskeratosis Congenita (Zinsser-Cole-Engman Syndrome, Sex-Linked)

Affected patients have reticulated hypopigmentation and hyperpigmentation of the skin, dystrophy of the nails, leukoplakia of the oral mucosa, thrombocytopenia, anemia, and testicular atrophy. Cancers include squamous cell carcinoma of the oral cavity, esophagus, nasopharynx, skin, anus, and cervix, as well as adenocarcinoma of the rectum.[46]

Bloom's Syndrome (Autosomal Recessive)

Cutaneous findings in this disease include skin photosensitivity. Systemic signs include dwarfism (low birth-weight type) and an increase in chromatid breaks. Cancers in this disease include leukemia, lymphomas, squamous cell carcinoma of the esophagus, and adenocarcinoma of the colon.[46]

Peutz-Jeghers Syndrome (Autosomal Dominant)

The cutaneous lesions are macular and pigmented with sharp margins and a color variation from brown through blue-black. These lesions appear in infancy or early childhood, and characteristically occur around the mouth, on the lips (especially the lower lip), and on the buccal mucosa. Pigmentation appears punctate and can occur on the fingers, hard and soft palates, tongue, and eyes. These patients also manifest generalized hamartomatous intestinal polyposis, although mixed hamartomatous-adenomatous and discrete adenomatous polyps have been observed. Adenocarcinoma of the colon and other areas of the gastrointestinal tract occurs, although ovarian cancer is more common, being seen in about 10% of affected women.[46]

REFERENCES

1. Cripps, W.H.: Two cases of disseminated polyps of the rectum. *Trans. Pathol. Soc. Land.* **33**:165-168, 1882.
2. Handford, H.: Disseminated polpi of the large intestine becoming malignant. *Trans. Pathol. Soc. Land.* **41**:133, 1890.
3. Lockhart-Mummery, J.P.: Cancer and heredity. *Lancet* **1**:427-429, 1925.
4. Dukes, C.E.: The hereditary factors in polyposis intestini or multiple adenomata. *Cancer Rev.* **5**:241-256, 1930.
5. Veale, A.M.O.: Intestinal polyposis. In: *Eugenics Laboratory, Memoir Series No. 40.* London, England: Cambridge University Press, 1965.
6. Bussey, H.J.R.: *Familial Polyposis Coli: Family Studies, Histopathology, Differential Diagnosis, and Results of Treatment.* Baltimore, MD: Johns Hopkins University Press, 1975, 104p.
7. Dukes, C.E.: Familial intestinal polyposis. *Ann. Eugen.* **17**:1-50, 1952.
8. McKusick, V.J.: Genetic factors in intestinal polyposis. *JAMA* **182**:271-277, 1962.

9. Gardner, E.J., and Richards, R.C.: Multiple cutaneous and subcutaneous lesions occurring simultaneously with hereditary polyposis and osteomatosis. *Am. J. Hum. Genet.* **5:**139-147, 1953.

10. Axelsson, C.K.; Clausen, B.; and Henriksen, F.W.: Gardner's syndrome: report of three cases and review of the literature. *Acta Chir. Scand.* **143:**121-125, 1977.

11. Danes, B.S.; Krush, A.J.; and Gardner, E.J.: Is Gardner's syndrome a distinct genetic entity? *Lancet* **1:**925, 1977.

12. Cohen, B.S.: Familial polyposis coli and its extracolonic manifestations. *J. Med. Genet.* **19:**192-204, 1982.

13. Woolf, C.M., and Gardner, E.J.: Carcinoma of the gastrointestinal tract (in a Utah family). *J. Hered.* **41:**273-276, 1950.

14. Woolf, C.M.; Richards, R.C.; and Gardner, E.J.: Occasional discrete polyps of the colon and rectum showing inherited tendency in a kindred. *Cancer* **8:**403-408, 1955.

15. Lynch, H.T.; Lynch, P.M.; Follett, K.L.; and Harris, R.E.: Familial polyposis coli: Heterogeneous polyp expression in two kindreds. *J. Med. Genet.* **16:**1-7, 1979.

16. Lindberg, T.R., and Kock, N.G.: A family with atypical colonic polyposis and gastric cancer: A three decade followup. *Cancer* **35:**255-259, 1975.

17. Morson, B.C., and Bussey, H.J.R.: Predisposing causes of intestinal cancer. *Curr. Probl. Surg.* **1:**1-50, 1970.

18. Swinton, N.W.: Polyps of colon and rectum. *JAMA* **154:**658-662, 1954.

19. Myers, T.B., and Bacon, H.E.: Adenomas of the colon and rectum. *Dis. Colon Rect.* **3:**523-532, 1960.

20. Oldfield, M.C.: The association of familial polyposis of the colon with multiple sebaceous cysts. *Br. J. Surg.* **41:**534-541, 1954.

21. Utsunomiya, J., and Nakamura, T.: The occult osteomatous changes in the mandible in patients with familial polyposis coli. *Br. J. Surg.* **62:**45-51, 1975.

22. Harned, R.K., and Williams, S.M.: Familial polyposis coli and periampullary malignancy. *Dis. Colon Rect.* **25:**227-229, 1982.

23. Ushio, K.; Sasagawa, M.; Doi, H.; Yamada, T.; Ichikawa, H.; Hojo, K.; Koyama, Y.; and Sano, R.: Lesions associated with familial polyposis coli: studies of lesions of the stomach, duodenum, bones, and teeth. *Gastrointest. Radiol.* **1:**67-80, 1976.

24. Denzler, T.B.; Harned, R.K.; and Pergam, C.J.: Gastric polyps in familial polyposis coli. *Radiology* **130:**63-66, 1979.

25. Lynch, H.T.; Ruma, T.A.; Albano, W.A.; Lynch, J.F.; and Lynch, P.M.: Phenotypic variation in hereditary adenomatosis: Unusual tumor spectrum. *Dis. Colon Rect.* **25:**235-238, 1982.

26. Weinberger, J.M.; Cohen, Z.; and Berk, T.: Polyposis coli preceded by hepatocellular carcinoma: Report of a case. *Dis. Colon Rect.* **24:**296-300, 1981.

27. Kingston, J.E.; Draper, G.J.; and Mann, J.R.: Hepatoblastoma and polyposis. *Lancet:* **1:**457, 1982.

28. Greenberg, M.S.; Anderson, K.C.; Marchetto, D.J.; and Li, F.P.: Acute myelocytic leukemia in two brothers with polyposis coli and carcinoma of the colon. *Ann. Int. Med.* **95:**702-703, 1982.

29. Veale, A.M.O.; McColl, I.; Bussey, H.J.R.; and Morson, B.C.: Juvenile polyposis coli. *J. Med. Genet.* **3:**1-76, 1966.

30. Sachatello, C.R.; Pickren, J.W.; and Grace, J.T.: Generalized juvenile gastrointestinal polyposis: *Gastroenterology* **58:**699, 1970.

31. Sachatello, C.R.; Hahn, I.S.; and Carrington, C.B.: Juvenile gastrointestinal polyposis in a female infant: Report of a case and review of the literature of a recently described syndrome. *Surgery* **75:**107-114, 1974.

32. Stemper, T.J.; Kent, T.H.; and Summers, R.W.: Juvenile polyposis and gastrointestinal carcinoma. *Ann. Int. Med.* **83:**639-646, 1975.

33. Grotsky, H.W.; Rickert, R.R.; Smith, W.D.; and Newsome, J.F.: Familial juvenile polyposis coli. *Gastroenterology* **82:**494-501, 1982.

34. Haggitt, R.C., and Pitcock, J.A.: Familial juvenile polyposis of the colon. *Cancer* **26:**1232-1238, 1970.

35. Rozen, P., and Baratz, M.: Familial juvenile colonic polyposis with associated colon cancer. *Cancer* **49:**1500-1503, 1982.

36. Goodman, Z.D.; Yardley, J.H.; and Milligan, F.D.: Pathogeneses of colonic polyps in multiple juvenile polyposis. *Cancer* **43:**1906-1913, 1979.

37. Barfknecht, T.R., and Little, J.B.: Abnormal sensitivity of skin fibroblasts from familial polyposis patients to DNA alkylating agents. *Cancer Res.* **42:**1249-1254, 1982.

38. Kinsella, T.J.; Little, J.B.; Nove, J.; Weichselbaum, R.R.; Li, F.P.; Meyer, R.J.; Marchetto, D.J.; and Patterson, W.B.: Heterogeneous response to X-ray and ultraviolet light irradiation of cultured skin fibroblasts in two families with Gardner's syndrome. *JNCI* **68:**697-701, 1982.

39. Danes, B.S.: Increased *in vitro* tetraploidy: Tissue specific within the heritable colorectal syndromes with polyposis coli. *Cancer:* **41:**2330-2334, 1978.

40. Perucho, M.; Goldfarb, M.; Shimizu, K.; Lama, C.; Fogh, J.; and Wigler, M.: Human tumor derived cell lines contain common and different transforming genes. *Cell* **27:**467-476, 1981.

41. Goldfarb, M.; Shimizu, K.; Perucho, M.; and Wisler, M.: Isolation and preliminary characterization of a human transforming gene from T24 bladder carcinoma cells. *Nature* **296:**404-409, 1982.

42. Lushbaugh, C.C.; Humason, G.L.; Swartzendruber, D.C.; Richter, C.B.; and Gengozian, N.: Spontaneous colonic adenocarcinoma in marmosets. In: *Primates in Medicine.* Vol. 10S (Goldsmith, E.I., and Mgor Jankowski, J., eds.). Basel: Karger, 1978, pp. 119-134.

43. Clapp, N.K.; Tomkersley, W.G.; Holloway, E.C.; Heukek, M.A.; Schroeder, E.C.; and Gillespie, D.: Antemortem double-air contrast radiologic diagnosis of spontaneous colon carcinoma in the cotton-topped Tamarin, *Saguinus oedipus oedipus. J. Am. Vet. Med. Asson.* **183:**1328-1330, 1983.

44. Miyamoto, M., and Takizawa, S.: Brief communication: colon carcinoma of highly inbred rats. *JNCI* **55:**1471-1472, 1975.

45. Oohara, T.; Ihara, O.; Saji, K.; and Tohma, H.: Comparative study of familial polyposis coli and nonpolyposis coli on the histogenesis of large-intestinal adenoma. *Dis. Colon Rect.* **25:**446-453, 1982.

46. Lynch, H.T., and Fusaro, R.M.: *Cancer-Associated Genodermatoses.* New York, NY: Van Nostrand Reinhold, 1982, 559p.

47. Turcot, J.; Despres, J.P.; and St. Pierre, F.: Malignant tumors of the central nervous system associated with familial polyposis of the colon: report of two cases. *Dis. Colon Rect.* **2:**465-468, 1959.

48. Baughman, F.A.; List, C.F.; Williams, J.R.; Muldoon, J.P.; Segarra, J.M.; and Volkel, J.S.: The glioma-polyposis syndrome. *N. Eng. J. Med.* **281:**1345-1346, 1969.

49. Lewis, J.H.; Ginsberg, A.L.; and Toomey, K.E.: Turcot's syndrome: Evidence for autosomal dominant inheritance. *Cancer* **51:**524-528, 1983.

13
The Process of Family Registration

Patrick M. Lynch, J.D., M.D.

The value of longitudinal surveillance of colon cancer-prone families was discussed at some length in Chapter 5. It was apparent that maintaining a resource of cancer-prone families might readily enable the investigator to determine whether a putative mode of genetic transmission of tumor susceptibility could be observed prospectively within a given family. Such follow-up would also serve to dispel concerns over biases inherent in the initial ascertainment cluster found in a given family. Moreover, follow-up of previously contacted families makes possible a varying degree of retrospective-prospective assessment of newly suspected clinical features or assessment of biomarkers that may be identified as being genotypically associated with colon cancer risk. The value of such endeavors has been seen in the discussions of natural history, including early age of onset, multiple primary malignancies, proximal colonic involvement, and extracolonic lesions.

CURRENT STATUS OF FAMILIES REPORTED IN INTERNATIONAL LITERATURE

While it has proven beneficial to longitudinally assess the kindreds in our own registry, we have often found it useful to compare clinical features in individual kindreds reported by other investigators. Identification of similar or differing patterns in colon cancer-prone families reported by international investigators would logically support or refute inferences made on the basis of data from families in our ongoing studies. Because not all details are provided in published accounts, inquiries to the authors themselves are pursued.

In a preliminary effort to assess the potential for retrospective-prospective evaluation, inquiries were directed to the authors of all known papers describing families with nonpolyposis, heritable colon cancer (NP-HCC).

Because of our early suspicion of a link between heritable colon cancer and Torre's syndrome (TS), case reports of the latter were similarly followed up. Among the inquiries directed to investigators were the following specific questions: Has the kindred ever been part of a registry organized to follow such families? With respect to colon cancer occurrences, what were the anatomic subsites within the colon where the tumors occurred? What were the ages of the affected patients? What was the frequency of multiple, primary malignancy? What was the pedigree relationship of newly diagnosed patients to previously affected patients? What biological–genetic marker or chromosome studies have been conducted on surviving cancer patients and their relatives? Has any other research in the field of colon cancer genetics been conducted at your institution?

Because many of these case reports were at least 15 years old, fewer than half of the investigators were still at the original institution. Information could rarely be retrieved regarding such cases. A capsulized overview of certain selected responses from these inquiries follows.

1. In one case, both authors had left the hospital where the propositus had been treated. The senior author indicated that he had unsuccessfully tried to trace members of the family approximately 10 years after the initial report.

2. In another case, an author was able to retrieve the records describing the site distribution of the tumors described in the initial report. He indicated that family members were rather widely dispersed geographically—frustrating an attempt at immunologic screening of asymptomatic members that had once been anticipated. He also indicated that because of the lack of cooperation of certain branches of the family, attempts at screening were not attempted. Because of the problems described, no further investigation of the family was planned.

3. A third author indicated that the family reported had not been part of any registry nor the subject of marker studies. No more recent cases were known to have occurred in the family, although, apparently, no follow-up had been attempted.

4. Another author indicated that no work beyond the initial report had been or could be performed. One reason for this was that the propositus had refused to allow the investigators to contact other members of his family. The report had been based in its entirety on history provided by the propositus, who had since died. No marker studies had been performed, and no other work with colon cancer-prone families had been conducted.

5. A fifth author suggested that because theirs was strictly a clinical department, they were not in a position to conduct further work of a research nature. It was stated that the necessity of visiting patients distributed over a large geographic area would more logically be the work of a

research department at a local university. There was no indication that any attempt had been made to collaborate with any such research institution.

Clearly, several factors hampered the potential for longitudinal evaluation and surveillance-management of the cancer-prone families reported in the literature. First and foremost, is the fact that most of these families were reported by clinicians who had the skill to recognize and adequately document a reported family history but who lacked either interest, funding, or other logistical support to maintain continuity of these efforts. The majority of these investigators also lacked adequate liaison with clinical genetics units. Such units, had they existed or been consulted, could have provided long-term follow-up, marker studies (when available), and feedback to those clinicians able to offer cancer screening. Another problem may have been that, at the time most of these reports were published, no one had much experience with the clinical features and inheritance patterns of these families. Thus, the now-recognized potential for establishing screening programs, an important justification for intensive follow-up, was not considered feasible or indicated. Similarly, the potential laboratory markers of high genetic risk that are currently being tested had not yet been refined at the time most early family studies were performed.

Establishment of a Registry of Cancer-Prone Families

Fortunately, systems for the storage of data on persons with genetic disease and their families were developed in recent years. The number of such registries, including those dealing with heritable cancer and precancer syndromes, is also on the increase. Regardless of the disease that is the focus of a given registry, the people operating the registry must decide whether the program's mission is to be primarily genetic counseling and disease management, clinical and basic scientific research, or a combination of both. Because it is difficult and usually undesirable to completely divorce treatment from research in clinical studies dealing with sensitive family issues, responsible genetic disease registries usually attempt to offer some degree of both management and research.

The registry of cancer-prone families that is housed at the Creighton University School of Medicine in Omaha, Nebraska is no exception. In addition to kindreds with hereditary colon cancer, (HCC) with or without polyposis, there are a number of families showing patterns of cancer expression consistent with autosomal-dominant inheritance of breast cancer, ovarian cancer, malignant melanoma, and much more complex multicancer syndromes. The total registry contains kindreds from virtually every state in the United States and several foreign countries. Accession of kindreds over the past 15 to 20 years has been from a host of sources including physician referral, patient self-referral, evaluations of family history in several hospital and community-based surveys, and most recently, family history interviews conducted on consecutively ascertained patients seen in the oncology clinics and related services at three teaching hospitals in Omaha (Creighton University-affiliated St. Joseph Hospital, the University of Nebraska Hospital, and the Omaha Veteran's Administration Hospital).

RECOGNITION OF RISK

With rare exception, the discovery of a family afflicted with an HCC syndrome requires much more than an exhaustive workup of any single patient since it is the *pattern* of cancer expression on which a diagnosis is made, particularly in the case of nonpolyposis HCC. Thus, there is a degree of feedback in which the initial history heightens the index of suspicion, leading to identification of additional affected patients through further information-gathering efforts. This in turn reinforces the initial suspicion enabling the identification of still more affected branches of the family. Ultimately, the diagnosis is established on the basis of a pattern observed over two, three, or more generations but with the continuing necessity of identifying collaterals for purposes of screening. The question of how much effort should be devoted to tracing collateral branches of the family depends to some extent on who has assumed the responsibility for doing so and the nature of that person's interest.

It is unreasonable to expect a primary care physician to work up a pedigree that may potentially reveal hundreds of family members extending over five, six, or more generations, much less attempt to organize a screening program for scores of high-risk persons scattered over a wide geographic area. On the other hand, given the increased interest in cancer genetics, there are insufficient referral centers capable of handling the growing number of high-risk families that are constantly being identified. Preliminary workup by the private clinician with ultimate referral of these extraordinary kindreds to research centers seems to be the most practical approach at this time.

Returning for a moment to the responsibilities of the individual practitioner, critical analysis necessitates that the issue be looked at somewhat legalistically. Clearly, every primary physician has a duty to perform a thorough history and physical on each patient. If that history reveals an obvious excess of early colon cancer in the immediate family, then at least two questions arise: What should the average practitioner be expected to know regarding the implications of such a history; that is, what are the prevailing standards of practice?; and supposing that the physician is, in fact, aware of the possibility of a heritable cancer syndrome, what is his responsibility for further workup, and does this responsibility extend beyond the immediate patient under his care? As to the first question, it is presently difficult to assess the standard of care since this depends on the geographic locality, practice specialty, and, of course, the customary practice of other physicians in the area. Certainly, as more and more knowledge is brought to bear in the general and specialty literature, such standards will become more clearly defined and, undoubtedly, they will be more demanding. As to the second question the scope of duty, relevant legal precedents can be cited in favor of the argument that the physician's responsibility extends beyond his immediate patient. An example of an expanded duty might include the patient who tells his psychiatrist he plans to kill his girlfriend and then carries out the threat. Here, the hotly debated questions are whether the psychiatrist had a duty to intervene on behalf of the girlfriend and what measures he might have taken. Another example might be failing to disclose the risk of Down's syndrome to pregnant mothers over age 35. In addition to the issue of required familiarity with such disorders, the question of duties to the unborn are also raised. Thus, it is not unreasonable to anticipate cases in the near future in which physicians are held liable for failing to identify and deal with risks to relatives of patients with diseases such as HCC, with or without polyposis coli.

Apparently, the primary care physician does have some duty to at least refer patients with suggestive family histories to specialized medical genetic centers or to obtain consultation from these centers. Unfortunately, though, few such centers exist. The National Foundation-March of Dimes International Directory of Genetic Services provides a listing of facilities offering such services, and "cancer genetics" was reported as an available service by 192 centers worldwide (22.8% of all genetic units responding). But because the directory lists services as they are volunteered by reporting units, no reliable assessment is available regarding the particular cancer genetics services offered. However, for our remaining discussion, we will assume that a center capable of dealing with the entire spectrum of issues is involved in a given situation.

Workup of Families: Initial Family History Screening Evaluation

Typically, a family physician reports a patient in his practice whose kindred resembles those previously documented in the literature, or, on rare occasions, a kindred that appears to manifest some previously undescribed syndrome. Whether the information is provided by a physician, concerned patient, or subject of a survey, an initial impression usually leads to one of three tentative classifications:

Random Cluster.   A random cluster is the chance aggregation of a few, late-age-at-onset tumors in sites not usually considered to have a significant hereditary component. Certainly, an occasional cluster may reflect a hereditary trait, but identification of clusters requires documentation of as yet unknown characteristics that are not evident from the obtainable family history.

Probable Syndrome.   Probable syndrome denotes a pattern of tumors of sufficiently high frequency within the kindred, with early onset, multiplicity of primary lesions in individual patients, or anatomic-site concordance, meriting more detailed genealogic investigation and pathologic verification of reported tumors. Obviously, such histories range from those that probably do manifest heritable cancer syndromes to those that may not. Further evaluation in all such cases is subject only to such factors as family size, cooperation by family members, availability of corroborating medical record data, and availability of resources.

Definite Hereditary Precancer Disease.   The Propositus is said to have definite, hereditary, precancer disease if he presents with incontrovertible physical signs or a compelling history of these signs in close relatives. Presuming that the physician recognizes such signs for what they are, (not always an easy task), the family workup focuses on identification of other similarly affected relatives and on a search for other signs or symptoms that may lead to subclassification of the syndrome through the contribution of newly recognized features of known disorders. Perhaps the classic example of this search was the recognition of soft tissue (epidermal cysts) and bony abnormalities (exostoses) in early reports of Gardner's syndrome (GS) supplemented in later years and in other families by the addition of features such as dental abnormalities and desmoid tumors.

The Ideal Setting

Accurate prediction of 50% cancer risk to a given patient requires a suitably large kindred that also shows an uncomplicated history of colorectal cancer with segregation, early onset, and the other salient characteristics previously described. Typically, the patient's direct genetic-line parent will have been afflicted with colorectal cancer at an early age. The younger the affected parent, the more credible the risk estimate.

Complicating Factors in Predicting Cancer Risk

Given the ideal circumstances just noted, the estimation of a 50% risk to offspring of affecteds consists of averaging the low (0–5%) risk to siblings who, in fact, are not gene carriers and the high risk (nearly 100%) to siblings who are gene carriers. The considerations cited below complicate the clinician's assessment of risk to any members of a given sibship, underscoring the value of identifying biological markers of gene-carrier status (see Chap. 6-10). Hopefully, comments regarding the common problems will enable the reader who has encountered such situations to approach the matter more pragmatically.

Small Family Size

Here, the issue is not so much whether risk for a particular patient can be estimated but, rather, the more fundamental question of whether the family as a whole is afflicted with the disease at all. Clearly, if only two or three relatives have been affected, genetic segregation cannot be demonstrated. If any relative had multiple adenomatosis coli, lack of segregation would normally not be a problem since the mode of inheritance is already established (autosomal dominant) and requires no proof of segregation. There is at least one exception to the axiom that polyposis always behaves as an autosomal-dominant trait; namely, TS (central nervous system tumors plus adenomatosis coli), which is thought to be inherited as an autosomal-recessive trait. As seen in Figure 13-1, the presence of a brain tumor in one sibling of a polyposis-affected patient and lack of signs in both parents would add considerable doubt to any estimate of risk to children in the next (third) generation. This problem of Turcot's alleged autosomal-recessive nature is compounded by the existence of several case reports of Gardner-like families in which brain tumors have been found, suggestive of the usual dominant inheritance.

Returning to the case of NP-HCC, small family size is a definite problem. However, even if only a few first-degree relatives are affected, with ages of onset sufficiently early (i.e., before 35 or 40), then the siblings and children of the affected should probably be screened according to a protocol nearly as rigorous as that employed in NP-HCC families. Certainly, in such cases, further investigation should be undertaken to identify collateral family branches to bolster the initial impression. In such a setting, further pedigree data can really only *substantiate* a syndrome diagnosis; negative findings in collaterals will not rule out a germinal mutation in the "high-risk branch". Longitudinal follow-up of the immediate offspring over a period of many years would offer a greater potential for supporting or refuting any tentative diagnosis and is, at present, probably the best approach.

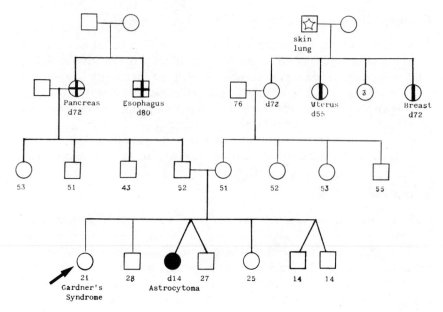

Figure 13-1. Pedigree of a family showing a 21-year-old woman with GS, including an intra-abdominal desmoid, whose 14-year-old sister had an astrocytoma. Both parents failed to show any evidence of GS. The possibility of TS has been advanced.

Late Onset in Parents

In this scenario and those that follow, one may assume we are describing a large, well-documented family in a typical sibship where colorectal cancer affects several siblings at an early age and leaves others unaffected at an advanced age. Add to this the diagnosis of colorectal cancer in another sibling at an advanced age, say, 70 or 80. Is this patient a gene carrier with reduced penetrance who simply did not express cancer until an advanced age, or is the patient a noncarrier whose disease was caused by the same (environmental?) factors that account for late-onset disease in the general population? Immediately before making such a diagnosis, we might have concluded that the patient's children are *not* at risk because the patient was asymptomatic at such a late age. Following the diagnosis, the risk to offspring may or may not be regarded as increased.

Such cases are not entirely hypothetical. In our largest family with site-specific colon cancer (C-198), there existed such a situation. Figure 13-2 shows relevant nuclear components of this large kindred.

Patient II-5 was diagnosed as having cecal cancer in 1972 at age 75. His father, three of seven siblings, and all three aunts and uncles had already had

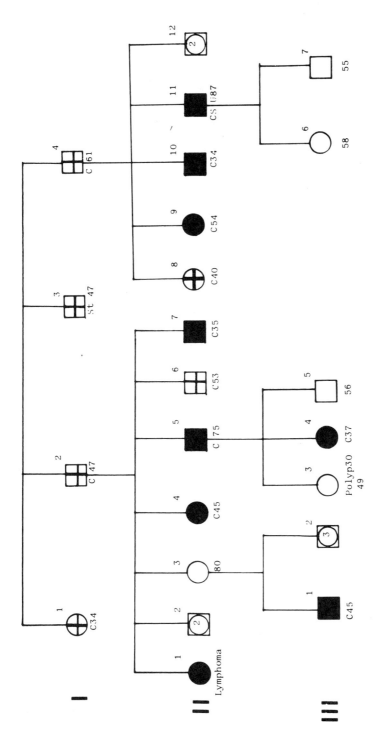

Figure 13-2. Pedigree of a family showing site-specific colorectal cancer. Note that patient II-5 had colon cancer at age 75 while his daughter had colon cancer at age 37. This shows the variable expression of this deleterious genotype.

colorectal (or in one case, possibly stomach) cancer at an average age of 46 years. By the time II-5 was found to have cancer, he had lost one 37-year-old daughter to colon cancer nine years previously. Another daughter, still cancer free, had had isolated adenomas removed at age 30. Had these daughters not already been affected, one might have concluded that patient II-5's case more likely represented a sporadic occurrence. On the other hand, given the fact of the daughters' involvement, patient II-5 would have to be regarded as an almost certain gene carrier whose ultimate affliction with colon cancer was nearly as certain, subject only to the possibility of earlier death from other causes.

Compare this circumstance to the case of patient II-11 (cousin of patient II-5), who himself had three colon cancer-affected siblings. In 1977 this patient died at age 87 of widespread abdominal carcinomatosis of uncertain primary origin. Of course, the uncertain primary diagnosis itself was a difficulty in this case. Assuming for the sake of argument that the primary lesion had been in the colon, then circumstances would have been identical to those of II-5, except that two children of II-11 are unaffected at ages 55 and 58. The key issue, then, becomes the risk to patients III-6 and III-7. No clear-cut answer based firmly on genetic interpretation can be given. Practically, however, patients in this position in the pedigree are customarily told that their risk is *probably* low (their father may not have had colon cancer; the cancer may have been "sporadic," anyway; they themselves are already beyond the age of greatest hereditary risk). Nevertheless, since any of the above considerations may be incorrect, surveillance is still recommended.

In summary, these observations clearly underscore the need for identification of one or more biomarkers of high sensitivity and specificity for discernment of genotype status.

Issues of Confidentiality and Privacy

Regardless of who assumes responsibility for identifying collateral relatives, a number of problems concerning patient privacy and record confidentiality are emerging. During the initial workup, it is difficult to acquire data and at the same time maintain the patient's and family's privacy. Suppose one provides an unsolicited notice to collateral relatives and their physicians regarding genetic risk information or attempts to seek background information for the family workup. Unless the original proband authorizes such activity, these efforts could technically be considered a breach of the confidential relationship between that patient and physician. However, this is rarely a problem if the patient is consulted as to the possible genetic etiology of cancer in his family and wants the workup performed. As a practical matter, the original patient must allow initial contact to be made with other family members or forsake his hope of obtaining the differential diagnosis required for effective counseling.

The setting in which problems more commonly arise involves the collateral relative who is contacted in the course of the workup of that branch of the family and responds negatively out of ignorance or fear. In this regard, a particularly unsettling example comes to mind. Several years ago, during the workup of an extremely large family with nonpolyposis, hereditary, site-specific colon cancer, a patient reported to us the existence of a large branch of the family located in another state, descended from a sibling of the patient's great-grandfather. Although there had been some exchange of correspondence in years past, little was known about the collateral relatives. We were encouraged by the patient to contact several of these collateral relatives, but when we attempted to obtain information from a distant cousin, she became noticeably upset and asked, "Where were you people when my father died?" Further discussion was abruptly terminated. Communication with other relatives eventually did reveal that this branch of the family had been as riddled with cancer as the initial cluster. The irate cousin's father had himself died of colon cancer many years before the initiation of our study.

Although this is a somewhat extreme example, it nevertheless points out the reactions that the well-intentioned investigator may encounter in the course of what would seem to be a necessary undertaking. Ideally, one would initially contact the physicians of collateral relatives before initial contact, but this is rarely possible because the patients themselves are the only source for identifying their physicians. Such considerations provide examples as to why extended pedigree analysis is usually not possible by an attending physician and why it requires the expertise of a cancer genetics team familiar with specific means of gathering data, preserving confidentiality, and doing patient–family counseling.

Financing

Reimbursement for services to cancer-prone families is not a matter of simply submitting a bill for diagnostic and therapeutic services rendered. With the increased expense of medical care, the role of third-party carriers in distributing such costs has become preeminent. Out-of-pocket payments could bankrupt even the well-to-do patients, and universal, governmental, health care programs are, for a variety of reasons, not acceptable to a majority of Americans or legislators. The problem with our existing dependence on commercial third-party carriers is associated with a preoccupation with acute care medicine. No one would argue that the sick patient at the hospital's door should be the top priority in any system. The extension of insurance payments to preventive medicine, would increase premiums across the board in exchange for benefits that are difficult to assess actuarially. The development of the detailed pedigree analysis, genetic-risk counseling, or cancer screening outlined earlier would not be covered by the typical insurance policy. Certainly, a physician could fabricate some reason for performing screening exams, and examples of this are known to us, but such practices border on insurance fraud and offer no long-term solution. Another part of the problem could be posed in terms of this question: Even if insurance covered screening of individual patients, to whose policy should the costs of working up the pedigree and identifying high-risk relatives be charged? On one hand, the benefits of the evaluation extend well beyond the Propositus, so it would be unfair for his policy to cover the expenses. On the other hand, the collateral relatives identified will not have solicited the effort already made on their behalf.

The circular reasoning described suggests that a somewhat different approach be taken altogether. Government- or foundation-research support of projects designed to carry out such work has been suggested, and indeed, clinical, research-counseling registries have existed for some time. Unfortunately, such schemes for support of centralized or local efforts could never reach the scale that solving the problem requires. Such sources would always be dependent on the caprices of private and governmental giving, and they are not the appropriate vehicles for handling essentially service-related work in the first place.

At this time, we can offer no panacea for resolving the dilemma that has been outlined. We can only emphasize that costs of implementing the comprehensive program must be distributed over a large population. Development of a mechanism for handling a multifaceted problem that is needed by large numbers of persons will test the ingenuity and creativity of workers in many disciplines.

Epilogue

Many physicians still do not recognize the existence of hereditary forms of colon cancer, at least not in the absence of polyposis. Although it was not our specific goal, we believe that this book has demonstrated that HCC, with or without diffuse adenomatosis, comprises clinical entities that may not only be recognized but may also be managed with reasonable success.

Evidence that HCC is a problem to be seriously addressed is further supported by the attention devoted to the disease at several recent conferences. In March 1981, the Second International Symposium on Colorectal Cancer held a series of workshops entitled "Risk Factors and Screening." One of the workshops was devoted primarily to inherited colon cancer without polyposis. The following excerpt is taken verbatim from the "Report of the International Workgroup on Colorectal Cancer," which summarized the findings from the workshops.

Risk

Number of Affected Relatives: If the risk of development of colorectal cancer in someone in a community who has no family history of colorectal cancer is taken as unity, the data collected from different centers suggests that the person who has one affected relative is between three and four times more likely to develop the disease than unity. The empiric risk probably increases with the number of affected relatives, but the data we have on this aspect makes it difficult to quantify. The risk is probably quite steep with increasing numbers of affected relatives until, with five or six affected, the risk probably approaches the 50% found in well-documented hereditary, colon cancer families.

Age at Onset and Multiple Primary Tumors: The risk is influenced by the age at onset of colorectal cancer in the affected relative, being particularly high if a first degree relative has had the disease below the age of 40 years. The data indicate that colorectal cancer may develop in 60% of first-degree relatives of people dying of early onset colorectal cancer.

There is an additional increase in risk if a first-degree relative has had multiple primary tumors. There is an association between early age at onset and multiple primary tumors, in that someone who had one colorectal cancer before the age of 40 years is at considerably greater risk of developing another primary colorectal cancer than the unity risk, though again, the data aren't sufficient to quantify the risk with precision.

Positive Family History: Medical geneticists often confine their analysis to first degree relatives, that is, parents, sibs, and offspring. In the context of colorectal cancer, however, with its preponderance of late onset cases, offspring are unlikely to be already affected, and many sibs who will develop the disease may still be unaffected when the family history is taken. A positive family history should therefore be one in which colorectal cancer has occurred in a first-degree relative or parental sib (an uncle or aunt). The workgroup was agreed that the family history taken by the average clinician is not of much value. Clinicians use family history as a guide to the degree of likelihood in differential diagnosis and to the priority to give to certain investigations. Once a diagnosis of colorectal cancer is made, the family history needs to be taken in great detail from the patient and verified by relatives, hospital records, and death certificates. The names and addresses of all living relatives at risk should be recorded. This is probably best done by someone specially trained in the technique. It might be a field worker attached to the interested clinician or perhaps someone from a medical genetics unit who collaborates with many clinicians.

Screening and Surveillance—Discussion and Recommendations

In familial adenomatosis coli, screening should start in the early teens. In a well-documented hereditary colon cancer family, with its apparent Mendelian dominant inheritance, it should probably start in the 20s. In the ordinary high-risk person who has one affected relative, the consensus of opinion was that 40 was a reasonable age to start screening. An earlier age might be indicated when several relatives have been affected or if the family history is of early onset and multiple or perhaps right-sided colorectal cancer.

The workgroup was in favor of testing for fecal occult blood as a primary screening technique and perhaps, that is all that is needed in the lower risk groups (negative family history or one affected relative). As the risk increases, an additional form of regular screening is needed. The workgroup considered that either barium enema or colonoscopy could be used, depending on local expertise. The frequency of such additional screening should depend on the degree of risk—from yearly colonoscopy in the very high-risk group of hereditary colon cancer family members to a screening of the whole colon for polyps once with a repeat perhaps every 5 years.

Markers

At present, there is no marker which can be used to detect which individual is more likely to develop colorectal cancer than another individual. There is certainly nothing as useful as the testing of serum pepsinogen-1 and serum gastrin as a pointer to future carcinoma of the stomach. There are, however, a great many tests and investigations which, in the opinion of the workshop members, may in the future be of practical value in predicting colorectal cancer. The different fields of ongoing research which were discussed were: chromosomal abnormalities; cytokinetic studies using tritiated thymidine labelling; studies of intestinal content of cholesterol and bile acids; and many aspects of immunology, including antigens, immunodeficiencies, viruses, and mixed leukocyte cultures.

Surgery

The workshop considered that the surgical treatment for patients after colorectal cancer has been diagnosed should be tailored to that patient's risk of developing further carcinomas of the colon. If the patient is under 40 years of age, there is a case for subtotal colectomy as an alternative to local resection and a long continued surveillance of the remaining colon. When a patient with the Cancer Family Syndrome presents with colorectal cancer, it seems wise to do a hysterectomy as well as subtotal colectomy.

Future Studies: Registries

The workgroup was almost unanimously against a national registry, principally because of confidentiality. Local registries maintained by clincians were, however, favored. In them, the patients should be subdivided into those with negative family histories whose relatives would therefore be at moderate risk and those with various degrees of positive family histories whose relatives would be at high risk. Details of the relatives, their degree of risk, and control of the screening program would be the most valuable features of such a registry.

There is little knowledge of the part played by heredity in the etiology of solitary colonic adenomata. In a few recorded families, there is a suggestion of an important hereditary component, but detailed study of the genetics of "small numbers of colonic polyps" might throw useful light on the problem of the polyp–cancer relationship and on the etiology of colorectal cancer.

The workshop considered the objectives of future workshop meetings and symposia. Even though there is need for further meetings to look into the genetics of colorectal cancer, it was felt that the geneticists should not meet in isolation, they should meet with the environmentalists and it was considered that a meeting to study the epidemiology and genetics of colorectal cancer could be very rewarding.

Critique of Workshop Report

Although this workshop was essentially directed towards consensus development, there were several issues with which we are forced to take exception. First, we are reluctant to encourage the use of empiric risk based solely on increasing numbers of affected first-degree relatives. As discussed in Chapters 4, 5, and 11, there are a plethora of factors that must be considered further before the initiation of any screening based on such empiric figures is undertaken. In this regard, the work group is to be commended for its recognition of early age at onset, multiple primary involvement, and right-sidedness as factors to be weighed in considering the significance of a given family history.

Second, the recommendation that hysterectomy be performed with subtotal colectomy in cases of Cancer Family Syndrome (CFS) should be carefully circumscribed. It must first be established that the family is indeed one in which endometrial carcinoma exists, not one with site-specific HCC in which endometrial carcinoma is absent. For reasons that remain elusive, ovarian carcinoma seems to occur excessively in certain CFS families but not in others, and because the increase in morbidity is negligible, oophorectomy at the time of hysterectomy and colectomy should be entertained.

Finally, we found ourselves in the minority for favoring a national, though not necessarily federally funded, registry. Although many obstacles do exist, and the concept must be dealt with very carefully and deliberately, alleged problems of confidentiality are by no means insurmountable. Indeed, it has been argued that greater centralization of any registry system fosters *preservation* of confidentiality, if only by virtue of the increased scrutiny that such a program would undergo before its initiation and throughout the course of its operation.

Not fully reflected in the report just explained was the intensive discussion devoted to the direction of future research. Because significant controversy surrounded the discussions of syndrome recognition, screening of known high-risk patients, and marker research, it was agreed that each factor should be more intensively and systematically studied so that more clinically useful recommendations might be offered.

Prevention of Hereditary Large Bowel Cancer

In June, 1982, the Comprehensive Cancer Center of Metropolitan Detroit, in conjunction with the Michigan Cancer Foundation, American Cancer Society Michigan Division, and the National Large Bowel Cancer Project sponsored a conference devoted entirely to the prevention of hereditary large bowel cancer. Speakers discussed the clinical features of the polypotic and nonpolypotic, hereditary, colorectal cancer syndromes, estimates of their incidence, methods for genetic linkage and clinical diagnosis, biochemical tissue-culture-assay methods for diagnosis, means for screening and treating high-risk and affected family members, genetic counseling, and legal issues in family studies. Two workshops were devoted to *in vitro* models for the study of malignant cell transformation and the potential for national, pedigree-linkage data banks of hereditary large bowel cancer.

In the brief span of a year, between the Washington and Detroit conferences, few concrete advances could be measured. There appeared to be an increasing consensus as to the clinical features that characterize nonpolyposis HCC, activity by investigators at centers not previously recognized for their work was apparent, and with respect to the use of centralized data banks, there appeared to be a moderate shift from the position taken at the Washington conference. Methodologies for computerization, linkage, and safeguarding were considered increasingly feasible, though obstacles were recognized as still being present.

There also seemed to be a greater willingness to use or recommend the use of specific risk-factor profiles in the clinical management of recognized high-risk families.

Multicentric Field Studies of Promising Laboratory Markers in a Large Sample of Nonpolyposis HCC

At the First International Symposium on Colorectal Cancer (New York, 1979), various investigators presented ongoing laboratory studies dealing with the polyposis syndromes. Others discussed the growing recognition of the nonpolyposis syndromes and the need for improved means of characterizing gene carrier status, as a prelude to interventional surgery and chemoprevention. During these meetings, an awareness emerged of the potential for laboratory investigation of the nonpolyposis syndromes using existing techniques. What was novel about the evolving project was the notion of simultaneously evaluating a battery of markers on the most informative members of large, thoroughly documented, cooperative kindreds.

We are now in the midst of a cooperative biomarker study of nonpolyposis HCC, with and without extracolonic malignancy. This study is being performed in collaboration with B. Shannon Danes, M.D., Ph.D. of Cornell University Medical College in New York City, Martin Lipkin, M. D. and Eleanor Deschner, Ph.D. of the Sloan-Kettering Cancer Center in New York City, and Avery A. Sandberg, M.D. of the Roswell Park Memorial Institute in Buffalo, New York.

To date, we have studied biomarkers in 11 extended kindreds from our resource. Preliminary findings suggest the following abnormalities in clinically affected and high-risk family members compared to low-risk members from unaffected family branches used as controls: increased *in vitro* tetraploidy in dermal monolayer cultures; increased ^{3}HTdR labeling in the upper compartments of the colonic crypts; high incidence of polymorphisms of centromeric heterochromatin, including complete inversion in stimulated lymphocytes; low serum IgA in 5 of 18 bloodline subjects from a single kindred; and linkage analysis showing possible linkage of Jk to the putative cancer-predisposing-gene locus (lod score 2.12). When increased *in vitro* tetraploidy and ^{3}HTdR uptake were incorporated in crude multivariate analyses, the lod score became 2.35. Although data continue to be collected on additional families and family branches, work to date emphasizes the advantages of integrating laboratory and clinical-genetic data for assessment of genotype status. The ultimate predictability of any one or several laboratory studies awaits the expression or nonexpression of cancer in the subjects of this investigation, all of whom will be followed prospectively.

Appendix
A Summary of Selected Pedigrees from One Registry of Cancer-Prone Families

FAMILY C-001 (PEDIGREE I)

The previously reported family that came to be known as "Family N," was discovered in 1963.[1] At that time, the 44-year-old proband (IV-33) was admitted to the Omaha Veterans Administration Hospital for recurrent right-upper-quadrant pain and a 30-pound weight loss. He was depressed and stated he was certain he had cancer and would die from it as had so many of his relatives. The patient underwent exploratory celiotomy, and the biopsy revealed cortical carcinoma of the right adrenal gland. The tumor was felt to be too large to be removed, and the patient died five months later.

The proband had reported that his mother (III-13) died of cancer of the liver. His maternal grandmother (II-3) died at an early age, supposedly of cancer. A brother (IV-24) underwent surgery at the age of 45, at which time a Grade 3 medullary carcinoma of the transverse colon was resected. At age 63 a diagnosis of inoperable carcinoma of the stomach was made. The brother's daughter (V-20) had a hysterectomy for noninvasive endometrial carcinoma at age 46. The daughter, who is now age 63, is receiving chemotherapy for a metastatic tumor in the liver. A colonscopy did not reveal a tumor, and the primary site remains undetermined.

One of the proband's sisters (IV-31) had a carcinoma *in situ* of the uterine cervix at age 41. At age 48, a resected segment of transverse colon revealed a Duke's Class-C adenocarcinoma. Approximately one year later, the sister was found to have a second primary tumor located in the cecum (mucinous adenocarcinoma, Duke's Class C). She expired four years later from metastatic disease.

At age 29, another sister (IV-30) presented to her physician with a history of irregular menses for approximately six months. Adnexal enlargements were found, and exploratory laparotomy revealed bilateral, Grade III carcinoma of the ovaries. Two years later, a dilitation and curettage yielded a

Pedigree I.

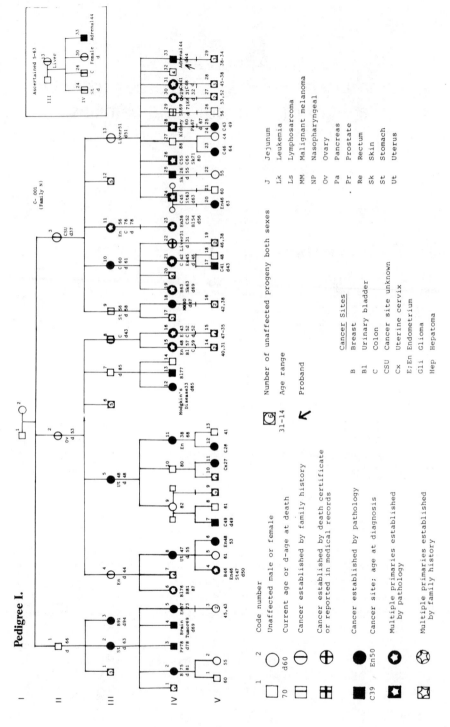

280

Grade IV carcinoma of the endometrium, believed to be a second primary tumor. The patient died a year later.

Prospective follow-up of this family over a 20-year span has revealed a number of new cancer diagnoses. To demonstrate their relatively consistent clinical presentations, these cases are summarized as follows.

At age 55, a second brother (IV-26) of the proband underwent a right hemicolectomy for a Grade III adenocarcinoma of the cecum. He remained well until age 65 at which time he noted rectal bleeding and abdominal tenderness. Surgery was performed, and he was found to have a Grade II adenocarcinoma of the sigmoid colon. He remains cancer free at the age of 80.

Patient IV-28 had a papillary, transitional-cell carcinoma of the kidney at age 60. Seven years later, he was admitted to the hospital for severe abdominal pain and weight loss. Laparotomy disclosed an unresectable, Grade III, pancreatic carcinoma. He died two months later. At age 43, his daughter (V-25) was found to have a Grade III adenocarcinoma of the cecum with extensive local invasion and metastasis in a single, small lymph node. She is alive and well at age 49.

Another brother of the proband (IV-29) died at age 71 of metastatic carcinoma of the stomach.

Patient V-17 underwent a right colectomy at age 41. A Duke's C adenocarcinoma (metastases to 1 of 13 lymph nodes) was diagnosed. He died in 1976 at age 43 from metastatic disease.

Patient IV-6 had tumors removed from the bladder at age 76. At age 81, a mass was noted in her left breast, which proved to be a poorly differentiated infiltrating carcinoma. She is alive and cancer free at age 87.

Patient IV-15 has had three, separate primary tumors. Because of postmenopausal bleeding, she had a total panhysterectomy, with a diagnosis of Grade II papillary adenocarcinoma of the endometrium. In 1972, at age 57, a defect in the left ureter was noted on intravenous pyelogram. She had a nephroureterectomy, and a transitional cell carcinoma, Grade III, of the ureter was diagnosed. In 1975, a barium enema was performed as part of a complete checkup. A filling defect at the hepatic flexure was found to represent tumor, which was resected. She is alive and well at age 67.

Patient IV-15's sister (IV-16), underwent a total hysterectomy in 1966 at age 43. A Grade III papillary adenocarcinoma of the endometrium was reported. At age 52, she was admitted to the hospital for evaluation of pedal edema, weakness, and chest pain. Barium enema revealed a lesion in the cecum. The surgical specimen showed a moderately well differentiated adenocarcinoma, Duke's B, with perforation of the intestinal wall. She died six months later.

Patient V-4 has had three separate primary carcinomas. At age 46, she underwent a radical mastectomy for carcinoma of the breast with metastasis to 4 of 16 axillary lymph nodes. A week later, a total hysterectomy was performed, and a well-differentiated adenocarcinoma of the endometrium was noted. Two years later, the patient presented with pyloric obstruction due to tumor; partial gastrectomy was performed.

At age 43, patient V-6 underwent a hysterectomy for well-differentiated adenocarcinoma of the endometrium. She is alive and well at age 53.

In 1970, patient V-7 was found to have a carcinoid tumor of the intestine with metastasis to the liver.

FAMILY C-025 (PEDIGREE II)

Family C-025 was discovered in 1969 by self-referral of the proband, II-6, who related her own history of breast cancer at age 56 as well as her immediate family history, as depicted in the inset. The history of the five members of this family known or supposed to have had colorectal cancer is as follows.

Patient II-10 had, in 1968 at age 64, a resection for an adenocarcinoma of the "left colon." The tumor measured 7 cm × 7 cm × 5 cm and extended into the pericolic fat. None of the six nodes examined were invaded by the tumor. No further details were available. Three months later, the patient underwent a left radical mastectomy for cancer. She is alive and well at age 76.

Patient II-9 had, in 1937, a total abdominal hysterectomy and bilateral salpingo oophorectomy for cancer of the "uterus," not otherwise specified. In 1964, she underwent radical excision and groin dissection for malignant melanoma over the tibia. In 1965, she had a mastectomy for infiltrating ductal adenocarcinoma of the right breast. And in 1970, at the age of 68, she was discovered to have a perirectal mass that, on biopsy, revealed anaplastic carcinoma consistent with metastases from the breast. However, invasive primary adenocarcinoma of the rectum could not be ruled out. The patient died several months later.

Patient II-3 had, in 1961 at age 69, an adenocarcinoma of the upper rectum measuring 5 cm × 7 cm and extending to the pericolic fat. All nodes were negative for cancer. Approximately 6 cm distal to this primary tumor a 4 cm × 3.5 cm adenoma was found with "atypical epithelim."

Patient II-2 had, in 1947 at age 56, an ulcerating adenocarcinoma of the cecum involving the ileocecal valve and extending to the serosa. No information regarding regional nodes was stated on the pathology report. This lesion had been an incidental surgical finding one month earlier when the patient was undergoing a total abdominal hysterectomy and bilateral salpingo oophorectomy for two, discrete, 1.5 cm adenocarcinomas of the endometrium.

Patient II-1 had, in 1948 at age 58, a carcinoma of the rectum with penetration of the bowel and involvement of the perirectal nodes. Two "benign mucosal polyps" of the rectum were removed at this time.

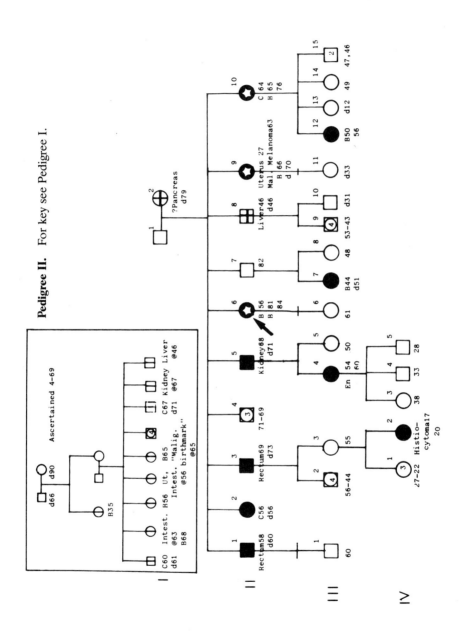

Pedigree II. For key see Pedigree I.

FAMILY C-050: (PEDIGREE III)

In 1980, Family C-050 was referred by a rural Nebraska pathologist who had performed autopsies on several family members. He had initially intended to work up the family himself, and had consulted us by telephone on several occasions regarding specific questions of logistics and syndrome characteristics. Following another death in the family, however, he decided to turn the investigation over to us for more detailed evaluation of the family history. The family history as known to him at that time is shown in the inset. Additional information was provided by the proband's widow and several other relatives over the following year. This family has been included in marker studies pursuant to ongoing laboratory investigations. Review of pertinent family medical history is as follows.

In 1964, at age 53, the proband (II-2) was hospitalized for severe headache. Past history included constipation for two years, a prior hospitalization for rectal bleeding with no final diagnosis being made, and removal of an abdominal skin cancer in 1962. Family history at this time revealed that the mother had died of uterine cancer, that one brother had died of generalized cancer, and that three other siblings were living and well. Physical exam revealed tenderness on palpation in the lower abdomen; sigmoidoscopy was negative. Details of further diagnostic tests were not described. At laparotomy, a right hemicolectomy with end-to-end ileotransverse anastomosis was performed. Tissue examination revealed a 2 cm $\times$ 2 cm $\times$ 1.5 cm polyp continuous with an annular carcinoma in the vicinity of the hepatic flexure, infiltrating through the wall of the colon and involving the serosa. A small, pedunculated polyp was also encountered near the ileocecal valve. No other mucosal abnormalities were found. Microscopically, the tumor tissue formed few glands and was comprised predominantly of anaplastic cells. Notably, the grossly described polyp in the cecum was comprised of similar anaplastic tissue. Regional nodes showed reactive changes only. The patient remained symptom free for several years; however, his death certificate five years later listed carcinoma of the stomach with metastases of five months duration as the cause of death.

Patient III-11, at age 34 (1968), had an abdominal-perineal resection and right hemicolectomy for synchronous tumors of the rectum and cecum. In 1980, the patient was admitted with abdominal pain and a right-sided abdominal mass. Barium enema showed carcinoma of the transverse colon, which proved to be unresectable at laparotomy. This tumor mass was located at the previous anastomotic line. Liver metastasis and adherence of tumor to the pancreas and duodenum were noted. A diversionary procedure was undertaken, but the patient continued on a downhill course and died four months later.

Patient III-5, at age 36 (1972), was admitted for severe cramps and diarrhea.

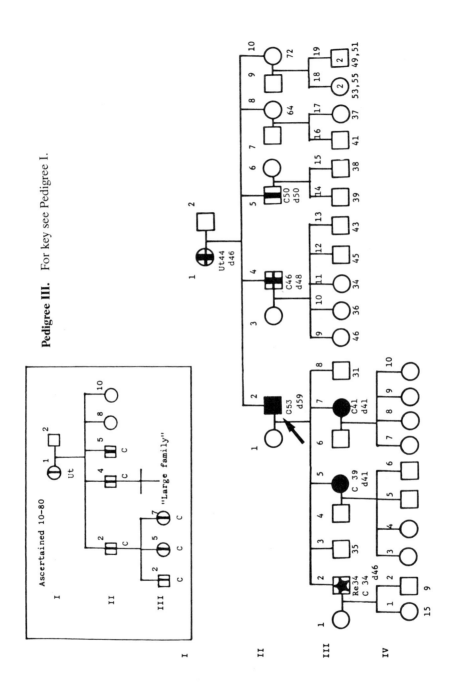

Pedigree III. For key see Pedigree I.

285

At that time, her reported family history of cancer included her father and brother. Other than stool for occult blood, no other gastrointestinal workup was performed. She was placed on intravenous fluids only and her symptoms subsided. Approximately four years later, she was admitted for increasing bulk of supposed uterine fibroids and anemia. At laparotomy, the suspected uterine fibroid was, instead, found to consist of a large carcinoma of the cecum, adherent to the bladder and uterus. A right hemicolectomy was performed. Pathology revealed mucinous adenocarcinoma with transmural extension involving three of six regional nodes. The following year was punctuated by recurrence of disease in the abdomen, and the patient died approximately one year following the initial resection.

Patient III-7 presented at age 41 (1979) with fatigue of five months duration. No weight loss or change in bowel habits was noted at that time. Family history included the cases just outlined and two paternal uncles. Barium enema showed a filling defect in the distal cecum. Segmental ileocolectomy was performed and revealed a moderately differentiated adenocarcinoma of the cecum with transmural extension. Ten of 15 nodes were positive for metastatic disease. Following surgery, the patient was begun on 5-fluorouracil (5-FU). Three weeks later she presented with diarrhea and nausea. Laboratory tests showed granulocytopenia (white count of 600 comprised of 90% lymphocytes). The white count did gradually rise over the following several days. Bilirubin was elevated at 14 mg%. Plain film of the abdomen showed dilated loops of small bowel suggestive of small bowel obstruction. Persistent gastrointestinal bleeding continued from the rectum. The patient was transfused and given broad-spectrum antibiotics, but she became hypotensive and died shortly thereafter.

Patient II-4 was diagnosed as having carcinoma of the transverse colon in 1959 at age 46, according to the death certificate. No medical records were available.

Patient II-5 is reported to have died at age 50 of colon cancer. No records were available.

Patient I-1 was diagnosed as having "cancer of the uterus and intestines" in 1927 at age 44, according to the death certificate. No primary medical records were available.

FAMILY C-113 (PEDIGREE IV)

Family C-113 was originally referred to us in 1968 by a pathologist who reported that the proband (IV-3) had recently been the subject of autopsy examination, having died of disseminated adenocarcinoma of the descending colon at age 34. Colonic cancer was reported to have occurred in other family members, but few details were known. Follow-up of the family led to

Pedigree IV. For key see Pedigree I.

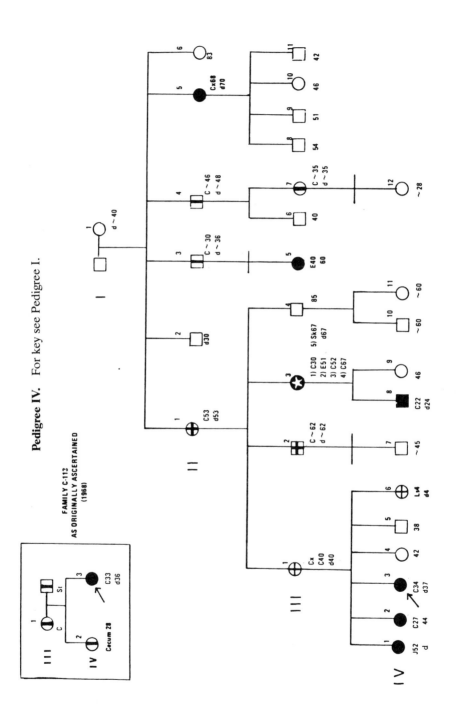

the identification of Torre's syndrome in patient III-3 (see Chap. 4). Patient III-3's son (IV-8) was hospitalized at age 22 for suspected acute appendicitis. At surgery, the appendix was inflamed due to obstruction at its base by a large, Duke's stage C, mucinous adenocarcinoma of the cecum. The son died 1½ years later with recurrent metastatic carcinoma. The proband's mother (III-1) was reported by death certificate to have died at age 40 from a mucoid carcinoma of the colon. A sister of the proband (IV-1) at age 52 was admitted to the hospital with a history of progressive, upper abdominal pain associated with nausea and vomiting. A laparotomy was performed, and a deeply infiltrating adenocarcinoma of the jejunum was found. A second sister (IV-2) had undergone a right hemicolectomy at age 27 because of an infiltrating, mucin-secreting adenocarcinoma of the cecum. To date, she remains cancer free.

The high frequency of mucinous adenocarcinomas in this family and several other kindreds is a subject presently under investigation by cooperating pathologists at our institution. The family is also notable for the unusually high numbers of members presenting below the age of 40 — younger even than customarily encountered in CFS.[2]

FAMILY C-115 (PEDIGREE V)

The previously described kindred known as Family C-115 is a small yet typical example of nonpolypotic HCC with extracolonic malignancies (CFS).[3] This family is noteworthy for the minimal yet classical findings that lead to its recognition and the short time frame within which three of the ten high-risk offspring in generation IV were prospectively found to have colorectal cancer.

The kindred was first ascertained in 1969, at which time the proband was referred to us by her family physician. Pedigree data disclosed at that time are depicted in the inset to the accompanying figure. Two of the proband's sisters had colon and endometrial cancer, while the brother and mother each had cancer of undetermined anatomic sites. The ages of onset were provided for only the proband and one sister. On the basis of this information, a thorough workup of the family was performed, revealing the characteristic clinical findings as described in the main body of the pedigree. The three patients whose malignancies were diagnosed subsequent to the initiation of the study are described next.

Patient IV-5, at age 38 (1970), following a two to three month history of rectal bleeding, had a 2.3 cm, pedunculated, benign adenoma removed by abdominal colotomy. At age 41, 40 cm of transverse colon were resected, and the specimen included a 4 cm, moderately differentiated adenocarcinoma, invading locally through the bowel wall. Regional nodes were tumor free. A

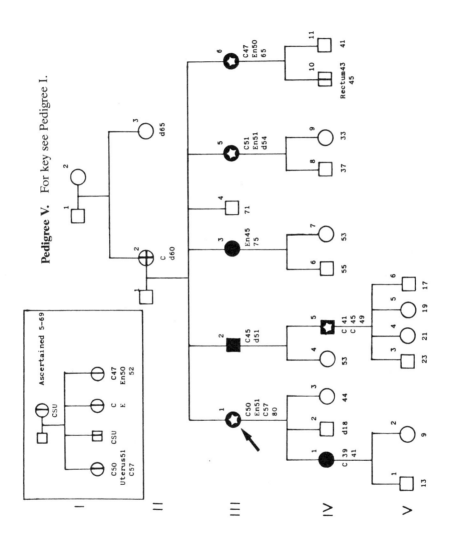

Pedigree V. For key see Pedigree I.

289

"small polyp" was found near one resection margin. At age 45, after three years of follow-up through fecal-occult-blood testing, successive heme-positive stools lead to colonoscopic biopsy of a polypoid cecal lesion that had not been apparent on barium enema. Because the significance of the family history of multiple primary cancer had been impressed on the attending physicians following the previous local resection, total abdominal colectomy and ileoproctostomy were performed. Pathologic evaluation revealed a 3 cm × 2 cm, well-differentiated adenocarcinoma of the cecum, 8 cm proximal to the previous anastomosis. Serosa and regional nodes were free of disease. The patient remains asymptomatic at this time.

Patient IV-1 is a 41-year-old female who, in 1979, showed colonoscopic biopsy evidence of adenocarcinoma in the ascending colon. The patient was asymptomatic and had been examined for several years by colonoscopy because of the then well-known family history. Before surgery, we were consulted for management recommendations. On the basis of these, total colectomy with ileorectal anastomosis was performed. The final diagnosis was well-differentiated adenocarcinoma of the ascending colon without serosal involvement. We know of no case of nonpolyposis HCC in which a more informed and compliant patient was cared for more successfully by physicians interested in carrying out a specifically tailored screening and treatment plan.

Patient IV-10 was diagnosed at age 43 (1978) as having an adenocarcinoma of the rectum, by reliable family history.

FAMILY C-164 (PEDIGREE VI)

The proband of Family C-164 (IV-9) was ascertained in the course of an epidemiologic–genetic survey of all patients diagnosed with colon cancer at the Omaha Veteran's Administration Hospital in the years 1964 to 1969.[4] In 1969, the 60-year-old patient was admitted for midabdominal pain radiating to the back over a period of months. Further workup of the abdominal mass revealed adenocarcinoma in the rectus abdominus, a probable recurrence from a 1966 carcinoma of the cecum. The 1966 colonic resection revealed a large (9 cm × 7 cm) ulcerating tumor with transmural invasion but no apparent metastases to regional nodes. A second, polypoid, adenocarcinoma of the cecum with invasion of the submucosa was located just distal to the first lesion. In addition, 15 adenomatous polyps ranging from 0.5 to 2.2 cm were identified. The patient died 14 months after the 1969 admission. During the 1969 hospitalization, an unusually detailed family history was taken by trained interviewers (medical students working summers) specifically inquiring as to history of cancer or other disease in mothers, fathers, brothers, sisters, and children of all the probands seen in this study. The

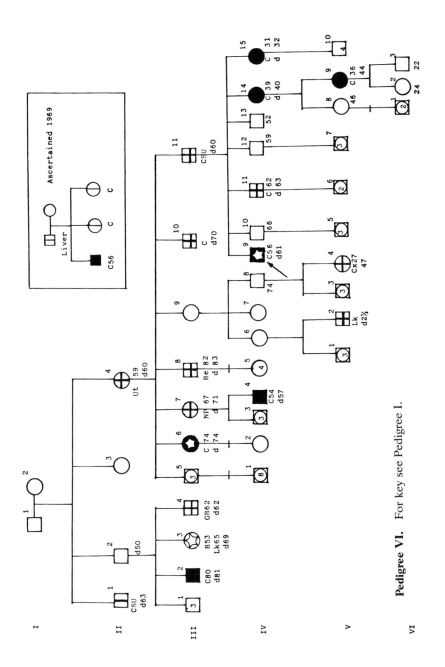

Pedigree VI. For key see Pedigree I.

proband reported that his father had had carcinoma in the liver that may have spread from the colon and two sisters who had died of colon cancer. Medical history regarding the patient's father and 2 sisters is as follows.

Patient III-11, father of the proband, at age 60 (1942) was admitted with pain, jaundice, and a palpable mass in the upper abdomen. At laparatomy, a large mass involving the liver, posterior wall of the stomach, and pancreas was found and considered inoperable. No biopsy was obtained at surgery, and following the patient's death a month later, no autopsy was performed. The operative diagnosis was carcinoma of the pancreas, stomach, and liver.

Patient IV-14, a sister of the proband, was admitted in 1949 (age 39) for weakness, abdominal fullness, and anorexia. Laparotomy revealed an intraperitoneal mass that on biopsy proved to be an adenocarcinoma, considered initially to most likely have been of ovarian origin. Upon reexploration a week later, an obstructing annular adenocarcinoma 5 cm × 3 cm × 1 cm of the transverse colon was found to involve muscularis, peritoneum, regional nodes, and a mesenteric vein. Local resection was performed, but the patient followed a downhill course and died approximately ten months later.

Patient IV-15, the second sister of the proband, was admitted at age 31 for cramping pain of the lower abdomen. At laparotomy, 18 cm of descending and sigmoid colon were resected. The sigmoid tumor penetrated bowel wall and invaded the serosa. Eleven of 17 regional nodes were involved. Four adenomatous polyps, ranging from 2-4 mm, were found between the tumor mass and distal resection margin. Prior barium enema with air contrast showed no proximal lesions.

The family pedigree known at the time of interview with the proband in 1969 is as shown in the inset.

Additional Affected Relatives

In addition to the immediate affected relatives reported by the proband that constitute the "ascertainment cluster," there are 14 additional cancer patients in the extended pedigree. These patients either were diagnosed before the ascertainment of the family or were earlier cases identified only by more exhaustive evaluation of the family history and identification of collateral family branches. The following are only those relatives expressing colonic cancer.

Patient III-2 was found at age 80 to have an infiltrating adenocarcinoma of the rectosigmoid colon. Only biopsy specimens were available. Clinically, extensive disease was identified in the peritoneum, and the patient died within 18 months of diagnosis.

Patient IV-4 was diagnosed at age 54 with a 5 cm × 5 cm adenocarcinoma of the sigmoid colon. "Few sessile polyps" were present in the immediate vicinity of the tumor. The tumor was fixed to the underlying muscle, but no metastases to the mesentery were observed. The tumor was moderately differentiated, extending on microscopic evaluation to the mesenteric fat with tumor thrombi in small veins of the advancing tumor margin. Three of 11 regional nodes were involved with tumor. The patient died three years later.

Patient III-8 died at age 83 of adenocarcinoma of the rectum, duration of 1 year (death certificate information only).

Patient III-6 had a right hemicolectomy at age 74 for an annular 7 cm × 3 cm adenocarcinoma of the cecum. Proximal to the main lesion were multiple polypoid lesions extending to resection margin. A few polyps exhibited malignant change. Multiple sessile polyps up to 1 cm were found at autopsy a few weeks later.

Patient III-10 was diagnosed at age 70 with "possible cancer of the right colon with hematogeneous spread" (death certificate information only).

Patient V-9 underwent a prophylactic subtotal colectomy at age 36. Multiple sections were taken for microscopic examination. Noted were five mixed adenomatous and villous polyps, and in one of the polyps a small superficial adenocarcinoma was found.

Comments

The problem of heterogeneity in polyp expression in colon cancer-prone families has been discussed in detail elsewhere. It was pointed out that classifying a given family as having a polyposis-like syndrome or being polyp free is not easy. Such classification requires meticulous documentation of any increase in number and size of polyps with advancing age in carefully screened high-risk patients. Family C-164 constitutes a somewhat typical example of a kindred in which numerous, previously unscreened patients present with advanced colon cancer. Information regarding polyps is limited to that described pathologically in resected colonic specimens and lacks quantitation of grossly evident polyps, much less microadenoma involvement. Several patients presented with adenoma expression that would tempt one to classify the family as having a polyposis syndrome. On the other hand, however, several colon cancer patients are documented as having a *lack* of multiple polyposis. Several of those patients who did present with multiple polyps did so at an age somewhat later than that normally encountered in classical polyposis.

Despite the difficulty in classifying this family with certainty and the variation in age at onset, a number of members of high- and low-risk branches of the family have had biological specimens obtained for evaluation of potential markers.

FAMILY C-196 (PEDIGREE VII)

The proband (III-17) was ascertained through a physician referral. She had multiple primary cancers (adenocarcinoma of the colon and endometrium, histologically confirmed). Her sister (III-15) also manifested carcinoma of the colon and endometrium. Another sister (III-18) had endocervical cancer, and a brother (III-19) had rectal cancer. Each of these cancers were histologically confirmed. The progenitor male of the pedigree (I-2) had children with cancer by two marriages. Vertical transmission of colon–endometrial cancer is evident through four generations in one branch. Since we initially published details of the family history,[5] patient IV-7 developed endometrial carcinoma at age 33, dying at age 35.

Patient II-1, apparently cancer free when she died at age 58, represents a recurrent problem in the interpretation of pedigree data. The patient's autopsy report provided no description of a uterus or ovaries. These organs may have been previously removed, thus precluding the expression of cancer. That five of her nine children were affected with colon cancer is typical of HCC and suggests that II-1 must have been an obligate-gene carrier. Such a statement, however, can only be made with confidence in the context of a large, otherwise classically affected kindred. Lacking such knowledge, the occurrences of colon cancer in her children would most likely have to have been attributed to chance.

FAMILY C-197 (PEDIGREE VIII)

The proband (III-2) received a diagnosis of endometrial carcinoma at the age of 40. Ten years later, because of the occurrence of adenocarcinoma of the colon in her 51-year-old brother (III-1), this patient requested that her physician perform appropriate diagnostic studies on her colon even though she was completely asymptomatic. Findings on proctosigmoidoscopy and barium enema revealed the presence of an early adenocarcinoma of the transverse colon, and colectomy was performed. Both of these patients (III-1 and III-2) had sebaceous tumors (see Chap. 4). The identical twin sister of the proband, asymptomatic at age 40, requested an evaluation of the uterus because of the occurrence of endometrial carcinoma in her twin. A diagnosis of early endometrial carcinoma was established, and a hysterectomy was performed.

The mother of the above siblings (II-2) had endometrial carcinoma at the age of 60 and adenocarcinoma of the rectum at age 77. A maternal uncle (II-1) died of cancer, primary site unknown and unconfirmed. An intracranial glioma developed in another maternal uncle (II-3) at age 49, and he died at age 50. A maternal first cousin (III-5) was diagnosed as having carcinoma *in situ* of the cervix.

Pedigree VII.

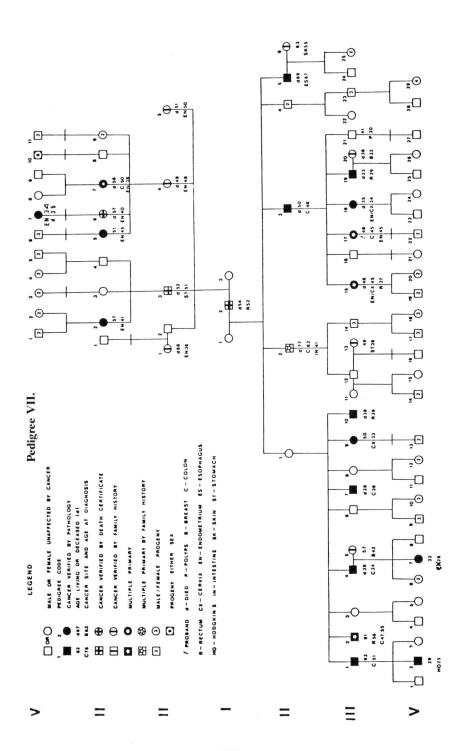

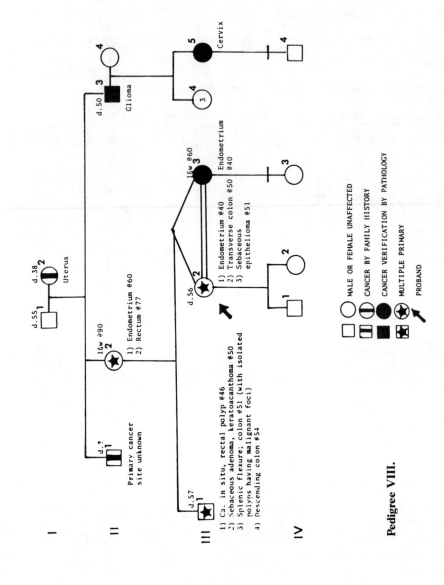

Pedigree VIII.

FAMILY C-198 (PEDIGREE IX)

The pedigree of Family C-198 has been published previously[6] and shows transmission of colon cancer on a site-specific basis through five generations. Early age of onset is also noted. One patient (III-13) had verified colon cancer at the age of 20 years, and 7 others were affected by the age of 35. Of the 25 patients for whom documentation of tumor sites was retrievable, 17 had at least one cancer of the cecum, and only three had cancer of the descending or rectosigmoid colon.

Fourteen members of the family were successfully treated for their initial colon cancer by local resection. In 11 of these persons, subsequent primary malignancies of the remaining colon developed from 2 to 23 years postoperatively with a mean of 8 years.

Two brothers (IV-6 and IV-8) with colon cancer at the ages of 41 and 39, respectively, were treated by hemicolectomy. Their mother (III-4) had cecal cancer at age 45 and subsequent primary malignancies of the colon at the ages of 47 and 48 years. Their brother (IV-5) had colon cancer at the age of 41. Because of the inordinately high frequency of subsequent primary malignancies of the colon in this family, these two brothers underwent prophylactic removal of their remaining colon segments. A small polypoid lesion was found in the colon specimen from patient IV-8. The diagnosis was low-grade primary adenocarcinoma arising in or about the villoglandular polyp.

FAMILY C-199 (PEDIGREE X)

Family C-199 was ascertained in 1976 by referral from a Pennsylvania physician. In 1975, at age 47, the proband (II-6) presented with melena and anemia. Further evaluation yielded a 10 cm adenocarcinoma of the splenic flexure and descending colon with mesenteric-node infiltration but without liver involvement. Microscopically, the tumor showed anaplasia with very little gland formation. Adjuvant therapy included 5-FU methotrexate, and CCNU. Barium enema and carcinoembryonic-antigen determinations one year later were negative. In 1981, a second lesion was detected during a routine barium enema. At surgery, an infiltrating adenocarcinoma of the sigmoid colon was found with extension to one local lymph node. The patient is currently asymptomatic.

Family history volunteered by the patient at the time of initial ascertainment revealed that his mother died in 1949 of breast cancer, at an unknown age. Two brothers and one sister had each had colon cancer at unspecified ages, although the eldest sibling was at that time only 60. A fourth sibling was

Pedigree IX.

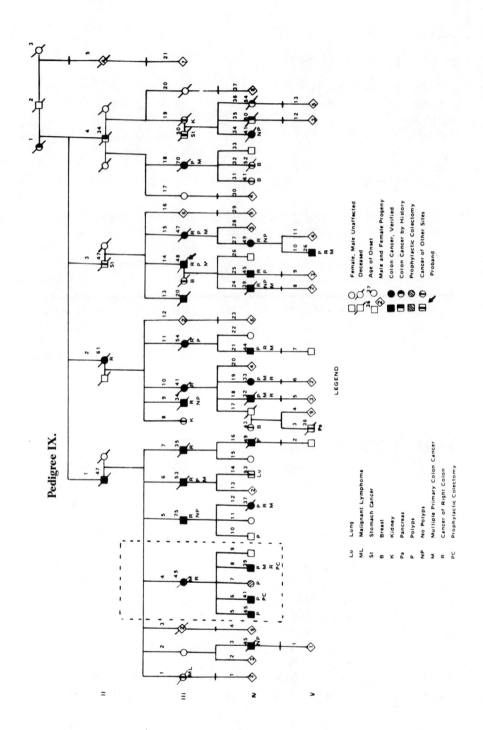

LEGEND

Female, Male Unaffected
Deceased
Age of Onset
Male and Female Progeny
Colon Cancer, Verified
Colon Cancer by History
Prophylactic Colectomy
Cancer of Other Sites
Proband

Lu   Lung
ML   Malignant Lymphoma
St   Stomach Cancer
B   Breast
K   Kidney
Pa   Pancreas
P   Polyps
NP   No Polyps
M   Multiple Primary Colon Cancer
R   Cancer of Right Colon
PC   Prophylactic Colectomy

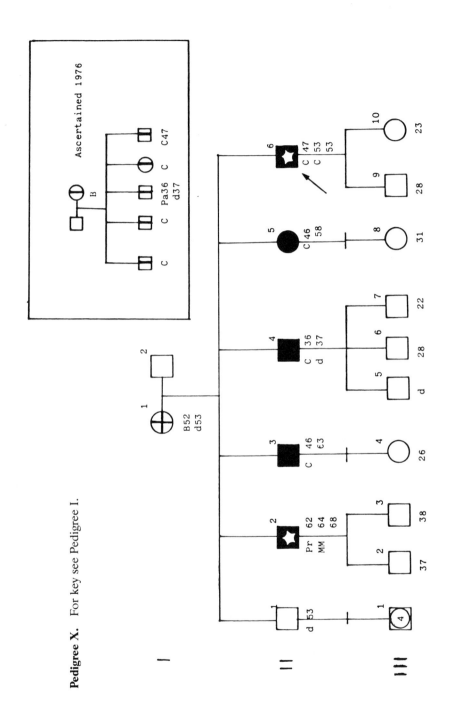

Pedigree X. For key see Pedigree I.

reported to have died of pancreatic cancer at age 37. Review of these cases follows.

Patient I-1's death certificate revealed that she died in 1945 at age 53 of breast cancer. No other details were available.

Patient II-3, the proband's brother, was diagnosed at age 46 (1966) as having an adenocarcinoma of the ascending colon, penetrating through the bowel and its subjacent mucosa. Histologically the tumor was poorly differentiated but did not involve local nodes or mesentery.

Patient II-4 had a cecostomy at age 36 (1958) and shortly thereafter had a right hemicolectomy for adenocarcinoma of the hepatic flexure. The tumor was an annular, poorly differentiated, mucoid adenocarcinoma with positive nodes. Later hepatobiliary involvement was responsible for jaundice, which led the family to believe the tumor had been pancreatic in origin.

Patient II-2, who had a history of adult-onset diabetes mellitus, was diagnosed at age 64 as having a Clark's Level-III, cutaneous, malignant melanoma. A prostatic cancer at age 62 was reported by patient history; further details are unavailable.

Patient II-5, the proband's only sister, was diagnosed at age 46 (1969) as having an infiltrating, ulcerating, partly gelatinous adenocarcinoma of the transverse colon. A villous adenoma of the sigmoid with marked atypia was also identified at this time. Five years later, an adenocarcinoma found near the hepatic flexure was considered to be a possible suture-line recurrence from the previous surgery, although the surgical report indicated the tumor to have been located 12 inches proximal to the suture line. A palliative resection was performed because of "large tumor masses adherent to the aorta." The patient is now living and well with no evidence of disease eight years later. A state tumor-registry report filed during the patient's 1969 admission specifically noted that there was no history of cancer in the family. But four years later, at the time of her second surgery, her history and physical performed by a medical student provided a detailed description of the cases diagnosed previously.

FAMILY 200 (PEDIGREE XI)

Family 200, previously published, is notable for the large number of cases prospectively identified and the emotional distress (denial) that has confounded management efforts in several high-risk branches of the kindred.[7]

The inset to the pedigree represents the ascertainment cluster. The family has been updated on several occasions and has recently been the subject of biomarker investigations described in previous chapters. In 1981, on initiation of the multiinstitutional laboratory studies of a number of families, we

Pedigree XI. For key see Pedigree I.

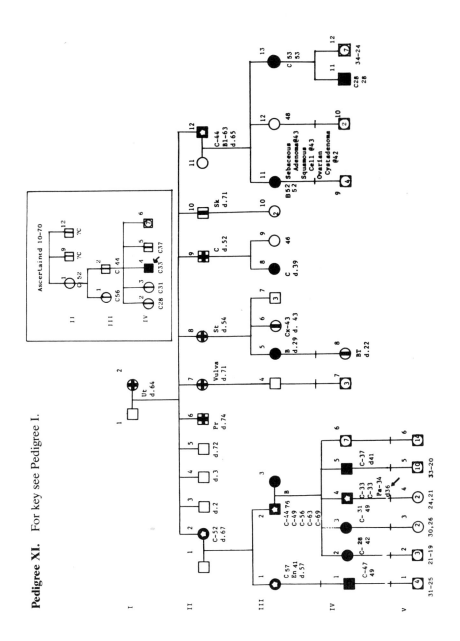

began contacting family members from high- and low-risk branches of this large kindred.

One high-risk member (IV-1) who was asked to participate in the marker studies expressed concern about the presence of melana and change in the character of his stools. He had apparently disregarded the symptoms up to this time since they had not been brought to the attention of his private physician. Eventually, barium enema was performed and revealed a mass in the cecum. When hospitalized in another city, this patient denied having a family history of cancer. However, following discussion with his wife, the surgeon contacted us to discuss the matter before the scheduled laparotomy. When informed of the high frequency of metachronous lesions in previously affected members of the patient's family, the surgeon elected to convert the contemplated right hemicolectomy to subtotal colectomy. The resected specimen revealed a primary cecal adenocarcinoma involving the entire colonic wall and superficial pericolic adipose. A second primary tumor was found distal to the larger cecal lesion. This was a small polypoid adenocarcinoma involving only the mucosa and submucosa. Two small adenomas were also present in the resected specimen.

Several months later, in the course of preparing for identical studies on a high-risk collateral branch of the same family, similar denial complicated not only the field studies, but management as well. Of the three offspring of patient II-12, two daughters (III-11 and III-13) and most of their children agreed to participate in the field studies. Patient III-12 and her children declined for reasons not specified, although all reside within ten miles of our clinic. Less than three months after our samples were obtained from the participating relatives, the 28-year-old son (IV-10) of patient III-12 presented to his local surgeon with an acute abdomen believed to be an acute appendicitis or cecal volvulus. Because of his young age and denial of a family history of cancer, colon cancer was not seriously considered in the differential diagnosis. However, at laparotomy, a large mass involving the ascending colon was found, and a right hemicolectomy was performed. The adenocarcinoma involved the entire colonic wall and superficially invaded the pericolic adipose tissue. Several lymph nodes contained metastases. No other mucosal abnormalities were evident in the resected specimen. The patient is currently receiving 5-FU chemotherapy.

As a consequence of this diagnosis, the previously uncooperative mother (III-12) became greatly concerned, expressing fear for herself and her other six children. She and several children agreed to participate in our research and surveillance program and were provided with the usual details: the natural history of nonpolyposis HCC, its mode of inheritance, their approximate personal risks based on pedigree analysis, and available methods for surveillance. By virtue of her position in the pedigree, patient IV-12 was informed that her risk of ultimately developing cancer approached 100%. Her children were told that their cancer risks were approximately 50%. The following week, colonoscopy was performed on the mother and three of her children. In the case of patient III-12, the colonoscope could be advanced no further than the splenic flexure due to the presence of a large mass, appearing to be a carcinoma. Biopsy revealed necrotic material considered nondiagnostic. The patient had specifically denied any symptoms of gastrointestinal tract disease.

The patient became visibly alarmed and refused further evaluation or surgery, despite the potential seriousness of the lesion and the risk of ultimate colonic obstruction and cancer death. Her fear of surgery was expressed in terms of a belief that "surgery would only spread disease like it had in so many other members of the family." For undisclosed reasons, the patient changed her mind and elected to undergo surgery. At laparotomy, a 5 cm × 6 cm lesion of the transverse colon was found and pathologically confirmed to be a well-differentiated adenocarcinoma with invasion of the muscle but without penetration of the pericolic fat. All regional nodes were negative. A solitary, sessile, polypoid lesion (1 cm × 1 cm) was discovered approximately 7 cm proximal to the initial lesion and was found to be an adenomatous polyp with epithelial atypia probably representing carcinoma *in situ*.

Despite or perhaps because of the presence of cancer in their mother and brother, several of III-12s children have persisted in their refusal to undergo colonoscopy or other diagnostic evaluation.

FAMILY C-220 (PEDIGREE XII)

Family C-220, an Italian–American family, is one of the most recent additions to our registry. In February 1982, we were telephoned by the proband (III-8) who related his concern about the strong family history of cancer. His wife, an office nurse, had recently discussed with her physician–employer a journal article of ours dealing with CFS. The physician suggested that III-8's family was a likely example of this syndrome. It was on the strength of this opinion that the proband assumed the initiative in contacting us and beginning the family investigation.

In 1980, in the course of one of many thorough physical examinations, patient III-8 was found to have a 0.2 cm × 0.3 cm sigmoid adenoma. He has had no further problems. A summary of the verified cases from his family follows.

Patient III-11, at age 54 (1980), was seen by his physician for undisclosed symptoms and found to have a cecal mass on barium enema. Colonoscopic follow-up revealed a second lesion of the transverse colon, malignant by

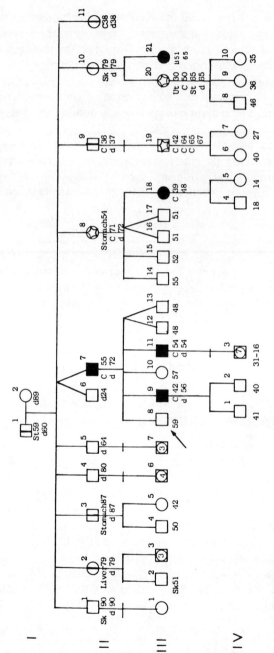

Pedigree XII. For key see Pedigree I.

biopsy. Total colectomy was performed. The cecal tumor was a 3 cm × 3 cm, mucinous, moderately well differentiated adenocarcinoma extending to the serosa. The transverse colonic lesion was a 4 cm, moderate to poorly differentiated adenocarcinoma that also extended to the serosa. Ninety-eight regional nodes were negative for malignancy. The patient is doing well 2½ years postoperatively.

Patient III-9, a brother of the proband, had, at the age of 42 (1963), 15 cm of ascending colon resected for a poorly differentiated, Duke's C carcinoma of the cecum. Two mesenteric nodes showed poorly differentiated adenocarcinoma and necrosis. Nevertheless, the patient did well postoperatively until 1973 when a polyp was removed from the stomach. In 1975, the patient was diagnosed as having membranous nephrosis, which was believed to be a possible autoimmune response to what was then believed to be a recurrence of the tumor in the right colon. However, the patient refused colonoscopic follow-up. In 1977, following a 35-pound weight loss, epigastric pain, and a palpable mass, the patient was finally admitted for evaluation, but he died less than 2 weeks after admission with no further tissue diagnosis having been made.

Patient II-7, the proband's father, had, at age 54 (1946), a hemicolectomy for removal of a large (approximately 18 cm diameter) adenocarcinoma of the cecum. Further pathologic details are unavailable. As in the case of III-9, the patient did very well postoperatively and died 17 years later of unrelated causes.

Patient III-18, is the proband's first cousin and the daughter of an affected sister of II-7. Patient II-18 is believed to have had carcinoma of the stomach at age 57 and a second primary tumor of the colon at age 71, although details have not yet been obtained. At age 39 (1973), the patient had a right hemicolectomy for carcinoma of the transverse colon. Though well differentiated, the tumor was quite necrotic and infiltrated the entire thickness of the bowel wall, involving the subserosal connective tissue but yielding only reactive nodes. She is doing well ten years postoperatively.

FAMILY C-250 (PEDIGREE XIII)

Family C-250 was referred to us by colleagues at the National Cancer Institute in 1979 following a preliminary evaluation. The family pedigree as it was then known constitutes the inset. The histories of syndrome-affected patients are summarized as follows.

Patient III-4, at age 44 (1977), presented to a local surgeon complaining of abdominal pain and was subsequently found to have obstructive carcinoma of the transverse colon. Thirty cm of transverse colon was resected revealing an annular, ulcerating, fungating tumor extending into adjacent pericolic

Pedigree XIII. For key see Pedigree I.

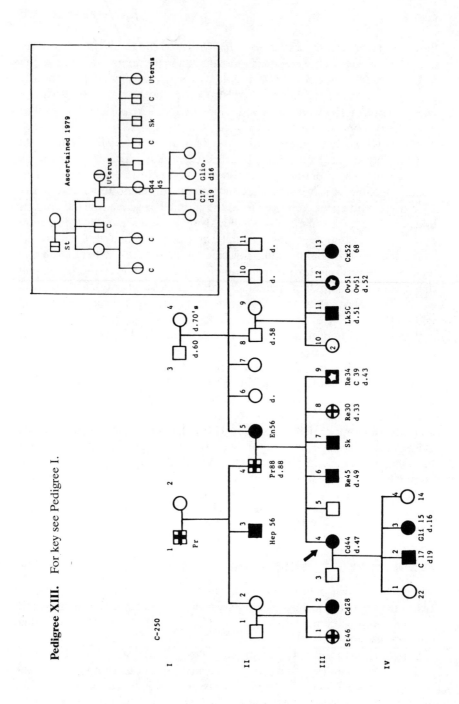

fat. Histologically, the nodule, a well-differentiated adenocarcinoma, was found to have extended into serosa and one small lymph node. Approximately 12 to 14 months later, discomfort and left-lower-quarter "firmness" led to abdominal biopsy and findings of infiltrated adenocarcinoma consistent with metastasis from the previous lesion. Irradiation reduced the tumor bulk, but the patient followed a generally downhill course and died 38 months after initial surgery.

Patient IV-2, the proband's son, was admitted to the hospital at age 17 (1976) because of massive gastrointestinal tract bleeding. He was worked up and at the time of surgery was found to have a moderately differentiated adenocarcinoma of the cecum with metastasis to the liver. He was treated with 5-FU without good short-term results and died two years later from extensive metastatic disease.

Patients III-6 and III-8, siblings of the proband, had carcinoma of the rectum at ages 45 and 30, respectively. Another brother (III-9) developed carcinoma of the upper rectum at age 34. At age 39, he was admitted to the hospital for anemia and given a series of transfusions before surgery. At exploration, he was found to have an infiltrating adenocarcinoma of the cecum without evidence of metastases. However, two years later, he was again admitted to the hospital for severe anemia. An exploratory laparotomy was performed and an inoperable metastatic tumor mass was found in the jejunum. He died six months later.

Patient III-2, a 28-year-old cousin of the proband, was admitted to the hospital with complaints of abdominal cramping, bloating, intermittent nausea, and vomiting for about three months, with a 20-pound weight loss. Sigmoidoscopy was unrevealing. Barium enema revealed a napkin-like constriction in the lower descending colon. The lesion was determined to be inoperable at the time of surgery. Biopsy of a portion of omentum showed undifferentiated metastatic carcinoma.

FAMILY C-251 (PEDIGREE XIV)

Family C-251, not previously described, is to our knowledge the first known American Indian kindred with CFS. The family was referred to us in early 1982 from a reservation in Arizona by a general surgeon. His interest and subsequent consultations with us were fostered by his anecdotal observation that most cases of the otherwise rare colon cancers diagnosed on this reservation were from a single large kindred. He further observed that the documented cases seemed to occur at an unusually early age.

Patient IV-1, the proband, was found at age 40 to have a solid adenocarcinoma of the right ovary, by histology a serous cystadenocarcinoma, Grade

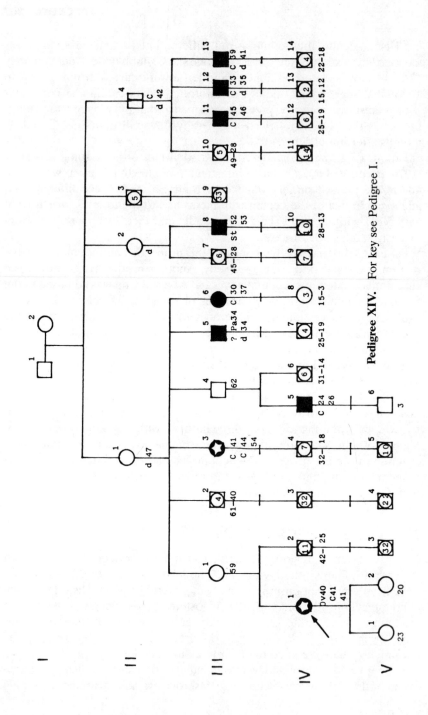

Pedigree XIV. For see Pedigree I.

II. At that time, the tumor was found to be metastatic to the uterus. A total abdominal hysterectomy and bilateral salpingo oophorectomy were performed. A second-look procedure performed five months later showed at least one lymph node positive for carcinoma. In February 1982, a right hemicolectomy was performed, revealing an annular mass 6 cm from the ileocecal valve (4.5 cm × 3 cm). The adenocarcinoma infiltrated the colonic wall to the superficial pericolic adipose. Histologically, the tumor appeared to be a well-differentiated, mucin-secreting adenocarcinoma. The immediately adjoining mucosae were free of tumor as were 33 pericolic nodes. The patient is asymptomatic at this time.

Patient III-3, currently age 54 and asymptomatic, is an aunt of the proband. In 1971, at age 44, the patient had a low abdominal resection and reanastomosis, coupled with total abdominal hysterectomy and bilateral salpingo oophorectomy for carcinoma of the sigmoid colon. The main tumor mass was a poorly differentiated adenocarcinoma with abundant mucus production that invaded the pericolic fat. A separate segment of nearby colonic mucosae showed two foci of the superficial carcinoma within an adenoma, the stalk being free of tumor. (A previous surgery for cancer was performed in 1968 and further details are being obtained.)

Patient IV-5 is a first cousin of the proband, related through the proband's asymptomatic 62-year-old uncle. At age 24, the patient presented with cramping abdominal pain and was found to have a positive Hemoccult. Barium enema demonstrated an annular lesion at the hepatic flexure. At laparotomy, the terminal ileum and proximal colon were resected up to the level of the splenic flexure and reanastamosed. Pathologic evaluation yielded a polypoid, annular tumor, 10 cm distal to the ileocecal valve and measuring 3 cm in diameter. The tumor histologically proved to be an adenocarcinoma moderately differentiated extending to the muscularis mucosae but not beyond. Twenty mesenteric nodes were free of metastases.

Patient III-6 presented with anemia and weight loss at age 30. Exploration and resection revealed a Grade II adenocarcinoma of the cecum. The tumor mass measured 8 cm × 6 cm × 6 cm and extended from the mucosa through the lamina propria and serosa. None of the nodes showed evidence of metastasis. She is now 37 and asymptomatic.

Patient III-11, a distant cousin of the proband, was found, at age 46, to have a filling defect at the splenic flexure on barium enema. Because of his family history of colon cancer, he was advised that the entire colon should be removed. Following laparotomy, the tumor was found to be a moderately differentiated, mucin-producing adenocarcinoma, extending through the full thickness of the bowel wall but not into the pericolic fat. No positive nodes were found. He is doing well one year postoperatively.

Patient III-12, at age 33, was having rectal bleeding and was found to have a moderately differentiated adenocarcinoma involving the entire wall of the transverse colon extending to the regional lymph nodes. He died two years later of metastatic disease.

Patient III-13 underwent a laparotomy for a 6 cm mass of the ascending colon at age 39. The tumor had infiltrated to the pericolonic fat. Several nodes from the right mesocolon were replaced by tumor and the liver was studded with multiple nodules. He expired 1½ years later.

REFERENCES

1. Lynch, H.T.; Shaw, M.W.; Magnuson, C.W.; Larsen, A.L.; and Krush, A.J.; Hereditary factors in cancer: Study of two large midwestern kindreds. *Arch. Int. Med.* **117:**206-212, 1966.
2. Lynch, H.T., and Lynch, P.M.: The cancer family syndrome: A pragmatic basis for syndrome identification. *Dis.Colon Rect.* **22:**106-110, 1979.
3. Lynch, H.T.; Lynch, P.M.; and Harris, R.E.: Minimal genetic findings and their cancer control implications. *JAMA* **240:**535-538, 1978.
4. Lynch, H.T.; Guirgis, H.; Lynch, J.; Brodkey, F.D.; and Magee, H.: Cancer of the colon: Socioeconomic variables in a community. *Am. J. Epidemiol.* **102:**119-127, 1975.
5. Lynch, H.T.; Harris, R.E.; Organ, C.H., Jr.; Guirgis, H.A.; Lynch, P.M.; Lynch, J.F.; and Nelson, E.J.: The surgeon genetics, and cancer control: The cancer family syndrome. *Ann. Surg.* **185:**435-440, 1977.
6. Lynch, H.T.; Harris, R.E.; Bardawil, W.A.; Lynch, P.M.; Guirgis, H.A.; Swartz, M.J.; and Lynch, J.F.: Management of hereditary site-specific colon cancer. *Arch. Surg.* **112:**170-174, 1977.
7. Lynch, H.T.; Swartz, M.; Lynch, J.; and Crush, A.J.: A family study of adenocarcinoma of the colon and multiple primary cancer. *Surg., Gynecol., Obstet.* **134:**1-6, 1972.

Index

About the Editors

PATRICK M. LYNCH is an internal medicine resident in the Department of Medicine at the University of Arkansas for Medical Sciences. He received the J.D. from Creighton University School of Law and the M.D. from Creighton University School of Medicine. Dr. Lynch is a member of the Alpha Omega Alpha honorary medical society. While *Colon Cancer Genetics* was in preparation, Dr. Lynch was an instructor in the Department of Preventive Medicine and Public Health at Creighton University, lecturing and conducting research in legal medicine and confidentiality in human subjects research. He worked with Dr. Henry Lynch on studies of families that now comprise the Creighton registry of cancer-prone kindreds. Dr. Lynch is a cofounder of the Hereditary Cancer Institute and is the author of more than fifty articles on cancer genetics.

HENRY T. LYNCH is professor and chairman of the Department of Preventive Medicine and Public Health and professor of medicine at the Creighton University School of Medicine, Omaha, Nebraska, and president of Creighton's Hereditary Cancer Institute. Dr. Lynch received the MA degree in clinical psychology in 1952 from Denver University. He did further graduate work in human genetics at the University of Texas at Austin, and received the M.D. in 1960 from the University of Texas at Galveston. Dr. Lynch completed a residency in internal medicine and was a senior cancer fellow in medical oncology at the University of Nebraska School of Medicine in Omaha between 1961 and 1966.

Dr. Lynch has authored more than 250 scientific articles on cancer genetics and has written eight books that deal with the general subject of cancer genetics. He has contributed chapters on cancer genetics to more than ten books and has served as a consultant to the National Cancer Institute and to the World Health Organization. He has been chairman of many scientific panels dealing with cancer genetics and has presented his work at many meetings worldwide.